Fibromyalgia & Chronic Myofascial Pain

A SURVIVAL MANUAL

Second Edition

Devin Starlanyl
Mary Ellen Copeland

Foreword by Christopher R. Brown, D.D.S., M.P.S.

New Harbinger Publications, Inc.

Except for the figures 3.1 and 8.28, all figures have been previously published in *Myofascial Pain and Dysfunction: The Trigger Point Manual, Volumes I and II* by Janet G. Travell and David G. Simons, 1983 (Vol. I), 1992 (Vol. II), Williams and Wilkins, Baltimore, MD, and are reproduced here with permission of the copyright holder. Figures 3.1 and 8.28 were previously published in *Travell and Simons' Myofascial Pain and Dysfunction: The Trigger Point Manual*, Second Edition. 1999. Williams and Wilkins: Baltimore, MD, and are reproduced here with permission of the copyright holder.

Copyright © 2001 Devin J. Starlanyl and Mary Ellen Copeland
New Harbinger Publications, Inc.
5674 Shattuck Avenue
Oakland, CA 94609

Text design by Tracy Marie Carlson

Distributed in Canada by Raincoast Books

Library of congress number: 01-132299

ISBN-13 978-1-57224-238-8
ISBN-10 1-57224-238-8

First Edition
Printed from April 1996 thru December 2000 totaling over 261,000 copies.

Second Edition
08   07   06
15   14   13   12   11   10   9

No Matter the Limits
by Rita Shaw (FMily member)

It is such a relief when you first find out
That the pain really does have a name,
And then you will ask (and everyone does),
"Just where can I place all the blame?"

No matter the limits, no matter the pain,
There's no evil, cruel "Master Plan,"
It just simply happens. It just simply is.
You adapt, and you change what you can.

But even with knowing the best and worst,
All the pitfalls the future could hold,
You still have a choice, you quit or you fight,
You determine the story that's told.

And every small step that we take, my dear friends,
Each battle that we slowly win,
Just credits the love and the caring we share
With the FMily that we call our friends.

To blaze a trail in science and medicine, no matter how small, one must stand on the shoulders of giants. I am deeply indebted to the memory of Janet G. Travell and to the presence of David G. Simons. They have held me so very high, enabling me to see what I would otherwise have missed. In addition, my husband, Rick, has provided my main life support throughout the writing of this edition, and that was no easy job. To the three of you, I dedicate this book.

—Devin J. Starlanyl

Contents

Acknowledgments

When we started planning this second edition with our publisher, we were faced with a dilemma. The studies of fibromyalgia and myofascial pain have been exploding with new research since the first edition. How could we fit in the new information, cover all that was covered in the first edition, and still produce a book of manageable size? I am grateful to the people at New Harbinger Publications who made this possible. Kristin Beck took on the project and Jueli Gastwirth helped us to begin.

Most of all, I am grateful for the support of one very special person who is dear to me, and who supplied wisdom, encouragement, wit, good humor, and understanding. There is a peril in close communications with high-level scientific and medical intellects. This communication often uses complex terminology, and often assumes as understood a vast knowledge in a variety of fields. There were times that I came from the rarefied heights of these scholarly interactions not only excited by what I had learned, but also communicating in a language that would not be understood by my readers. It was the task of my editor, Kayla Sussell, to see that I translated this knowledge into text that was not only scientifically correct but also understandable. She is responsible for the smooth flow of this book, and any success we have had in communicating its wide variety of complex medical and scientific concepts in a comprehensible manner. She has been a blessing to me.

I have been extraordinarily honored by frequent dialogue with amazing scholars who think on a very rarefied plane. Most especially, I have been given the great gift of many years of communication with David G. Simons, one of the founders of myofascial medicine. It is a source of wonder and delight that he has taken so much time to discuss issues and ideas with me, shepherd me through the painstaking task of writing medical journal articles, and, in general, being my mentor for so many years. He is a warm and wonderful teacher, full of understanding for the limitations these chronic pain conditions have placed on me, yet always encouraging me to stretch them as far as I can.

I am very grateful that Williams and Wilkins again allowed the use of the wonderful illustrations by Barbara Cummings from *The Trigger Point Manual*s.

I give thanks to all those who have contributed material to this book, especially to my co-author Mary Ellen Copeland for providing chapters 16, 18, and 25 through 27; Chris Brown, John Barnes, Eduardo Barrera, Hal Blatman, Neal Clark, Jim Clements, Camilla Cracchiolo, Judith Day, Mary Lee Esty, Richard Finn, John Giltinan, Melissa Hays, Kathleen Janel, Julian Jonas, John Lowe, Claudia Marek, Carolyn McMakin, Dameron Midgette, Len Ochs, Allie Powers, Bonnie Prudden, Craig Ryan, Wesley Shankland, Rita Shaw, Tasso Spanos, R. Paul St. Amand, Andrew Waldie, Mary Wright, and Samuel Yue.

In addition, I have been privileged to share communications with other doctors and researchers who also know how to think creatively, and are in the business of expanding the envelope of knowledge that I share with you in this book. They have given freely of themselves, both their time and their wisdom, in spite of overwhelming schedules. In appreciation for much kindness, I thank Jan Dommerholt, Jean Bernard Eisinger, Richard Garrison, Robert Gerwin, Chang-Zern Hong, Pat Joyce, Lewis Mock, Trent Nichols, Salih Ozgocmen, Marco Pappagallo, Denise Park, George Roentsch, I. Jon Russell, Michael Schneider, Lois Simons, and Jacob Teitelbaum. In addition, I am grateful to the many researchers who sent their papers to me.

My gratitude goes out to my friend and research assistant, Lanice Aldridge, who appeared when I needed her, with all the talents that I required. I also thank medical librarian Marty Fenn, as well as the very special people at Brooks Memorial Library who managed to come up with all sorts of information I requested.

FMily and friends who sent me information and provided support include Blondilou, Chip Davis, Paul Gallagher, Julia Gauvin, Bonnie Heintskill, Jane Kohler, John Labby, Ann LeBlanc, Tammie Liller, Ed O'Keefe, Sharon Palmer, Leza Raymond, Nancy Solo, Mother Theodora, and Rob Zilin. In addition, Chip and Jane managed to keep my Web site in good operation, in spite of my computer illiteracy. Thank you all.

I have great praise for my own health team: Carolyn Taylor Olson, Craig Anderson, Lynne August, Artie Carrasquillo, Joe Carroll, Al Cramer, Lindsay Crossman, Julie Emond, Bob Fagelson, Debbie Feiner, the Hotel pharmacists, Dana McGinn, George Roentsch, Jeff Wallace, and especially Justine Jeffrey, who relocated in time to become my TrP myotherapist through much of this work. It is a tribute to their abilities that I finished this eighteen-month marathon of research and writing with my myofascia in better shape than when I began.

I am grateful for the support of my church family, especially for the guidance and care of Rev. Jean Jersey and Rev. Thomas Brown, and that of my local support group. I also thank the FMily on the Internet support group FIBROM-L, who have been patient with my absence during the last part of the writing.

Day-to-day computer gremlins were defeated by my husband, Rick, who is developing greater understanding of the path I travel (along with a few trigger points), as well as patience with my long run of medical projects, endless emails and phone calls, and occasional attempts to travel in the name of medical education. The struggle to complete this book has brought us closer together. I wouldn't have made it without him.

In many ways, this is the most difficult part of the book to write, due to my concern that fibrobefuddlement might cause me to forget all those I wish to thank. Now that the book is done, I promise I will pace myself better. Overwork is a preventable perpetuating factor, so it's time for me to prevent it. There have been so many people who took part in the creation of this book. For those whom I haven't mentioned by name here, please forgive me. I thank you all, and thank God for bringing us together on this awesome path.

—Devin J. Starlanyl

Foreword

Chronic pain is a world unto itself. The simple things in life are no longer simple. In fact, life itself is no longer simple. Pain moves from being an unwanted, occasional guest intruding in one's life to being the driving force behind nearly all decisions. Daily choices are governed by the need to survive mentally, physically, and emotionally from day to day. Ordinary life becomes a battlefield. And too often the losers in this battle are those who suffer and their families and friends.

Acute, short-term pain has a face we recognize. A slip of a knife leaves a gaping wound. A bump on the head leaves a bruise and a lump. A broken bone is signified by a limb in a cast. The agony of an abscessed tooth fills all around with sympathy. These injuries hurt but they will heal and, most importantly, the sufferers have directions for seeking help. You cut yourself? Go to the emergency room. You have an abscessed tooth? Go to a dentist. In these and many other instances the sufferers do indeed have a cross to bear but they also have hope. Billions of dollars are spent on advertising all kinds of pain relief for these situations, convincing most people in our society that relief is just a swallow, a rub, or an injection away. Cause and effect. If it hurts, use our product and your pain will go away.

But what about the patient who suffers from fibromyalgia or chronic myofascial pain. Where is the source of the pain? It has to be something! After all, other types of pain go away. If it doesn't go away, maybe it's the sufferer's fault. Maybe you did something to deserve this pain. At least, that's what some may think.

Chronic pain is exhausting in every way: physically, mentally, emotionally, spiritually, and financially. It robs the sufferers of their families, friends, jobs, and relationships, even their life force. Pain is suppose to be a warning to tell our brains that there is a problem needing to be corrected. Chronic pain, however, becomes the problem in and of itself. Acute pain protects life. Chronic pain destroys it.

Chronic pain also brings isolation, both real and perceived. It may be brought on by the victims themselves, a careless word dropped by a family member exhausted by the struggle, or by a noncaring, miseducated health care professional. Being alone violates the basic need all humans have for the company of others. "Misery loves company" may be true about short-term pain, but chronic misery can build a wall that sometimes will keep even the most caring people at a distance, sending the sufferer further and further away from human solace.

In my eighteen years of practice in the field of head, neck, and facial pain and my role as President of the American Academy of Pain Management, the largest multidisciplinary pain organization in the world, I have come to appreciate both the complexities in the study of chronic pain and the anguish of those who suffer its effects.

Healing always begins with careful listening. All good treating doctors realize early in their practice that they must become eternal students, and that the best teachers are our patients. I also have had the honor of learning a great deal from fellow professionals from all walks of life. No one discipline has the complete answer to chronic pain. Those of us who are privileged to treat patients must acknowledge this, accept our roles, and realize that often the best health care advice we can provide is to refer the patient to another professional who treats in a complementary manner to our training. We are all team members. The team must always include the patient.

This second edition of *Fibromyalgia & Chronic Myofascial Pain Syndrome: A Survival Manual* serves as a beacon of light in the dark world of chronic pain. It shines light to all those who must deal daily with the effects of chronic pain: the victims, their families, and their treating clinicians. All readers, no matter what their calling, can learn more about chronic pain and immediately apply that knowledge for the betterment of all. No matter where you are in the journey of life, this book can serve as a benchmark for a new beginning. A beginning of hope, help, and the satisfaction of knowing you are not alone.

> —Christopher R. Brown, D.D.S., M.P.S.
> Immediate Past President
> American Academy of Pain Management
> cbrown@hsonline.net
> www.aapainmanage.org

Introduction

If you are reading this book, you are probably part of the world of fibromyalgia (FMS) and chronic myofascial pain (CMP). You may have lived in this world for some time without knowing its name, and you may have felt lost and confused. You may be experiencing many symptoms for which you don't have an explanation, and for which you have not found relief. This is about to change. Many of the answers you seek are found inside the covers of this book. Welcome to the FMily. The term "FMily" is a name I invented some time ago. It describes the special bond we share.

This is the second edition of the *Survival Manual*, but the material inside is quite new. This material updates all the information in the first edition; it also brings you the latest in research findings. This second edition has been documented much more thoroughly than the first one, and the style of documentation has changed to make the book more reader-friendly. Instead of a separate reference section at the end of the book, the chapters provide individual "endnotes" for those who need to look up the sources. Two terms are employed in these endnotes with which you might not be familiar. The first is *Ibid.*, which means "in the same place" and refers to the endnote immediately preceding it. The second term, *Op. cit.* means "in the work cited." That means the source you are looking for was cited earlier in the endnotes. If you look for it by the name of the author(s) and the date, you will be sure to find it. Some of these *Op. cit.* sources also show different page numbers. That is to aid in finding quoted material.

Some of the ideas in this book are years ahead of the medical establishment's theories. Many of the people I work with and whom I respect are trailblazers in medical science. Somebody has to go first. But those who follow need to know why we are going in the direction we are taking. The facts are the facts, and the "disbelievers" will have to get over it.

Recently, there has been an explosion of research in the study of FMS and CMP. As I was working on this edition, I was in personal communication with researchers concerning still unpublished papers. I will do my best to cover the new research and make it as understandable as possible, without being too tedious. I will explain all new terms and concepts as I go. Note that some doctors don't understand them either. That's why we have endnotes at the end of every chapter. Today, we should all take heart at the quantity and quality of the research that is being done in myofascial medicine, fibromyalgia, and related medical fields.

Those of you who have read the two other books in this series will notice a basic change in terminology. The phrase "myofascial pain syndrome" (MPS) is no longer used, because myofascial pain due to trigger points is now considered a true disease, and is no longer called a syndrome. In this book, we call it "chronic myofascial pain" (CMP).

The first edition of the *Survival Manual* was all about introducing you to the conditions of FMS and CMP, and this edition will repeat the fundamental concepts for new readers. Its companion book, *The Fibromyalgia Advocate*, focused on self-advocacy, on providing you with the information you need to get the services you need. This edition of the *Survival Manual* is focused on getting you to the point of *self-sustaining function*. A lot of the material is heavily documented because there are still those who "don't believe in" these conditions. Until they do, they cannot help you. Each of us has a unique set of needs. You will require a medical team designed to meet your own individualized requirements. See chapter 24 for a discussion of the different kinds of practitioners who should be on your team.

When the first edition of the *Survival Manual* came out, several medical experts told me that reactive hypoglycemia did not exist. It is now well documented. These days, all you have to do is conduct a search of established medical journals under "insulin resistance" to find that it does indeed exist, and in epidemic proportions. Reactive hypoglycemia is often coupled with insulin resistance (see chapter 28).

I want to help educate the medical world as well as my FMily, so I have provided the documentation you need to be taken seriously by your medical and legal teams. There are still doctors and others who "don't believe in" fibromyalgia, myofascial pain, and many of the complexities that may accompany both conditions. You are about to embark on a journey of discovery. You will learn how to recognize myofascial pain trigger points, FMS, and CMP. You will also find many steps you can take to manage your symptoms successfully.

Chronic noncancer pain costs the American economy $40 billion a year.[1] One main reason for the high cost is that most doctors are untrained in the diagnosis and treatment of fibromyalgia and chronic myofascial pain. Thus, many people are put through many unnecessary tests and procedures all of which exhaust them physically, emotionally, and financially. Some of these inappropriate treatments may even worsen their conditions.

In the world of fiction, most people love a mystery. They search for clues and eventually find out "who done it." In real life, when "who" turns out to be FMS and/or CMP, the real mystery remains: What can you do about all your mysterious symptoms, many of which are frightening, not to mention disabling?

In the case of CMP, the map leading to diagnosis and treatment is specific and accurate, thanks to the medical texts written by Drs. Travell and Simons.[2, 3] This book refers to these doctors and their texts often. They have profoundly affected the measure by which you can raise the quality of your life. Unfortunately, many members of the medical profession have not read these medical texts, nor have they been trained in the diagnosis and treatment of trigger points (TrPs). For this lapse in their medical education, their patients pay. With your help, this book can lead such doctors to these invaluable manuals. One of my great desires is to see that Travell and Simons' dream remains alive. I need your help in this task. We are making progress.

Many readers don't know how to approach their doctors with new information. Ideally, this book will already be on your doctor's bookshelf, along with Travell and Simons' manuals. If it is not, the next time you visit your doctor go with your own copy in hand, and say something like, "There's a lot of detailed information in here about trigger points, and I don't understand it all. I'd appreciate it if you would take a look and help me out." Or you could ask, "Have you ever heard of this treatment (or symptom)? Will you help me find out more about it?"

New ideas are important. You need to know when to go out on a limb with them, and when to levitate beyond that limb. Have faith. You may fall, but you may also learn to fly. The difference is faith and perseverance. Writing four articles for medical journals and doing one clinical study in 2000, preparing this new edition, *and* coping with FMS and CMP has been a true learning experience. But I have found that the center of the whirlwind can be a very serene place, if you don't fret about the storm.

I am not a practicing physician, and neither is Mary Ellen Copeland. My formal training was in emergency medicine, not myofascial medicine, although I have learned a considerable amount since then. When I discuss FMS and CMP "patients," I am speaking of those who have FMS and CMP. I have spoken with thousands of these patients personally, and thousands more over the Internet. I refuse to speak of my FMily as "victims." Words are powerful, and we need to use them wisely.

Neither Mary Ellen nor I are wizards capable of working endless long days. We cannot interact with each of you on a one-to-one basis. We both have severe FMS and CMP. We cannot give specific medical advice by correspondence, do not serve as expert witnesses, and attempt only to teach guidelines. What we know we have put into our books and tapes. It is our hope that this edition of the *Survival Manual*, used properly, will fill your needs and answer your questions.

—Devin Starlanyl   http://www.sover.net/~devstar

Endnotes

1. Sheehan, J., J. McKay, M. Ryan, N. Walsh, and D. O'Keefe. 1996. "What cost chronic pain?" *Ir Med J* 89(6):218-219.

2. Simons, D. G., J. G. Travell, and L. S. Simons. 1999. *Travell and Simons' Myofascial Pain and Dysfunction: The Trigger Point Manual*. Second edition. Baltimore: Williams and Wilkins.

3. Travell, J. G., and D. G. Simons. 1983. *Myofascial Pain and Dysfunction: The Trigger Point Manual, Vol. I*. First edition. Baltimore: Williams and Wilkins.

CHAPTER 1

Fibromyalgia 101: A Disturbance in the Force

Fibromyalgia (FMS) is the commonest cause of widespread pain,[1] yet it may remain undiagnosed for a long time. The number of people who have FMS is unknown, but uncertainty and frequent misdiagnosis cause considerable havoc in the lives of many patients. Every expert in the field seems to have his or her own estimate of how many people actually have FMS. This confusion will remain until doctors are trained in comprehensive differential diagnosis. Most FMS patients are female, but again, experts disagree on the percentage.

Fibromyalgia Syndrome is pronounced FIE-bro-my-AL-jia SIN-drome. The word "fibromyalgia" is derived from the Greek "algia," meaning pain, "myo," indicating muscle, and the Latin, "fibro," meaning the connective tissue of tendons and ligaments. The word "syndrome" means a group of signs and symptoms that occur together and that characterize a particular abnormality. Fibromyalgia is not a new "fad disease." For many years the medical profession called it by many different names, including "chronic rheumatism" and "fibrositis." Because we did not understand what was causing FMS, it was thought to be psychological. There now is sufficient *evidence* to show otherwise. In this edition, we are supplying numerous medical journal references that should convince even the most obstinate of footdraggers.

The American Medical Association (AMA) recognized FMS as a true illness and a major cause of disability in 1987, even though most physicians today still lack the skills to diagnose and treat it effectively. Fibromyalgia, like many other conditions, is not *curable* right now, but it is very *treatable*, and there are quite a few ways in which you can improve your health and quality of life considerably. You will learn about many of those ways in this book.

It's not unusual for FMS patients to feel a profound sense of relief when they finally learn they have a recognized illness, and they come to understand that it isn't progressive. Self-doubt is then replaced with appropriate therapies and self-care. Admittedly, if your doctor has no specific training in FMS, getting an initial diagnosis can be extremely difficult. You may come to your doctor with symptoms that seem unrelated that can run the gamut from mental confusion to burning feet, but are usually accompanied by an overall flu-like feeling that impacts on every aspect of your life.

Kristin Thorson, the editor of *The Fibromyalgia Network Newsletter*, points out that just because the mechanisms of FMS aren't fully understood doesn't mean that it is less real.[2] Our symptoms are no less difficult to endure because they have complex causes. If your doctors cannot help you, they should promptly send you to people who can. There are *always* options. This book provides information on many of those options. Just because there is no *one* way that helps everyone doesn't mean that each of us can't find ways to feel a whole lot better.

What Fibromyalgia Is

Fibromyalgia is real. Research supports FMS as a "distinct clinical syndrome deserving of informed medical care and continued research to better understand chronic widespread pain."[3] The American College of Rheumatology, the American Medical Association, the World Health Organization, and the National Institutes of Health have all accepted FMS as a legitimate clinical entity. There is no excuse for doctors "not believing" in its reality. If your doctor "doesn't believe in FMS," you are going to the wrong doctor.

At the Travell Focus on Pain Seminar 2000, Dr. I. Jon Russell, editor of the *Journal of Musculoskeletal Pain*, mentioned the use of the Functional MRI, which shows the brain in action. In a healthy individual, when a tender point was pressed, there was minimal response, but in a patient with FMS, "the result was wild. The whole brain went crazy." Clearly, something is happening in the central nervous system of those who have FMS that is not happening in healthy people.

Fibromyalgia can be a source of substantial disability.[4] This is especially true if you have had it for a long period of time without adequate medical support. FMS can add stress to everything you do. For example, many of us cannot sit still or maintain any other position for longer than twenty minutes without becoming stiff. Nearly everyone with FMS exhibits reduced coordination skills and decreased endurance abilities, although some of this may be due to coexisting chronic myofascial pain (CMP). FMS can be as disabling as rheumatoid arthritis, and about 30 percent of FMS patients cannot continue in their customary occupations due to their chronic, unrelenting symptoms.[5]

The "Irritable Everything" Syndrome

Fibromyalgia is a complex syndrome characterized by pain amplification, musculoskeletal discomfort, and systemic symptoms. In FMS, there is a generalized disturbance of the way in which pain is processed by the body.[6] I think the definition of FMS as widespread allodynia and hyperalgesia[7] describes it very well. "Allodynia" means ordinary nonpainful sensations are experienced as pain sensations. "Hyperalgesia" means that pain sensations are intensified and amplified. The combination can be disastrous. If there is a physically traumatic initiating event, these changes in the way your central nervous system processes pain seem to worsen.

You may be sensitive to odors, sounds, lights, and vibrations that others don't even notice. The noise emitted by fluorescent lights might drive you to distraction. At times, your body may interpret touch, light, or even sound as pain. Sleep, or the lack thereof, plays a crucial role in FMS. You may not be getting enough sleep, or the right quality of sleep. Sleep disturbances, a swollen feeling, and exercise intolerance are significantly related to FMS.[8]

In addition to specific tender points, the essential symptom of FMS is pain, except in the case of older patients. Seniors are more troubled by fatigue, soft-tissue swelling, and depression.[9] In younger people, discomfort after minimal exercise, low-grade fever or below-normal temperature, and skin sensitivity are also common.[10] So many FMS patients say, "I feel like I was hit by a Mack truck" that one study referred to this as the "18-wheeler sign,"[11] although these researchers did indicate that the make of the truck was not significant.

Central Nervous System Sensitization

"It is now firmly established that a central nervous system (CNS) dysfunction is primarily responsible for the increased pain sensitivity of fibromyalgia."[12] There is a generalized CNS-mediated deep tissue sensitivity in FMS that includes the muscles, which is why so many people mistakenly believe that it is a muscular condition. Anything that results in tissue injury, whether from obvious physical trauma like an auto accident or from subtler biochemical damage, can cause hypersensitivity at the site of the injury. If there is repeated or continued trauma, other areas may develop the hypersensitivity.[13] This can lead to a state of "central sensitization," as your nervous system reacts to chronic, long-term pain in several different ways. For example, more nerve connections develop in your spine as a response to the chemical damage caused by chronic pain. This is called *neural plasticity*, and it multiplies the number of pain-carrying channels you have. Neurotransmitters associated with transmission of pain also increase in number. And pain signals coming from outer areas are amplified.

In FMS, you have delayed, inappropriate, and exaggerated autonomic nervous system responses to an external or internal stimuli that has long passed. Argenine vasopressin (AVP) is a biochemical that may be important in FMS, although most researchers have ignored it. Argenine vasopressin may be a key biochemical that prevents the "fight or flight" stress response from turning off in FMS patients once the reason for its activation has passed. Your mind is constantly told that your body is being damaged, and it won't stop feeling the pain until you do something about it. Because any number of neurotransmitters and pain receptors may be involved, you may have to try many different medications (and therapies) before finding a combination that works well for you. Many physicians give up too soon. Pain is a major perpetuating factor for FMS, and you *need* pain relief so that your body and mind have a chance to work on feeling better. Otherwise, pain itself can consume your life. You can't concentrate on stretching exercises when someone is chewing off your leg.

The tendency to develop FMS may be inherited. Many mothers with FMS have children with FMS. Because psychological and familial factors were not different in children with or without FMS, this tendency may be due to genetics.[14] In 1989, Pellegrino, Waylonis, and Sommer[15] found that FMS might be inherited on an autosomal dominant basis, with a variable latent phase. This means that approximately half of the children of an FMS parent will eventually develop FMS. The sooner FMS is recognized and treated, the more easily symptoms can be controlled. (See chapter 12, which deals with age-related issues, from infancy to old age.)

What Fibromyalgia Isn't

Fibromyalgia is not a musculoskeletal disorder.[16] It should have been called "Central Nervous System-myalgia" (see chapter 15). That is where the dysfunction is located. It has nothing to do with the fibers of your muscles. In FMS, muscle fibers are not causing the problem, although there may be cellular changes caused by the biochemical FMS dysfunction. Fibromyalgia is a biochemical disorder, and these biochemicals affect the whole body. You can't have FMS only in your back or in your hands. You either have it all over or you don't have it at all. If you have localized complaints, they are probably not caused by FMS, although FMS may be *amplifying* the local symptoms.

Fibromyalgia is not progressive.[17] If your illness becomes significantly worse over time, then there is some perpetuating or aggravating factor or some coexisting condition that has not been addressed. If you identify that factor and deal with it thoroughly and promptly, your symptoms should ease considerably. Fibromyalgia is not a diagnosis of exclusivity. You may have coexisting conditions, such as multiple sclerosis, arthritis, and/or myofascial pain, and still have FMS pain amplification.

Fibromyalgia is not a catchall, wastebasket diagnosis. It is a specific, chronic non-degenerative, noninflammatory *syndrome*. It is not a disease. Diseases have known causes and well-understood mechanisms for producing symptoms. A syndrome is a specific set of signs and symptoms that occur together. Rheumatoid arthritis, lupus, and many other serious conditions are also classified as syndromes.

Fibromyalgia is not the same as chronic myofascial pain.[18] It is fundamentally different in an important way.[19] *There is no such thing as a fibromyalgia trigger point.* Mention of *"FMS trigger points"* by your doctor or physical therapist should be a warning that there is a serious lack of understanding. Trigger points (TrPs) are part of myofascial pain, not FMS, and your care provider must understand this.

Fibromyalgia is not the same as Chronic Fatigue Immune Dysfunction Syndrome (CFIDS), although they may be part of the same family of central nervous system dysfunctions. Most patients with FMS show increased amounts of substance P in their cerebrospinal fluid. But when levels of substance P were examined in the cerebrospinal fluid of fifteen patients with CFIDS, all values were within normal range. The results of this study support the hypothesis that FMS and CFIDS are different disorders in spite of overlapping symptoms.[20] Another study points out that "In FMS, there is a condition of physiological hyperarousal. In CFIDS, a blunted response, the exact opposite, occurs."[21]

Healthy cerebrospinal fluid (CSF) is clear and colorless, forming a liquid cushion for your brain. Molecules in the CSF can penetrate your brain, as well as bathing it and your spinal cord with nutrients. The CSF helps carry information within your central nervous system. Chemicals in the CSF may help in causing sleep, stimulating appetite, and may affect reproduction. Studies have shown that some of the biochemical levels in the CSF of patients with FMS are not normal.[22]

Fibromyalgia is not just widespread pain or achy muscles. In the general population, adults who meet the American College of Rheumatology (ACR) definition of FMS appear to have distinct features compared to those with chronic widespread pain who do not meet those criteria.[23] There are many conditions that cause widespread pain besides FMS. Chronic myofascial pain (CMP) can cause widespread pain due to trigger point cascades, for example. Side effects of some medications can do the same. Widespread pain is also common in Lyme disease, HIV, hypothyroid and other endocrine abnormalities, and in some genetic diseases.[24]

> I coined the word "FMily" to describe the special bond those of us who have fibromyalgia all share. We often have more in common with our fellow fibromyalgia patients than we do with members of our family.
>
> D.J.S.

Fibromyalgia is not a homogenous condition. The cause of muscle pain and allodynia may not be the same in all persons fulfilling the ACR criteria for FMS.[25] There are many subsets of FMS. Fibromyalgia seems to include patients with different pain processing mechanisms.[26] One study has separated some subsets into meaningful categories,[27] and this separation may help decide which treatment regimens are more likely to help specific patients.

Fibromyalgia is not an autoimmune condition.[28] The presence of antinuclear antibodies and other connective tissue disease features is similar in patients with fibromyalgia and healthy control subjects.[29] Some FMS patients may develop coexisting autoimmune conditions, and patients with immune conditions may develop

FMS, but this does not show a causal relationship. There is a subset of people with FMS who test positive for antinuclear antibodies.[30] We don't yet know what this means. A response to antipolymer antibodies is associated with a subset of patients with FMS.[31]

Fibromyalgia is not a mental illness and must not be categorized as such. Some people with FMS also have mental illness. Some people with flu have mental illness, too, but that doesn't mean that flu is caused by mental illness. Studies have shown that the incidence of mental problems is no higher with FMS patients than with any other type of chronic pain syndrome.[32] There is now clinical evidence that FMS represents a distinct rheumatic disorder and should not be regarded as a somatic illness secondary to psychiatric disorder.[33] Psychiatric Diagnostic Interview data failed to discriminate in any major way between primary fibromyalgia syndrome (a disorder with no known organic etiology) and rheumatoid arthritis (a disorder with a known organic etiology). Therefore, these data do not support a psychopathology model as a primary explanation of the symptoms of primary fibromyalgia syndrome.[34]

Fibromyalgia is not infectious. Infection from many causes can start the neurochemical cascade of FMS. This does not mean that FMS itself is infectious. Both FMS and CMP can be brought on by specific triggers, such as stress, infections, pollution, and diet. Because there is a great deal of financial and other stress when dealing with a chronic illness, it is not surprising that some partners of those with FMS develop the same illness.

An Official Diagnosis

FMS has been around for a long time, under a variety of names. In 1990 a group of physicians tried to clarify matters after a clinical study when they published a consensus description of FMS.[35] To do this study, two groups of doctors separately evaluated patients with widespread pain who had also been diagnosed as having FMS by experts. The most consistent finding by both groups of doctors was the eighteen diagnostic tender points. Unfortunately, these doctors and this study have been widely misunderstood. This was a description of FMS for *research purposes*. In other words, patients chosen for inclusion in a clinical study for FMS must have eleven of the eighteen tender points to be absolutely sure that the patients in the studies have FMS, and thus that the research conclusions will describe FMS. Unfortunately, this definition did not explain that coexisting CMP can complicate and skew the research, and I believe that has happened in a great number of studies. Regardless, "eleven of eighteen specific tender points" was *initially* not meant to be the criterion for *diagnosis* of FMS.

Widespread hypersensitivity and allodynia can be present with fewer than eleven tender points. The patients in this study were all picked for their widespread pain, so we aren't even sure that is always a condition of FMS. Presently, the tender points are what we have as characteristic for FMS. The official definition of FMS came about as a result of the Copenhagen Declaration, which established FMS as an officially recognized syndrome on January 1, 1993, for the World Health Organization. This definition was presented at the Second World Congress on Myofascial Pain and Fibromyalgia, which was held in Copenhagen in 1992. (See the Consensus Document on Fibromyalgia.)[36]

Tender points hurt where pressed, but they do not refer pain. In other words, pressing a tender point does *not* cause pain in some other part of the body. The examiner must use enough pressure to whiten the thumbnail, which is about 4 kg pressure. The official definition further requires that tender points must be present in all four quadrants of the body, that is, the upper right and left and lower right and left parts of your body. (See figure 1-1.) Tender points occur in pairs, so the pain is usually distributed equally on both sides of the body.

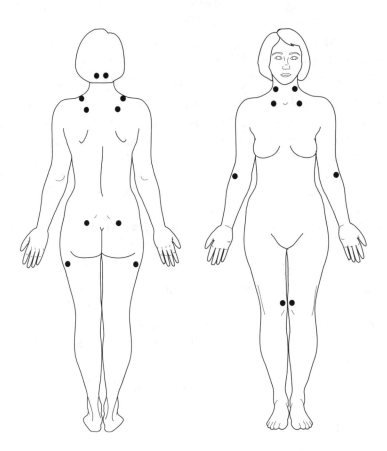

Figure 1-1: Fibromyalgia tender points

On the back of your body, tender points are present in the following places:

- Along the spine in the neck, where the head and neck meet;
- On the upper line of the shoulder, a little less than halfway from the shoulder to the neck;
- About three finger widths, on a diagonal, inward from the last points;
- On the back fairly close to the dimples above the buttocks, a little less than halfway in toward the spine;
- Below the buttocks, very close to the outside edge of the thigh, about three finger widths.

On the front of your body, tender points are present in the following places:

- On the neck, just above inner edge of the collarbone;
- On the neck, a little farther out from the last points, about four finger widths down;
- On the inner (palm) side of the lower arm, about three finger widths below the elbow crease;
- On the inner side of the knee, in the fat pad.

The tender point count may decrease with proper medical treatment and self-care, but that doesn't mean that the FMS has been *cured*. It simply means that you have learned to deal with the perpetuating factors and coexisting conditions and have them under control.

Initiating Events

In FMS, we believe that there is often an initiating event that activates biochemical changes, causing a cascade of symptoms. For example, unremitting grief of six months or longer can trigger FMS. In many ways, FMS is sort of like survivor's syndrome. Cumulative trauma, protracted labor in pregnancy, open-heart surgery, and even inguinal hernia repair have all been initiating events for FMS. The start of each case of FMS probably has multiple causes.[37] Not all cases of FMS cases have a known triggering event that initiates the first obvious flare. During a flare, current symptoms become more intense and, frequently, new symptoms develop.

Many patients, when questioned carefully, reveal that their symptoms began at an early age. Pain is often the most obvious symptom of FMS, but there are other symptoms too. There are no common specific diagnostic tests for FMS, but demonstrable biochemical differences do exist. The tests are very expensive, some require a research laboratory, and the results are not specific to FMS. Here are some of these tests:

- There are reduced high-energy phosphate levels in the muscles of patients with primary fibromyalgia.[38]

- Levels of phosphocreatine and adenosine triphosphate (ATP) are lower at rest as well as during exercise.[39] ATP is the prime source of cellular energy.

- Fibromyalgia is associated with metabolic abnormalities.[40]

- Increased concentrations of homocysteine[41] and nerve growth factor are found in the cerebrospinal fluid of FMS patients.[42]

- Fibromyalgia may be due to dysfunctional thyroid regulation of the genetic code information transfer between types of nucleic acids. This may be due to mutation of the c-erbaA beta gene, as well as to thyroid deficiency. The result would be tissue-specific hypothyroid-like symptoms despite normal circulating thyroid hormone levels, and thus normal thyroid test results.[43]

- A subset of FMS patients have low levels of insulin-like growth factor 1 (IGF-I).[44]

- Abnormal cerebral blood flow in the caudate nucleus[45] and thalamus[46] have been found in FMS.

- In FMS there is dysfunction at least at the brain stem level. The cerebrospinal fluid showed discrete changes in cell differential count.[47]

This is a small sample of the many research papers available on FMS. Why are there still some doctors who "don't believe in" FMS? One reason is that we don't yet have a common, cheap, sensitive, and specific test for FMS. We must be very careful not to take something that may be a "finding," like a specific blood value found in *some* but not all patients, and assume it can be used as a *specific* test for FMS. This simply adds to the confusion.

FMS has a major effect on direct health costs.[48] It is in the interest of many insurers, at least in the short term, to deny patients the health care they need. "It's All In Your Head" is a cheaper diagnosis for the insurance companies and HMOs. In the long term, this attitude costs the health care system more by creating sicker patients who require more extensive services, further stressing medical resources.

Fibromyalgia seems to be the result of many neurotransmitter cascades.[49] A neurotransmitter cascade is like a waterfall that starts at the top and bounces off rocks and ridges on the way down, wearing down the rock, moving the gravel, and changing the river as it goes. The neurotransmitter cascade can cause changes throughout your body, and many of these changes may start cascades of their own. Once these cascades get moving, a combination of peripheral and central factors join in to make the changes chronic, and the result is what we call fibromyalgia. Every patient may have different neurotransmitters and other biochemical "informational substances" disrupted in different ways.

Note that the term *informational substance* is a relatively new, broad term that includes peptides, neurotransmitters, neuromodulators, growth factors, hormones, interleukins, cytokines, and similar substances. These are the biochemicals in your body that convey information from one part to another. Each informational substance may be used in many different ways in your body and brain, and may affect many other informational substances. You could think of yourself as a vast network of messages traveling in three dimensions at all times, even when you are asleep.

The Fun Stuff

Some of us can create complex meals, organize households, or run businesses. (Or at least we could before FMS.) But few of us understand how our own bodies and minds work. You *need* to understand some basics to have a better relationship with your own self. If you have FMS, something—or more likely several somethings—have gone wrong. These somethings have become your perpetuating factors: components or elements in your life or lifestyle that perpetuate your illness(es) and will continue to do so until you change them. You need to set as many of them right as possible.

To do this, you *need* to understand how you are supposed to function as the complex and wonderful being that you are. Which is why I did not title this section "Basic Biochemistry," as most of you would skip it until "later," later being synonymous with the end of the world or the next time the ice cap overruns your neighborhood, whichever comes first. For the reasons stated above this is important information, and I will make it as easy to understand as is possible. You need to become your own best friend. In the cause of enlightened self-interest, read on. It will be worth the effort.

Just as a group of people can often become more efficient if they learn to work as an organized team, so it is with the biochemicals of your body. Unfortunately, when FMS steps in, the coach goes on vacation, and a state of hyperarousal develops. In this state, the brain releases more of the neurotransmitter acetylcholine. This chemical causes every sense to go on alert. This is the stress response; the "flight or fight" response. There are also "startle" and "freeze" responses among the options as well. Some of us overreact to a sudden noise or event, and go into panic or "startle" mode. Then again, some of us may "freeze" like deer in the headlights of a car.

The Hypothalamus-Pituitary-Adrenal Axis and Other Balancing Acts

Now we have some axes to grind. An *axis*, in medical terms, is a balance between one informational substance and another. Neuroendocrine axes provide communication between the brain and body, using informational substances as the messengers. When you have too much of one biochemical, another is produced which will result in a decrease of the first, if all is going well. In FMS, all is not going well.

The hypothalamic-pituitary-adrenal (HPA) axis seems to be one of the first axes to become dysfunctional in FMS. It is the main stress-responder. The HPA axis affects the immune system, the gonadal axis hormones, the growth hormones, and the thyroid axis. These axes all loop back to exert influence on the HPA axis. All of these axes can be profoundly influenced by insulin resistance, which is an extremely common perpetuating factor.

The hypothalamus is a small gland in your brain. It regulates eating, drinking, and sexual urges. It's one of your main regulatory centers. The hypothalamus helps determine your emotional behavior. It also helps regulate your autonomic nervous system, which controls many of the automatic functions of your body. This includes the rate at which your heart beats, digestion, and how widely your blood vessels dilate at any given time. If this sentinel gland receives certain signals, it interprets them as threats to your body. It will then signal your pituitary gland, which is located close to the hypothalamus in the brain, to prepare your body for some kind of action to reduce the danger.

The pituitary gland is a sort of central control in the body, and regulates many other glands, including the thyroid and the adrenals. When the pituitary is signaled by the hypothalamus that the body is threatened, it sends an emergency message to the adrenal glands to jump (figuratively, of course) into action.

The adrenals are a pair of tiny glands perched on top of the kidneys like little triangular caps. They influence almost all of the body systems. They produce adrenaline and many other biochemicals that the body uses in stressful situations. The balance and relationship among these three glands is called *the HPA axis*. In healthy people, when the stress or threat is removed, the adrenals signal the pituitary that it's time to relax again. Unfortunately, one of the problems in FMS is the hormone balance between these three glands does not work properly, and something happens to disrupt the feedback loop. This means that the fight or flight response system is always on a hair-trigger alert. Your body and mind cannot maintain this state of alert readiness indefinitely, and the system begins to break down.

Cells and Energy

When I was a student, one of the most exciting things I learned about in biochemistry was the Krebs cycle. Well, I admit it wasn't exciting to me at the time. It is now. The Krebs cycle is the name of the basic biochemical cycle that explains how you turn "dinner" into "you," and how you generate the energy you need to keep going. This energy production takes place in little "factories" in your cells, called mitochondria (MY-toe-KON-dree-ah). The mitochondria depend on many biochemicals to function efficiently. Many FMS abnormalities may be related to abnormal mitochondria.[50]

There is a theory that, a *very* long time ago, way before the age of dinosaurs, during the time cells were first developing nuclei, mitochondria were actually viruses or viruslike particles that invaded early cells and developed a mutually beneficial relationship with them. During the course of evolution, mitochondria became an integral and very interesting part of our mammalian cells. We have taken these little invaders for granted far too long, and if our hard-working little factories become polluted, or start to fail in other ways, they and we become fatigued and produce excess lactic acid, which causes muscle pain.

In some cases, the mitochondria may no longer be able to receive and process the amounts of fuel we give to them. They might even use neurotransmitters to signal you to breathe more shallowly, because they can't use the oxygen they would use to burn that fuel. Unfortunately, at this time it is impossible to send a health inspector to check out these tiny biofactories and get them up to code, but we're working on it.

Low Growth Factor

Some studies have indicated a subset of patients with FMS has low levels of insulin-like growth hormone one (IGF-1).[51] Women with FMS and low IGF-1 levels improved and the number of their tender points were reduced after nine months of daily hormone growth therapy. IGF-1 is expensive, but it provided symptom relief for this subset of patients. There may be many pain generators leading to central sensitization, and it is important to address them with as many methods as possible. IGF-1 is known to improve glycemic control.[52] If you have insulin resistance as a perpetuating factor, this may be a helpful therapy. It is important, however, that you first be tested for your insulin base level.

Microcirculation may cause some of the pain and dysfunction in FMS. Your body is on alert, and your muscles demand more oxygen to move. Transcapillary permeability is significantly reduced in FMS, so your muscles receive less oxygen than those of a healthy person.[53]

From what we can tell, FMS occurs in all races and ages. Some age or racial groups may have more FMS because they may have a greater incidence of a specific perpetuating factor. As we age, for example, there is a greater drift to dysfunction of informational substance axes. During menopause, there is a greater chance of hormonal change. In some Native American tribes, there is a tendency toward reactive hypoglycemia/insulin resistance leading to abdominal obesity and type II diabetes. These can all contribute to or perpetuate FMS. That does not necessarily mean that these groups might have a greater incidence of FMS if the perpetuating factors were brought under control.

As more people understand that FMS is a real illness, and the public begins to recognize the term "fibromyalgia" and all that it signifies, we won't feel so isolated. Studies show that having others believe the pain of FMS is real is crucial to patients' quality of life and to their ability to cope.[54]

In one study, the researchers stated, "Scientific breakthroughs in FM research are likely to occur soon due to the combined efforts of multiple investigators from different disciplines working on what now appear to be isolated phenomena or events, but which may prove to be intertwined. As our understanding of the etiopathogenesis of FM improves, more rational and effective therapeutic programs will be developed."[55] The next step is learning how to put it right again. FMS *amplifies* pain, myofascial trigger points *cause* pain–and many other symptoms. In the next chapter we will take a close look at myofascia and see what it is, what it does, and why it can cause us so much grief.

Endnotes

1. Bennett, R. M. 1995. Fibromyalgia: The commonest cause of widespread pain. *Frontiers* 21(6):269-275.

2. Thorson, K. 1999. Is fibromyalgia a distinct clinical entity? The patient's evidence. *Baillieres Best Pract Res Clin Rheumatol* 13(3):463-467.

3. Russell, I. J. 1999. Is fibromyalgia a distinct clinical entity? The clinical investigator's evidence. *Baillieres Best Pract Res Clin Rheumatol* 13(3):445-454.

4. Kaplan, R. M., S. M. Schmidt, and T. A. Cronan. 2000. Quality of well being in patients with fibromyalgia. *J Rheumatol* 27(3):785-789.

5. Wolfe, F. 1989. Fibromyalgia: the clinical syndrome. *Rheum Dis Clin North Am* 15(1):1-18.

6. Morris, V., S. Cruwys, and B. Kidd. 1998. Increased capsaicin-induced secondary hyperalgesia as a marker of abnormal sensory activity in patients with fibromyalgia. *Neurosci Lett* 250(3):205-207.

7. Russell, I. J. 1998. Advances in fibromyalgia: possible role for central neurochemicals. *Am J Med Sci* 315(6):377-384.

8. Jacobsen, S., I. S. Petersen, and B. Danneskiold-Samsoe. 1993. Clinical features in patients with chronic muscle pain—with special reference to fibromyalgia. *Scand J Rheumatol* 22(2):69-76.

9. Yunus, M. B., G. S. Holt, A. T. Masi, and J. C. Aldag. 1988. Fibromyalgia syndrome among the elderly. Comparison with younger patients. *J Am Geriatr Soc* 36(11):987-995.

10. Reiffenberger, D. H., and L. H. Amundson. 1996. Fibromyalgia syndrome: a review. *Am Fam Phys* 53(5):1698-1712.

11. Sigal, L. H., D. J. Chang, and V. Sloan. 1998. 18 tender points and the "18 wheeler" sign: clues to the diagnosis of fibromyalgia. *JAMA* 279(6):434.

12. Simons, D. G., J. G. Travell, and L. S. Simons. 1999. *Travell and Simons' Myofascial Pain and Dysfunction: The Trigger Point Manual,* Second edition. Baltimore: Williams and Wilkins, p. 17.

13. Yaksh, T. L., X. Y. Hua, I. Kalcheva, N. Nozaki-Taguchi, and M. Marsala. 1999. The spinal biology in humans and animals of pain states generated by persistent small afferent input. *Proc Natl Acad Sci* 96(14):7680-7686.

14. Yunus, M. B., M. A. Kahn, K. K. Rawlings, J. R. Green, J. M. Olson, and S. Shah. 1999. Genetic linkage analysis of multicase families with fibromyalgia syndrome. *J Rheumatol* 26(2):408-412.

15. Pellegrino, M. J., G. W. Waylonis, and A. Sommer. 1989. Familial occurrence of primary fibromyalgia. *Arch Phys Med Rehabil* 70(1):61-63.

16. Simms, R. W. 1998. Fibromyalgia is not a muscle disorder. *Am J Med Sci* 315(6):346-350.

17. Wolfe, F., J. Anderson, D. Harkness, R. M. Bennett, X. J. Caro, D. L. Goldenberg, I. J. Russell, and M. B. Yunus. 1997. Health status and disease severity of fibromyalgia: results of a six-center longitudinal study. *Arthritis Rheum* 40(9):1571-1579.

18. Gerwin, R. D. 1999. Differential diagnosis of myofascial pain syndrome and fibromyalgia. *J Musculoskel Pain* 7(1-2):209-215.

19. Simons, D. G., D. G. Travell, and L. S. Simons. 1999. *Op. cit.,* p.18.

20. Evengard, B., C. G. Nilsson, G. Lindh, L. Lindquist, P. Eneroth, S. Fredrikson, L. Terenius, and K. G. Henriksson. 1998. Chronic fatigue syndrome differs from fibromyalgia. No evidence for elevated substance P levels in cerebrospinal fluid of patients with chronic fatigue syndrome. *Pain* 78(2):153-155.

21. Crofford, L. J. 1998. Neuroendocrine findings and patients with fibromyalgia. *J Musculoskel Pain* 6(3):69.

22. Russell, I. J. 1998. *Op. cit.*

23. White, K. P., M. Speechley, M. Harth, and T. Ostbye. 1999. The London Fibromyalgia Epidemiology Study: Comparing the demographic and clinical characteristics in 100 random community cases of fibromyalgia versus controls. *J Rheumatol* 26(7):1577-1585.

24. Soppi, M., and E. Beneforti. 1999. Muscular pain in some rheumatic diseases. *J Musculoskel Pain* 7(1-2):225-229.

25. Henriksson, K. G. 1999. Is fibromyalgia a distinct clinical entity? Pain mechanisms in fibromyalgia syndrome. A myologist's view. *Baillieres Best Pract Res Clin Rheumatol* 13(3):455-461.

26. Sorensen, J., A. Bengtsson, J. Ahlner, K. G. Henriksson, L. Ekselius, and M. Bengtsson. 1997. Fibromyalgia—are there different mechanisms in the processing of pain? A double blind crossover comparison of analgesic drugs. *J Rheumatol* 24(8):1615-1621.

27. Eisinger, J., D. Starlanyl, F. Blotman, L. Bueno, E. Houvenagle, R. Juvin, P. Kaminsky, K. Lawson, X. Le Loet, J. Lowe, P. Manesse, et al. 2000. [Protocole d'informations anonyme sur les fibromyalgiques.] *Medicine du sud-est Lyon Mediterranee Medical.* 1:9-11. [French]

28. Wittrup, I. H., A. Wiik, and B. Danneskiold-Samsoe. 1999. Antibody profile in patients with fibromyalgia compared to healthy controls. *J Musculoskel Pain* 7(1-2):273-277.

29. Yunus, M. B., F. X. Hussey, and J. C. Aldag. 1993. Antinuclear antibodies and connective tissue disease features in fibromyalgia syndrome: a controlled study. *J. Rheumatol* 20(9):1557-1560.

30. Smart, P. A., G. W. Waylonis, and K. V. Hackinshaw. 1997. Immunologic profile of patients with fibromyalgia. *Am J Phys Med Rehabil* 76(3):231-234.

31. Wilson, R. B., O. S. Gluck, J. R. Tesser, J. C. Rice, A. Meyer, and A. J. Bridges. 1999. Antipolymer antibody reactivity in a subset of patients with fibromyalgia correlates with severity. *J Rheumatol* 26(2):402-407.

32. Goldenberg, D. L. 1989. Psychological symptoms and psychiatric diagnosis in patients with fibromyalgia. *J Rheumatol* Suppl 19:127-30; Merskey, H. 1989. Physical and psychological considerations in the classification of fibromyalgia. *J Rheumatol* Suppl 19:72-79.

33. Dunne, F. J., and C. A. Dunne. 1995. Fibromyalgia syndrome and psychiatric disorder. *Br J Hosp Med* 54(5):194-197.

34. Ahles, T. A., S. A. Kahn, M. B. Yunus, D. A. Spiegel, and A. T. Masi. 1991. Psychiatric status of patients with primary fibromyalgia, patients with rheumatoid arthritis, and subjects without pain: a blind comparison of DSM-III diagnoses. *Am J Psychiatry* 148(112):1721-1726.

35. Wolfe, F., H. A. Smythe, M. B. Yunus, R. M. Bennett, C. Bombadier, D. L. Goldenberg, et al. 1990. The American College of Rheumatology 1990 Criteria for the classification of fibromyalgia. Report of the Multicenter Criteria Committee. *Arth Rheum* 33(2):160-172.

36. Consensus Document on Fibromyalgia: The Copenhagen Declaration. Issued by the Second World Congress on Myofascial Pain and Fibromyalgia meeting August 17-20, 1992. Published *Lancet*, vol. 340, Sept. 12, 1992, and incorporated into the World Health Organizations 10th revision of the International Statistical Classification of Diseases and Related Health Problems, ICD 10, Jan. 1, 1993. Also can be found in the *Journal of Musculoskeletal Pain*, vol. 1, no. 3/4, 1993.

37. Bennett, R. M., and S. Jacobsen. 1994. Muscle function and origin of pain in fibromyalgia. *Baillieres Clin Rheumatol* 8(4):721-746.

38. Bengtsson A., K. G. Henriksson, and J. Larsson. 1986. Reduced high-energy phosphate levels in the painful muscles of patients with primary fibromyalgia. *Arthritis Rheum.* 29:817-821.

39. Park, J. H., P. Phothiamat, C. T. Oates, M. Hernanz-Schulman, and N. J. Olsen. 1998. Use of P-31 magnetic resonance spectroscopy to detect metabolic abnormalities in muscles of patients with fibromyalgia. *Arth Rheum* 41(3):406-413.

40. Eisinger, J., A. Plantamura, P. A. Marie, and T. Ayavou. 1994. Selenium and magnesium status and fibromyalgia. *Magnes Res* 7(3-4):285-288.

41. Regland, B., M. Andersson, L. Abrahamsson, J. Bagby, L. E. Dyrehag, and C. G. Gottfries. 1997. Increased concentrations of homocysteine in the cerebrospinal fluid in patients with fibromyalgia and chronic fatigue syndrome. *Scand J Rheumatol* 26(4):301-307.

42. Giovengo, S. L., I. J. Russell, and A. A. Larson. 1999. Increased concentrations of nerve growth factor (NGF) in cerebrospinal fluid of patients with fibromyalgia. *J Rheumatol* 26(7):1564-1569.

43. Lowe, J. C., M. E. Cullum, L. H. Graf, Jr., and J. Yellin. 1997. Mutations in the c-erbA beta gene: do they underlie euthyroid fibromyalgia? *Med Hypo* 48(2):125-135.

44. Bennett, R. M., D. M. Cook, S. R. Clark, C. S. Burckhardt, and S. M. Campbell. 1997. Hypothalamic-pituitary-insulin-like growth factor-I axis dysfunction in patients with fibromyalgia. *J Rheumatol* 24(7):1384-1389.

45. Bradley, L. A., A. Sotolongo, K. R. Alberts, G. S. Alarcon, J. M. Mountz, H-G Liu, et al. 1999. Abnormal regional cerebral blood flow in the caudate nucleus among fibromyalgia patients and non-patients is associated with insidious symptom onset. *J Musculoskel Pain* 7(1-2):285-292.

46. Mountz, J. M., L. A. Bradley, and G. S. Alarcon. 1998. Abnormal functional activity of the central nervous system in fibromyalgia syndrome. *Am J Med Sci* 315(6):385-396.

47. Johansson, G., J. Risberg, U. Rosenhall, G. Orndahl, L. Svennerholm, and S. Nystrom. 1995. Cerebral dysfunction in fibromyalgia; evidence from regional cerebral blood flow measurements, otoneurological tests and cerebrospinal fluid analysis. *Acta Psychiatr Scand* 91(2):86-94.

48. White, K. P., M. Speechley, M. Harth, and T. Ostbye. 1999. The London Fibromyalgia Epidemiology Study: direct health care costs of fibromyalgia syndrome in London, Canada. *J Rheumatol* 26(4):885-889.

49. Starlanyl, D. 1998. *The Fibromyalgia Advocate*. Oakland, CA: New Harbinger Publications. Chapter 2.

50. Olsen, N. J., and J. H. Park. 1998. Skeletal muscle abnormalities in patients with fibromyalgia. *Am J Med Sci* 315(6):351-358.

51. Bennett, R. M., S. C. Clark, and J. Walczyk. 1998. A randomized, double-blind, placebo-controlled study of growth hormone in the treatment of fibromyalgia. *A J Med* 104(3):227-231.

52. Morrow, L. A., M. B. O'Brien, D. E. Moller, J. S. Flier, and A. C. Moses. 1994. Recombinant human insulin-like growth factor-I therapy improves glycemic control and insulin action in the type A syndrome of severe insulin resistance. *J Clin Endocrinol Metab* 79(1):205-210.

53. Grassi, W., P. Core, G. Corlino, F. Salaffi, and C. Cervini. 1994. Capillary permeability in fibromyalgia. *J Rheumatol* 21(7):1328-1331.

54. Seers, K. 1996. The patients' experiences of their chronic non-malignant pain. *J Adv Nurs* 24(6):1160-1168.

55. Alarcon, G. S., and L. A. Bradley. 1998. Advances in the treatment of fibromyalgia: current status and future directions. *Am J Med Sci* 315(6):401.

CHAPTER 2

Myofascia 101: What It Is, What It Does, and What You Need to Know

Myofascial pain is probably the most common cause of musculoskeletal pain in medical practice.[1] It is a vital factor in the practice of internal medicine, physical medicine and rehabilitation, gynecology, rheumatology, neurology, pediatrics, gastroenterology, proctology, cardiology, and just about any other specialty you can think of. Pain from myofascial dysfunction is probably the source of many of *your* symptoms. So why is there so little common knowledge about the myofascia?

"Fascial" and "facial" are similar words with two different meanings. In the United States, the word "fascia" is usually pronounced *fashia*, similar to *fashion*. In other English-speaking countries, the word is often pronounced *fassia*. Many doctors prefer to avoid mentioning the word entirely. Most doctors don't know a lot about the workings of the myofascia. That's because one of the chief ways that doctors learn about anatomy is through cadaver dissection. Dead, embalmed fascia has little in common with living fascia. The magic is gone.

The Importance of Myofascia

A small change in the myofascia can cause great stress to other parts of your body. Restriction of one major joint in a lower extremity can increase the energy expenditure of normal walking by as much as 40 percent, and, if two major joints are restricted in the same extremity, it can increase by as much as 300 percent.[2] Multiple minor restrictions of movement, particularly in the maintenance of a normal gait, also may have a detrimental effect upon total body function.

One of the problems in discussing myofascia is that there is no familiar metaphor to help you visualize what and where it is. Recently I saw a three-dimensional IMAX theater presentation on the undersea world, and that is the sort of thing I wish I could show you about myofascia. There are no three-dimensional movies about the myofascia, so you will have to use your imagination and stretch your visualizing skills.

In the first edition, we described the myofascia as the thin and almost translucent film that wraps around muscle tissue. It's that sticky white film you see covering some of the chicken parts you buy at the grocery. It gives shape to and supports all of your body's musculature. All of that is true, but it is only part of the picture.

One of the local FMily members told me a good story. Her seven-year-old son was at the pediatrician with leg pain. The doctor condescendingly told the boy he might have FMS like his mother. The boy was scornful. "You stupid head!" he replied. "It's myofashion! Don't you even know the difference!" His mother then handed the doctor some information on myofascial pain.

Visualize a gauzelike network that shapes your entire body. Make that network three-dimensional, covering your entire interior, and then fill the gauze with structures including blood vessels, nerves, and lymph. Remember to put your organs into this image. They are held in place with fascial scaffolding. Then, add your muscles, which are permeated with their own myofascial network. Finally, position your bones to anchor your muscles, and cover it all with skin. And that's still only part of *where* your myofascia is.

Myofascia 101

In *Principles of Manual Medicine,*[3] the author finds it convenient to separate fascia into three layers, but remember as you read that it is all continuous and three dimensional. *Superficial fascia* is attached to the underside of your skin. Capillary channels and lymph vessels run through this layer, and so do many nerves. The subcutaneous fat is attached to it. If your superficial fascia is healthy, your skin can move fluidly over the surface of your muscles. In fibromyalgia (FMS) and chronic myofascial pain (CMP), the superficial fascia is often stuck. In this layer of the fascia, there is a great potential to store excess fluid and metabolites, the breakdown products of informational substances and other chemicals in your body. This is the area of fascia that often is the easiest to palpate. *Palpation* is the art and skill of applying the hands or fingers to the external surface of the body for examination purposes; in other words, to palpate means "to touch meaningfully," to interpret what the skin and fascia can indicate about the state of health of the person being palpated.

Deep fascia is a much tougher and denser material. Your body uses deep fascia to separate large sections, such as the abdominal cavity, from each other. Deep fascia covers some areas like huge sheets, protecting them and giving them shape. Deep fascia also separates your muscles and organs. The baglike covering around your heart (the pericardium), the lining of your chest cavity(the pleura), and the area between your external genitals and your anus (the perineum) are all composed of specialized deep fascia.

There is a third layer of fascia, called *sub serous fascia*. This loose tissue covers your internal organs and holds the network of blood and lymph vessels that keep them moist. It is important for you—and for your doctor—to understand that sub serous myofascia surrounds the blood vessels, lymph vessels, and nerves. Changes of pressure due to compression by tightening myofascia can affect the cells that lie within the blood and lymph vessels and nerves. The dural tube is another form of fascia. This tube surrounds and protects your spinal cord, and contains the cerebrospinal fluid. This tube is connected to the membranes surrounding your brain. Together, they hold and protect your craniosacral system.

Cells are not simply empty sacs filled with fluid. Each cell has a support structure called a *cytoskeleton*. About 25-35 percent of all cellular protein is part of this cytoskeleton.[4] The cytoskeleton and associated proteins control the flow of ionic minerals, such as calcium and magnesium; the movements of functional units such as mitochondria inside the cell; cell division; movements of the chromosomes, and movements of the cell itself.[5] You will learn more about the cytoskeleton later in chapter 15.

Part of the organization of the cell has a very important and complex name, but that's okay, because it is important and complex. A *reticulum* is a network formed by cells, or structures within cells, or of connective fibers between cells. The *endoplasmic reticulum* is the network found in the *endoplasm*, or inner part of the cell, but outside of the nucleus. It often contains many microfilaments that provide support for the cell membrane. Nucleoproteins, which contain DNA, are present in both the nucleus and the cytoplasm. The endoplasmic reticulum synthesizes proteins. In liver cells, it helps to metabolize glycogen to produce energy.[6] In the glands, it helps to secrete hormones.[7]

Other structures in the cell include the mitochondria. They are mobile and flexible structures that produce adenosine triphosphate (ATP). They are self-reproducing, because they have their own form of circular DNA. Each DNA molecule of your body is enclosed in a nuclear envelope that separates the DNA from the rest of the cell. The outer membrane of the envelope is physically connected to the endoplasmic reticulum.[8] Most physicians don't understand the significance of these connections. The next time your physician, your insurance company, or other care provider tries to deny the importance of bodywork, especially fascial work, to the state of your health, teach them what they need to know. Bodywork can affect your health at the cellular level.

John Barnes, master of Myofascial Release (see chapter 19), explains the continuity and pervasiveness of the myofascia in the following way:

> "Every muscle of the body is surrounded by a smooth fascial sheath, every muscular bundle of fibrils is surrounded by fascia, every fibril is surrounded by fascia, and every microfibril down to the cellular level is surrounded by fascia. Malfunction due to trauma, poor posture, or inflammation can bind down the fascia. Restrictions of the fascia can create pain or malfunction throughout the body, sometimes with bizarre side effects and seemingly unrelated symptoms. At the cellular level, fascia creates the interstitial spaces. [See chapter 5 on the lymph.] It has extremely important functions in support, protection, separation, cellular respiration, elimination, metabolism and fluid and lymphatic flow. It can have a profound influence on cellular health and the immune system.
>
> If fascia is restricted at the time of a trauma, the forces cannot be dispersed properly and areas of the body are then subjected to an intolerable impact. The forces do not have to be enormous; a person who just does not have enough "give" can be severely injured. Fascia reorganizes along the lines of tension imposed on the body, adding support to misalignment and contracting to protect the individual from further trauma (real or imagined). This has the potential to alter organ and tissue physiology significantly. Over time, the tightness spreads like a pull in a sweater or stocking. Flexibility and spontaneity of movement are lost, setting the body up for more trauma, pain, and limitation of movement."[9]

Fascia is also the material that forms adhesions and scar tissue.

Ground Substance

In the myofascia, there is a material called *ground substance*. This material can change its form from liquid to solid and back again. When you are healthy, your ground substance has a gelatinous consistency so that it can absorb the forces that are created when you move. It is also a shock absorber if you are involved in trauma. The ground substance can resemble gelatin that has not yet set, or seem like a firm gelatinous slurry, or even harder, like sprayed-on Styrofoam insulation. When the ground substance hardens, it is as if it has turned to glue or cement.[10] When ground substance changes from a liquid to a gel, and then into its more solid form, the myofascia tightens. It won't reverse to its previously more liquid state without outside intervention.

One of the main jobs of the ground substance is to transfer nutrients from the parts of the body where they are broken down into usable materials to the places in the body where they will be used; and to remove the waste products from those areas of use.

Another important job the ground substance does is to maintain the distance between connective tissue fibers. This prevents micro-adhesions from forming, and keeps the tissues supple and elastic. When the critical distance is not maintained, the fibers become cross-linked by newly synthesized *collagen*, which is also part of the fascia. Collagen cross-links are arranged haphazardly, unlike healthy linkages, and they are hard to break apart. When the ground substance has hardened, it isn't enough for the therapist to break up the cross-linkages. The ground substance must be returned to its healthy, more fluid state.

Normal muscle action is the *patterned response of groups of muscles*. This means that no muscle works alone. For every muscle that stretches, another one must contract. Muscle function depends on groups of muscles working together. Your muscles must stay active to remain healthy and responsive. Activity helps to ensure that the fluids in the body keep moving. Anything that interferes with muscle activity, such as FMS or CMP, interferes with the health of your muscles.

The majority of connective tissue consists of fluids and fibers. The constituents of the fluid are constantly changing. Because bodywork and other therapies move toxins and wastes out of the intercellular fluids and into the bloodstream, it is not uncommon for nausea or headaches to result. This movement is a necessary step in ridding yourself of these chemical toxins and wastes,[11] so it is a good sign, even though it doesn't feel good at the time.

Muscles and Wastes

The products of your body's cellular factories, as well as the wastes from its cellular processing, must pass through the ground substance to reach the lymph and later be processed for removal. When the myofascia is "gunked up" (sorry, I have to use *some* medical terms) and stuck together, informational substances, those biochemical messengers that run the body, can't work properly. When wastes and chemical toxins back up in the tightened muscle, local nerve endings become irritated. These irritated nerves tell your brain to activate its arousal system, so your body knows something is going wrong. The ground substance becomes more solid because the fight or flight response is activated when the body mobilizes to rid itself of irritation.[12]

Fibrous myofascial adhesions can form anywhere along nerves and block normal healthy function. Too often, fascia has been considered by the medical world as merely packing material, simply a connective tissue between areas of function. The mobility, elasticity, and slipperiness of living fascia can never be appreciated by dissecting embalmed cadavers in medical school.[13]

As your fascia twists, turns, and tightens, due to the stressors of life, long threadlike structures called *myofascial trains* can develop. These will restrict your movement. Fascial construction is basically vertical, except for areas of transverse fascial planes at joints like the pelvic and shoulder girdles. Dysfunctions don't show up in most exams, unless range of motion studies are included. Even then, the blame for dysfunction is too often placed on bony irregularities, which may show up on X-ray and other tests, even though they may not be the cause of the dysfunction itself.

Fascia not only binds and supports, it is a primary communication channel in the body. In ancient Chinese and Tibetan texts there are allusions to *chi* or *qi* (energy) moving through the fascia. In some ways, the myofascia may function as an independent nervous system. It has electrical, magnetic, and crystalline qualities. The crystalline structures may store memory as the brain does, only as a form of cellular tissue memory, which must be released before the tissue can become functional again.

Trauma and Immobilization

As you heal from a trauma, your body may be involved in two myofascial processes resulting in a loss of ability to stretch. Scars occur in the areas of direct trauma, and are part of the body's healthy response to repair the damage. Scar formation is a localized response and is a self-limiting condition. *Fibrosis* is a homogenous change in the fabric of the connective tissue. Fibrosis can occur as a reaction to the biochemicals created in the area of trauma. Fibrotic change also can take place as a result of low-grade irritation from poor posture, repetitive motions, or movement dysfunctions.

If you are relatively immobile after a trauma, microadhesions will form. The biochemicals released when there is trauma promote the formation of microadhesions during immobility. These adhesions become progressively more fibrotic with increased length of immobilization.[14] If you can get moving again in a short period of time, this effect will reverse. If you don't move, your muscle can become increasingly firm and tight, so that muscle definition and mobility are lost and the muscle appears to be cast in concrete. Muscle fibrosis occurs as a change in the texture of the whole muscle tissue, and is not the same as the lumps and bumps and taut ropy bands of myofascial trigger points.

A contractured muscle is not the same as a tense muscle. When you voluntarily relax your muscles, you can reduce the number of nerve signals transmitted by that muscle. If the muscle is only tense, it will be able to relax. If the muscle is contractured, it will stay contractured until it is treated. A contracture may loosen up when you stretch or instinctively massage the problem muscles, but specific intervention is the only way to treat multiple contractures.

Attachments

Where muscles and tendons, bones, and ligaments come together—these are areas of attachment. The cellular membranes in these attachment areas can become extremely convoluted, which increases the surface area and changes the angle of force. This increases the potential for tissue to get stuck together, and causes the tissue there to become more easily torn.[15]

Trigger points (TrPs) are extremely sore points that can occur in the myofascia in taut, ropy bands throughout the body. They also can be felt as painful lumps or nodules. When you have a TrP in your muscle, it causes pain at the end of your range of motion when you attempt to stretch that muscle. The TrP weakens that muscle. You begin to avoid stretching that muscle because it hurts when you do. Your muscles are designed to work their best when they move freely, so as you move the TrP-laden muscle less frequently, it becomes less healthy. Circulation in your smallest capillaries, the *microcirculation*, becomes impaired in the area of the TrP. Nutrients and oxygen cannot reach the area easily, and wastes cannot easily be removed. Your lymph system (see chapter 5) depends on the movement of the muscles to move the lymph fluid, so that system begins to stagnate as well. Finally, because some of your other muscles have to do the work of the muscle that is weak, these overworked muscles start developing TrPs.

Trigger points can occur in the myofascia, skin, ligaments and tendons, bone lining, and other tissues. In chapter 8 you will find diagrams of many of the common TrPs and their pain-referral patterns, along with explanations of their symptoms and what to do about them. You may immediately recognize some of the TrP pain patterns as your own. This pattern recognition is one thing that should alert your medical team to the presence of TrPs, but they must be educated to recognize the patterns themselves. It is important that you do more than just look at the pictures in that chapter. You need to know why they are causing you pain before you can understand how to relieve those symptoms.

Endnotes

1. Imamura, S. T., A. A. Fischer, M. Imamura, M. J. Teixeira, T. Y. Lin, H. S. Kaziyama, et al. 1997. Pain management using myofascial approach when other treatment failed. Myofascial pain—update in diagnosis and treatment. *Phys Med Rehab Clin North Am* 8(1):179-187.

2. Greenman, P. E. 1996. *Principles of Manual Medicine*. Second edition. Baltimore: Williams & Wilkins.

3. *Ibid.*

4. Sperelakis, N. (Ed.) 1998. *Cell Physiology Source Book*. Second Edition. San Diego: Academic Press, p. 85.

5. *Ibid.* p. 532.

6. *Ibid.* p. 79.

7. *Ibid.* p. 81.

8. *Ibid.* p. 62.

9. Barnes, J. 1990. *Myofascial Release*. MFR Seminars, 10 S. Leopard Road, Suite One, Paoli, PA 19301.

10. *Ibid.*

11. Juhan, D. 1987. *Job's Body*. Barrytown, NY: Station Hill Press.

12. *Ibid.*

13. Leahy, M., and L. E. Mock III. 1992. Myofascial release technique and mechanical compromise of peripheral nerves of the upper extremity. *Chiro Sports Med* 6(4):139-140.

14. Cantu, R. L., and A. J. Grodin. 1992. *Myofascial Manipulation: Theory and Clinical Application*. Gaithersburg, MD: Aspen Publishers, Inc.

15. Simons D. G., J. G. Travell, and L. S. Simons. 1999. *Travell and Simons' Myofascial Pain and Dysfunction: The Trigger Point Manual, Volume I*, Second edition. Baltimore: Williams and Wilkins, p. 17.

CHAPTER 3

One Little, Two Little, Three Little Trigger Points

It is a source of frustration that so many readers have written telling me that once they saw the first edition, they *knew* they had fibromyalgia (FMS), because they recognized the patterns on the cover as their own. The diagrams on the cover, with the exception of one showing the fibromyalgia tender points, do not illustrate FMS! They are diagrams of myofascial trigger points (TrPs) and the pain-referral patterns that those TrPs create. So what are these things called TrPs, and why do they make our lives so miserable?

Until recently, we had no scientific and understandable cause for the existence of TrPs, and they had no officially recognized diagnostic criteria. Because of this, physicians and therapists, for the most part, have not been trained to recognize and treat them. Lack of understanding on the part of insurance carriers and the Social Security Administration has made some lives even more difficult. All this is about to change.

We now have facts that cannot be disputed. Myofascial pain caused by TrPs is a *true disease*. We now know what creates a trigger point, what causes those taut bands that constrict our muscles, and why our muscles become so tight that they hurt. Fibromyalgia and chronic myofascial pain (CMP), as far as we know, occur in people all over the world. Trigger points have even been found and treated in dogs, cats, and horses. "Myogenic (muscle-generated) pain is badly neglected by medicine. . . . Myofascial trigger points are one of the most common and most neglected sources of musculoskeletal pain."[1]

A myofascial TrP is a hyperirritable area of skeletal muscle. Trigger points exist in association with hypersensitive contraction nodules, which feel like rock-hard lumps in your muscle. You may be able to feel the taut ropy band of tense muscle fibers that extends from the TrP to the area where your muscles attach to other structures. Your anatomy changes in response to the biochemical stressors that cause the TrP, even before your pain receptors are sensitized. This means that you develop the taut band even before you feel the pain.

These changes, and the myofascial TrPs, are caused by a *thousandfold* increase in the release of acetylcholine, an important neurotransmitter. This release of acetylcholine is a response to the release of greater-than-normal amounts of calcium in the area of the muscle where nerves end, called a motor endplate.[2] The cause of TrPs appears to involve serious disturbances of these nerve endings.[3] In this chapter, you will find out what this means for you.

Latent Trigger Points

Almost anyone can get TrPs, but if nothing perpetuates or aggravates them, they become latent. The latent TrP doesn't hurt at all, unless it is being pressed upon. It does cause increased muscle tension and muscle shortening, and uses extra energy while doing so. The latent TrP restricts movement, and weakens and prevents full lengthening of the muscle in which it is located. A latent TrP may be activated by perpetuating factors (conditions or circumstances that aggravate and thus perpetuate the TrP). People who don't exercise regularly have a greater chance of developing latent TrPs than those who do. If latent TrPs are treated immediately, and perpetuating factors are avoided or remedied, they can be eliminated. If TrPs are left untreated, or are inappropriately treated, they will remain. When a stressor comes into your life, a latent TrP can become activated. A perpetuating factor increases the likelihood of latent TrPs becoming active.

Active Trigger Points

If you force your muscle to work in spite of pain, especially if perpetuating factors exist, your TrPs will become active. This can be quite dramatic if you have accumulated many latent TrPs over time, and suddenly they are all activated. This may happen due to an auto accident, fall, infection, or other stressor. Active TrPs cause referred pain and other symptoms in expected pain pattern locations whenever you move the muscle. If you keep using the muscle and push it to work harder, the pain may remain even when the muscle is at rest.

Some TrPs lie within a pain pattern and refer pain in that general area, and some TrPs refer pain to an area quite distant from that TrP. Some do both. Unless your medical team members are trained to recognize these patterns and the TrPs to which they belong, they will be mystified. Their lack of training doesn't mean that your pain isn't real. "The intensity of myofascial pain due to TrPs should not be underestimated, as it has been rated by patients as equal to or slightly greater than pain from other causes."[4] The effects of low-back pain of myofascial origin can be as bad as or worse than low-back pain from a herniated disc.[5]

Pain from trigger points is usually steady, dull, deep, and aching. The intensity can range from mild discomfort to incapacitating torture. If a nerve is trapped in tightened, inflexible myofascia, the pain can become burning, sharp, and lightning-like. Note that trigger point pain, unlike the tender point pain of FMS, is rarely distributed equally on both sides of the body unless it has become chronic.

Satellite and Secondary TrPs

A satellite TrP develops in a muscle because that muscle is located in the primary TrP's referred pain area. A secondary TrP develops in a muscle that is overloaded because it is compensating or substituting for a muscle that contains the primary TrP. These concepts explain how TrPs spread. There is an important difference between a condition that is worsening and a progressive illness. Symptoms from a true progressive condition cannot be reversed, whereas symptoms from TrPs definitely can be. Commonly applied therapies for myofascial pain cause *substantial abrupt reduction* in pain intensity.[6] If your symptoms are getting increasingly worse over time, it is a sign that there is at least one hidden perpetuating factor and/or coexisting condition that has not been addressed.

Here is an example of how TrPs can spread: Suppose you work at a desk alongside an air-conditioning vent, and the cold air blows directly onto your neck on your right side. This constant chilling of your neck will stress your scalene muscles (see chapter 8) on the right side.

Trigger points in the scalene muscles cause you to tilt your head slightly, which sets up stress on the left side of your neck to compensate for the unequal weight distribution. This causes secondary TrPs on the left side of your neck to develop, and may cause more TrPs to form on the right side as well, as other muscles try to take up the slack caused by the weak scalenes. Stresses caused by pain in the referral pattern of the right scalenes cause levator scapulae TrPs to develop on the right, causing a stiff neck on that side. It hurts to lengthen muscles with TrPs, so the muscles in the right side of your neck contract and pull your shoulder upwards, forcing you to lean to the left.

The muscles in your left abdominal area under your ribs become compressed, and you develop secondary latissimus dorsi trigger points on that side. These TrPs cause you to breathe in a shallower pattern, thus setting up TrPs in your other respiratory muscles. Your spine develops a twist to protect these painful muscles, as your lower spine twists one way and your upper spine twists the other way. This is called *rotoscoliosis*, which activates a compensatory rotation of your pelvis. This process can continue until your entire body is covered with trigger points. This process is reversible.

Recognizing Trigger Points

The fact that referred pain patterns are very similar from patient to patient with TrPs helps the physician to make a diagnosis, if that physician is familiar with the patterns. An educated doctor will know where to look for TrPs before the physical exam begins. Trigger points can vary in irritability from hour to hour and day to day. The amount of stress needed to activate a latent TrP depends on the conditioning of the muscle, and that also varies. If you have stubborn chronic pain, you probably have multiple causes and perpetuating factors.

For many years, the emphasis has been on the pain caused by myofascial TrPs, because the pain can be so prominent. Even more significantly, *trigger points cause muscle weakness and restricted range of motion*. Physical and occupational therapists, as well as doctors, often recommend strengthening exercises without understanding that the TrP is inhibiting the muscle. **You cannot strengthen a muscle with a trigger point**. If you try to strengthen such a muscle, the TrPs then worsen and develop satellite and secondary TrPs. *Improper physical therapy can be a prime perpetuating factor.*

Trigger points can slowly accumulate through life. As you age, you may notice that one muscle will "give out" from time to time, or there may be an old fracture or strain that has "never quite healed." Once a fracture has healed, there should be no muscle weakness. If there is weakness, there is probably a TrP causing it, and that TrP can be treated. It is never acceptable for a doctor to suggest that you have to live with TrPs because "anyone can get them." This attitude puts you on a path toward iatrogenic (physician-caused) chronic myofascial pain. Trigger points cause weakness and muscle dysfunction. If you don't deal with them promptly, they can develop satellites and secondary TrPs, and *you* will be the one dealing with the consequences, not the doctor.

One of the most common causes of developing a TrP is to hold a muscle in an awkward position. That forces the sustained contraction of other muscles to maintain that posture. This happens regularly to auto mechanics, dental hygienists, ceiling painters, and postal workers, and it can happen to you, too. Emotional stress can cause this contraction. If you constantly hold your muscles tight in a fight-or-flight stress response, this will change your body's musculature patterns. Become aware of how you use your body. Trigger points also form as a result of other medical conditions. For example, a case of arthritis may be otherwise well managed, but the accompanying TrPs could be overlooked. The arthritic patient's pain load could be substantially lessened if the associated TrPs were treated successfully.

Central TrPs are usually in the belly of muscle, are associated with dysfunctional motor endplates, and are located near the center of the muscle fibers.

Attachment TrPs occur in areas of tenderness where the muscle attaches to other structures. These may result from the sustained tension from the taut bands of central TrPs. Some of us feel that attachment TrPs may be TrPs in the tendons. They often respond well to ice, whereas central TrPs, unless there is associated nerve entrapment, often respond better to moist heat.

Remember, *there is no such thing as a fibromyalgia trigger point*. Trigger points are part of myofascial pain. Unlike FMS tender points, TrPs can and do refer pain to other parts of the body. Referred pain is not unique to TrPs. Most people have heard of the referred pain radiating down the arm during a heart attack. Furthermore, many women have experienced pain radiating down their thighs during painful menstrual periods.

Trigger Point Symptoms

Often, TrPs can be felt as painful lumps of hardened fascia. It is often easier to feel ropy bands in an arm or leg if you extend it about two thirds of the way out. The band is often easier to palpate when the muscle is neither fully lengthened nor fully shortened. As you progress through successful trigger point therapy, older TrPs become revealed, layer by layer. This can be frustrating at times, because you eliminate one TrP only to have another one surface as your tissues release. Your muscles can get so tight that you can't feel the lumps or the tight, ropy bands, but that doesn't mean the TrPs aren't there. It may mean that your muscles have become fibrotic. This is exceedingly difficult to reverse. It takes time and patience.

When a nerve passes through a muscle between the ropy bands, or when a nerve lies between the ropy band and bone, the pressure on the nerve can produce numbness, but only in the area of compression. That's called *nerve entrapment*. You may have observed that when one part of your body turns over and rests on another part while you are sleeping, the part being compressed goes numb. For example, if you sleep on your side and your body is resting on an arm, that arm will likely go numb. Trigger points can also constrict fluid flow in the body, entrapping blood and lymph vessels and ducts.

Trigger Points: The In-Depth Scoop

Trigger points are not homogenous knots in the myofascia. Each TrP is a cluster of abnormal spots called *loci* (pronounced low-sigh) that are scattered throughout each knot or nodule.

The taut, ropy band is the initial response to stressors that produce the TrP. This happens independent of pain sensations. The development of pain is a separate step involving activation of peripheral pain-sensing receptors, called *nociceptors* (see chapter 9).

Myofascial Pain from Trigger Points: A True Disease

Myofascial TrPs can be identified and have been *documented* by characteristic *spontaneous electrical activity* (SEA).[8] Doctor Robert Gerwin made an ultrasound video of a TrP local twitch response.[9] Biopsies of myofascial TrPs show contraction knots and giant rounded muscle fibers. The structure of the cells has changed microscopically, forming *contraction knots*—the lumps and bumps we know only too well. "The endplate dysfunction characteristic of MTrPs involves both the nerve terminal and the postjunctional muscle fiber. This relationship identifies MTrPs as a neuromuscular *disease*."[10] This doesn't mean that everyone needs a biopsy or an ultrasound

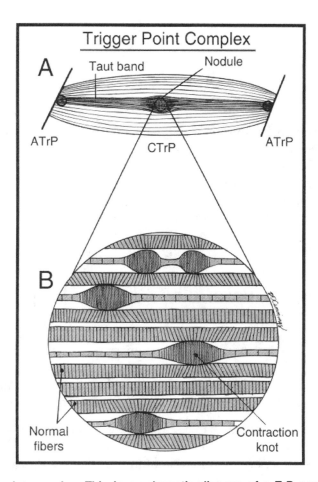

Figure 3-1: The Trigger point complex. This is a schematic diagram of a TrP complex showing the pathophysiology as we believe it to be at this time. This view, and our knowledge of TrPs, is still developing. This diagram is from *Travell and Simons' Myofascial Pain and Dysfunction: The Trigger Point Manual*[7] and it is printed with permission of authors and publisher.

video of her or his TrPs. It *does* mean that doctors and other care providers who "don't believe in" myofascial trigger points had better become educated.

Doctor Chang-Zern Hong, a presenter at the Focus on Pain Seminar, believes that the sensitive locus in a myofascial TrP region is probably related to a sensitized nerve fiber. Sensitive loci can be widely distributed in the whole muscle, but are highly concentrated in the TrP region. The sensitive loci may also be found in some tender points in FMS patients. The TrP is a common pathogenic pathway of muscle pain from different causes.[11] Dr. Hong has found that a calcium channel blocker, such as propranolol, can block the characteristic spontaneous electrical activity of a TrP. He mentioned a paper presently under review about calcium channel blocker effects at the neuromuscular junction.

I have been testing a topical (transdermal) form of calcium channel blocker for use on specific resistant TrPs. If we can find a way to block the excess calcium release, we may be able to defuse the TrPs, but we must be careful. Calcium channels are in use throughout the body. It is a mechanism that is involved in heart muscle and other smooth muscles, as well.

The sensitive locus in a myofascial TrP region is probably related to a sensitized nerve fiber. Theoretically, referred pain can be caused by sufficiently intense stimulation at any site containing nociceptors (peripheral pain receptors), but greater pressure is required to elicit a referred pain from a less sensitive site. Sensitive loci can be widely distributed throughout the whole muscle, but they can be highly concentrated in the TrP region. Sensitive loci may also be found in some tender points in some FMS patients.

Autonomic Nervous System Trigger Point Symptoms

Sensitization of autonomic nerves in the myofascial TrP can be the cause of autonomic nervous system symptoms. These include abnormal sweating, tearing of the eye, persistent runny nose, excessive salivation, and "goose bumps" on your skin. Trigger points may also have related *proprioceptive* disturbances. Proprioceptors are receptors that govern spatial awareness. This includes knowing where you are in relation to objects in the world around you, as well as the relationships between one part of your body and another. Proprioceptor dysfunctions can include imbalance, dizziness, ringing in your ears, and a distorted perception of the weight of objects.

Chronic Myofascial Pain: The Shrink Wrap, Not the "Shrink Rap"

When the myofascial nature of pain is unrecognized, such as the pain caused by TrPs in the pectoral muscles that mimics cardiac pain, the symptoms are likely to be diagnosed as neurotic, psychogenic, or behavioral. This adds frustration and self-doubt to the patient's misery and blocks appropriate diagnosis and treatment.[12]

In myofascial pain, local tissue changes are very similar to mechanically induced muscle damage. In acute stages, such changes are accompanied by edema, and in chronic forms by local fibrosis.[13] *Fibrosis* means an abnormal formation of fibrous tissue as a reaction to a stimulus, such as trauma or infection.

Nonmyofascial TrPs are not caused by the same mechanism that causes myofascial TrPs. Trigger points in the skin often cause sharp, moderately severe stinging, prickling, or numbness. Trigger points that occur in scars can cause burning, prickling, or lightning-like jabs. "A considerable portion of the chronic pain due to myofascial TrPs could have been prevented by prompt diagnosis with appropriate treatment. . . . When the myofascial nature of pain is unrecognized . . . the symptoms are likely to be diagnosed as neurotic, psychogenic, or behavioral. This adds frustration and self-doubt to the patient's misery and blocks appropriate diagnosis and treatment. . . . The total cost is incalculable, but enormous, and most of it is unnecessary."[14]

Chronic Myofascial Pain

Some medical and dental practitioners use the term "myofascial pain syndrome" to refer to a TMJ (temperomandibular joint) dysfunction. This use is both confusing and obsolete. TMJ dysfunction may be caused by TrPs, but chronic myofascial pain can be bodywide. When chronic myofascial pain develops, overlapping pain patterns may cause confusion even for care providers experienced with single muscle TrPs. Because myofascial pain is no longer classified as a syndrome, we prefer the term "CMP" to indicate this widespread condition.

Once doctors and therapists learn to recognize CMP, they are surprised to see how very common it is. One reason CMP develops is that single TrPs have gone unrecognized and untreated. Early, aggressive treatment of myofascial pain gives the patient a much better chance to improve.[15] Even with CMP, as progress is made in resolving the perpetuating factors, the involved muscles become increasingly treatable.

Other Interactions

Joint dysfunction can interact strongly with TrPs. This can be in the form of joint hypomobility that must be mobilized, or joint hypermobility that must be stabilized.

Myofascial pain modulation disorder can develop. In this disorder, one area is hypersensitized and other TrPs in the region refer pain to this one area. Generally, this is the site of previous trauma or other intense pain. The nerve path is like a road well traveled; it is the easiest place to reach. Not only TrP pain, but even other sources of pain can refer to this hypersensitized area. For example, if your knee is hypersensitized, not only can a TrP in your hip or foot refer pain to your knee, but if you stub your toe, that pain can be felt in your knee as well.

Algometry

There is a way to measure the TrP area using a handheld instrument. The tissue compliance meter can measure both local tenderness and the alteration of tissue consistency, and this can be documented quantitatively.[16] We used one of these instruments in our recent clinical study (see chapter 15), and found that you must assess muscle guarding and startle reactions if you are testing patients with both FMS and CMP.

Diagnostic Criteria

A Special Interest Group for Certification in Myofascial Trigger Point Pain Diagnosis and Treatment has been formed this year (2000) within the International Myopain Society. There are also plans underway to ensure that separate special medical codes for fibromyalgia and for myofascial pain are created (for insurance and other purposes). Please urge your doctors to join this organization (see Resources). A subscription to the *Journal of Musculoskeletal Pain* comes with the membership.

Dr. I. Jon Russell, the editor of this journal, proposed a study to establish reliable classification criteria for myofascial pain in the upper torso.[17] Once this is established, it can be applied with a high degree of sensitivity and specificity for research and clinical purposes. This will establish, in turn, a model for developing diagnostic classification, criteria for myofascial pain.

Endnotes

1. Simons, D. G. 2000. Focus on Pain Seminar. Mesa City, AZ.

2. Gerwin, R. D. 1999. Myofascial pain syndromes from trigger points. *Pain* 3:153-159.

3. Hong, C-Z. 1999. Current research on myofascial trigger points: pathophysiological studies. *J Musculoskel Pain* 7(1-2):121-129.

4. Simons, D. G., J. G. Travell, and L. S. Simons. 1999. *Travell and Simons' Myofascial Pain and Dysfunction: The Trigger Point Manual*. Second edition. Baltimore: Williams and Wilkins.

5. Cassisi, J. E., G. W. Sypert, L. Lagana, E. M. Friedman, and M. E. Robinson. 1993. Pain, disability, and psychological functioning in chronic low back pain subgroups: myofascial versus herniated disc syndrome. *Neurosurgery* 33(3):379-385.

6. Skootsky, S. A., B. Jaeger, and R. K. Oye. 1989. Prevalence of myofascial pain in general internal medicine practice. *West J Med* 151(2):157-160.

7. Simons, D. G., J. G. Travell, and L. S. Simons. 1999. *Op. cit.* page 70.

8. Hubbard, D. R., and G. M. Berkoff. 1993. Myofascial trigger points show spontaneous needle EMG activity. *Spine* 18(13):1803-1807.

9. Gerwin, R. D., and D. Duranleau. 1997. Ultrasound identification of the myofascial trigger point. *Muscle Nerve* 20:767-768 (letter).

10. Simons, D. G. 1999. Diagnostic criteria of myofascial pain caused by trigger points. *J Musculoskel Pain* 7(1-2):112.

11. Hong, C-Z. 1996. Pathophysiology of myofascial trigger points. *J Formos Med Assoc* 92(2):93-104.

12. Simons D. G., J. G. Travell, and L. S. Simons. 1999. *Op. cit.*, p. 76.

13. Pongratz, D. E. and M. Spath. 1998. [No title available]. *Fortschr Med* 116(27):24-29. [German]

14. Simons D. G., J. G. Travell, and L. S. Simons. 1999. *Op. cit.*, p. 14.

15. McClaflin, R. R. 1994. Myofascial pain syndrome. Primary care strategies for early intervention. *Postgrad Med* 96(2):56-59.

16. Fisher, A. A. 1999. Algometry in diagnoses of musculoskeletal pain and evaluation of treatment outcome: an update. *J Musculoskel Pain* 6(1):5-32.

17. Russell, I. J. 1999. Reliability of clinical assessment measures for the classification of myofascial pain syndrome. *J Musculoskel Pain* 7(1-2):309-324.

CHAPTER 4

Fibromyalgia and Chronic Myofascial Pain: The Double Whammy

Now that you know *what* a trigger point (TrP) is, you will learn how it can work in concert with other TrPs to cause you so much grief, and some of the reasons why fibromyalgia (FMS) and chronic myofascial pain (CMP) together cause more trouble than just the sum of their symptoms would indicate they could.

Fibromyalgia and CMP both share muscle pain as a symptom. This has resulted in many persons with bilateral or widespread muscle pain being diagnosed as having FMS when, in fact, the pain is from CMP or some other source. Right now there is no cure for FMS, although there are many treatments that help. There *are* cures for many of the other causes of widespread pain, but your doctor must understand that *all widespread pain is not FMS.*

Widespread Diagnostic Confusion

"The fibromyalgia literature remain stuffed with references to myofascial pain as a regional syndrome in contrast to fibromyalgia as the widespread syndrome. This is a particularly dangerous concept in chronic pain, where myofascial pain is more likely to be generalized."[1] It is important to study *individual* TrPs to learn their referral patterns, but it is also important for medical team members to understand that complex overlapping pain patterns exist in chronic pain patients. As the perpetuating factors are addressed and the TrPs are adequately treated, the single muscle pain patterns eventually will become apparent again, and then those TrPs can be treated.

You may have FMS and CMP, as well as joint dysfunction and other perpetuating factors. Each condition requires separate attention. People with FMS and CMP face more than just the two sets of symptoms of both conditions. Physical therapy and other forms of treatment must proceed carefully. Any treatment tried will be both more complicated and less successful than if the patient had only one of the two conditions.

We didn't ask for complex invisible illnesses that so far have no easy diagnostic tests. No matter how complex it is for the doctor (and everyone else) to deal with, it is infinitely more complex for us, as patients. We must deal with a bewildering array of symptoms, often with a malfunctioning brain and body that do not communicate well with each other. We must learn to manage our lives and do the best we can with what we've got. That's all any of us can do. It is our medical team's job to support us. That means they need to supply more than a cheery hello and a pat on the back. We need guidance and direction. We need help to search out the perpetuating factors and coexisting conditions. Myofascial TrPs need to be treated locally, and their perpetuating factors need to be addressed. Fibromyalgia needs to be treated systemically, and its perpetuating factors need to be addressed.[2]

Sorting It Out

Making a diagnosis of FMS and CMP can be complicated. The symptoms of each person can vary in many ways. In the CMP component, not only is there a wide variety of combinations of TrPs, there may also be different nerves, blood and lymph vessels, and ducts entrapped. There may be many kinds of perpetuating factors and many different kinds of initiating events.

Some doctors will tell you that they never saw a patient with just FMS, or just CMP, so they must be the same condition. Unless you understand the concepts behind each, that may *seem* true, because it takes a great deal of training and experience to palpate TrPs and the patient's muscles may be guarded or fibrotic. You can't get palpation experience just by looking at diagrams. Too many doctors do not have this skill, which is why it is often easier for bodyworkers to palpate TrPs. Robert Gerwin is a doctor who *does* understand these conditions. He was one of the first doctors to grasp the significance of Travell and Simons' work.

In a study of ninety-six patients, Gerwin found that 74 percent of the patients had only myofascial pain. Thirty-five percent of the myofascial pain patients had generalized TrP pain in three or four quadrants. (The quadrants of the body are the upper right, upper left, lower right, and lower left.) In other words, even though these patients had CMP and not FMS, they had widespread pain. They had the symptoms of CMP, but they did not have the generalized hypersensitivity and tender points of FMS. Among the FMS patients in this study, 28 percent had only FMS. Among the FMS patients, 72 percent had both FMS and CMP.[3]

Dr. Gerwin has a marvelous series of tapes on the diagnosis and treatment of TrPs (see Resources). One article[4] he wrote explains the differences between FMS and CMP very clearly. If you have both of these conditions, their coexistence will have a direct impact on every phase of your treatment.

I have seen or heard of far too many cases where a patient with both FMS and CMP had one or the other condition undiagnosed. Some people have suffered needlessly for years because of this and were often given inappropriate therapy. Some had coexisting conditions that were missed because their doctors attributed all of their pain to FMS. The same TrPs were treated over and over without any attempt to find the hidden perpetuating factors. In some cases where there was cancer or other life-threatening illnesses, this lack of understanding on the doctor's part proved deadly.

Fibromyalgia is a chronic illness that can be controlled. Chronic myofascial pain is a condition that is potentially curable, unless there is a fixed, uncorrectable underlying cause. The focus of treatment for both conditions is to restore more normal functioning with minimized pain.[5]

Some Practical Differences

1. Restricted motion is not a part of FMS. Generalized fatigue is, but not the specific muscle weakness that is caused by TrPs.

2. With CMP, there is no pain in the areas of the muscle that do not have TrPs or their referral patterns, unless FMS or something else is causing generalized pain.

3. Disturbed nonrestful sleep is found in both conditions, due to different causes (see chapter 10).

4. If you have only FMS, you are not going to find hard lumps and bumps and ropy bands in your muscles. Those are part of the TrPs that characterize CMP.

5. You are not going to find a generalized hypersensitivity to pain and/or allodynia (feeling pain from nonpainful stimuli) in CMP. That is characteristic of FMS. If you have both symptoms, you *may* have both conditions.

Other conditions can cause bodywide pain, so you need a doctor who knows how to make the diagnosis. This is not the same as having a doctor who has *heard* of these conditions. If your doctor doesn't understand this, take in these medical references. If s/he won't look up the references, and won't listen and won't learn, document it in writing. Then get another doctor. Even if you are in an HMO, you can make a good case for your need to have a doctor and physical therapist who recognize, understand, and can treat your illnesses.

FMS *and* CMP: Why They Are More Than Double the Trouble

The proper treatment of patients with both FMS and CMP requires special skills. In CMP, a chronic pain condition exists with many different symptoms, TrPs, and perpetuating factors that will be magnified by the pain amplification aspect of FMS. Furthermore, some of the treatments normally prescribed for FMS patients can harm CMP patients, and the reverse is also true.[6]

Fibromyalgia patients can tolerate slow and gentle strengthening of muscles. Chronic myofascial pain patients can't. You *cannot* strengthen a muscle that harbors a trigger point. If you have FMS and CMP, you are not as likely to experience pain relief from TrP injections. Some people do receive temporary pain relief from the injections, but some get none at all. Even if you do receive some relief, you may have severe postinjection soreness.

Theories About the FMS/CMP Connection

To understand what happens when FMS and CMP combine, we need to look at the big picture. Most of the body's processes rely on the unobstructed movement of fluids throughout the various systems. Blood circulates, carrying food, fuel, oxygen, and other materials. It also carries away wastes. Lymph circulates, carrying fats, salts, proteins, white blood cells, and other substances. Ducts release biochemicals, and these ducts can become constricted, too.

On the microscopic level, every cell in the body depends on the motion of liquids from outside to inside the cell, and back. In one *Star Trek* episode, an alien described humans as bags of dirty water. That description, while unsavory, is quite correct. Your body depends on the motion of this dirty water in and out of its cells. When there is impaired microcirculation, which happens in both FMS and CMP, this motion is restricted.

In CMP, the layers of fascia tend to stick to other fascial layers as well as to other tissues. The fascia loses elasticity. This compromises function and may cause added pain. In FMS, the neurotransmitter balances are out of whack. Neurotransmitter activity determines the elasticity of the tissues.[7] Connective tissues become stiffened, shortened, and tightened, and fluid exchange is disrupted.

FMS perpetuates CMP and the reverse is also true. You can't get rid of the CMP until you successfully treat the FMS, and you can't successfully treat the FMS until you get rid of the CMP.

Then, too, chronic pain, all by itself, causes stress, which can create TrPs. That's another reason why so many cases of FMS are accompanied by CMP.

Don't despair. A lot can be done to relieve CMP and to lighten the pain load. Many therapies are helpful for FMS. What you do to help your FMS will indirectly help the CMP, and the reverse is also true. Note, however, that many traditional TrP therapies may need to be modified because of the FMS sensory amplification. Severe pain may be caused by some forms of bodywork, TrP injections, electronic stimulation, and other therapies that could be well within the tolerance level of patients who do not have hypersensitization and allodynia. These therapies may cause sensory overload and, as described in chapter 8, can further sensitize the nervous system. They can even produce a shocklike state that can be frightening to patient and therapist alike, which requires an immediate reduction in the stimuli.

Tolerance to therapy can vary considerably. For example, during times of high stress and/or a heavier workload, a longer recovery may be needed between therapy sessions.

Physical Examinations

With FMS and CMP, even a physical examination can be extremely painful and have lasting repercussions. Extra medication may be needed before the examination to minimize discomfort. If there is a great deal of pain following a physical exam, extra supportive therapy may be required in the week after the exam in the form of more medication. After a painful physical, the patient should try to do less work than usual and also try to minimize painful stimuli. Often, much examination pain can be avoided by taking a careful history.

For a patient with severe FMS and CMP, any new therapy, or new area of bodywork, should be tried with caution. At times, therapies that might prove beneficial in the long term may cause extra symptom load in the short term. Go into every new therapy with the knowledge that no matter how gentle it seems, it may provoke a flare response if too many toxins and wastes are released.

The Geloid Mass

In patients with coexisting FMS and CMP, we have discovered the presence of multiple geloid or hard, clearly definable, measurable masses that seem to overlie TrPs. These are very sore and add to the pain burden. They also make bodywork very difficult. They are accompanied by a specific type of swelling (see chapter 5) and by extremely taut areas of dense tissue. We think we know why they occur in patients with both of these conditions, and what causes them, as well as what to do about them. (See chapter 15.) The geloid mass may be one of the first objective indications that FMS and CMP together form a separate illness that is more than the sum of the two.[8]

What You Can Do

If you have CMP and FMS, your body and mind may seem to be at war but, in reality, peace talks are progressing! Armed with what you already know and with what you will learn in the rest of this book, you can take responsibility for managing your own treatment. It won't be easy and it takes an intensely concentrated focus to change the habits of a lifetime. Get as much help as you can. The task may seem overwhelming right now, but we'll break it up into small segments and take it one at a time.

Endnotes

1. Gerwin, R. D. 1999. Differential diagnosis of myofascial pain syndrome and fibromyalgia. *J Musculoskel Pain* 7(1-2):209-215.

2. Borg-Stein, J., and J. Stein. 1996. Trigger points and tender points. *Rheum Disease Clin North Am* 22(2):305-322.

3. Gerwin, R. D. 1995. A study of 96 subjects examined both for fibromyalgia and myofascial pain. *J Musculoskel Pain* 3(Suppl 1):121 (abstract).

4. Gerwin, R. D. 1999. Differential diagnosis of myofascial pain syndrome and fibromyalgia. *J Musculoskel Pain* 7(1-2):209-215.

5. Gerwin, R. D. 1998. Myofascial pain and fibromyalgia: diagnosis and treatment. *J Back & Musculoskeletal Rehab* 11:175-181.

6. Starlanyl, D. J. 1997. Fibromyalgia and myofascial pain syndrome: a special challenge. *Clin Bull Myofas Ther* 2(2/3):75-89.

7. Starlanyl, D. J. 1998. *The Fibromyalgia Advocate*. Oakland, CA: New Harbinger Publications.

8. Starlanyl, D., and J. Jeffrey. 2001. The presence of geloid masses in a patient with both fibromyalgia and chronic myofascial pain. *Phys Ther Case Rep* 4(1):22–31. (January/February).

CHAPTER 5

The Lymph System and the Immune Connection

You may not have heard of interstitial fluid and other subjects you will be reading about in this chapter, but it is important that you understand them. They may have a direct impact on your health. At school, you may or may not have learned about the lymph system. It's spread out in many layers all over the body, not compact as some other organ systems are. I have observed that many people with fibromyalgia (FMS) have a condition called interstitial edema, and many experts in the field have noted this as well. If you have been troubled by a diffuse swelling that seems to spread across your body, unseen by others but certainly felt by you, this could be interstitial edema. If the clothes that fit you in the morning are too tight by afternoon, we think we know why. The answers are to be found in this chapter. Let's dive into the lymph system and discover its connection to FMS and chronic myofascial pain (CMP).

Interstitial Space

Interstitial space, sometimes referred to as *"Third Space,"* is the space in your body that is defined as what it is not. It is not intracellular (within the cell) space, nor extracellular (outside of the cell) space, but something else entirely. It is the "Third Space." Honest. That's how the medical world refers to it, so it's no wonder that others might find the term, and the concept, strange. Interstitial fluid isn't even what we generally think of as fluid. Most interstitial fluid is trapped in the gelatinlike ground substance. As you know from chapter 2, ground substance is an integral part of the myofascia.

Under normal conditions, it's very hard for interstitial "fluid" to flow from one interstitial space to another. That is quite fortunate for us, because this fluid would rapidly pool in our lower body and we would not survive. In abnormal conditions, such as some types of shock, this fluid does migrate rapidly through the interstitial spaces, and the results can be disastrous. Doctors and nurses elevate the legs of patients in shock. This helps prevent pooling of blood in the legs. Part of this fluid comes from the interstitial areas.

As blood flows through capillary walls, there is a transfer of informational and other substances between the blood and the interstitial spaces. Material diffuses through the interstitial spaces from the blood to the lymph. These biochemicals move along through the ground substance of myofascia (see chapter 2), and these movements are affected by the ground substance's consistency. The blood carries nutrients and biochemicals to where they are needed, and the lymph carries them away. These exchanges take place in interstitial space.

The Lymph Fluid

Lymph is composed of interstitial fluid, but interstitial fluid is not consistent. In its composition, lymph resembles whatever interstitial tissue it came from just before it diffused into the lymphatic system. For example, lymph formed in intestinal cells is high in fat content, absorbed during digestion. Much excess fat exits your body through the lymph. In cases of reactive hypoglycemia or insulin resistance, some of this fat may be deposited in a fat pad on the belly. Abdominal obesity commonly coexists with insulin resistance, and the two may be linked with an HPA (hypothalamic-pituitary-adrenal axis) dysfunction.[1] (See chapter 1.)

There are valves in the veins that prevent blood from flowing the wrong way. This is necessary because the blood in the venous system doesn't have the direct force of the blood pump, the heart, which pushes blood through the arteries. There are similar flap-like one-way valves in the lymphatics, spaced about 1½ inches apart. These valves ensure that the clear, yellowish-to-white lymph does not flow backwards. Lymph pressure is very low compared to blood pressure. The movement of muscles propels the lymph along, including the muscles of respiration.

Every day, a little over five gallons of lymph move through the average adult lymphatic system. This fluid comes from the bone marrow, thymus, spleen, and intestines, and constantly bathes the body's cells and tissues. It carries substances that the tissues need, and, at the same time, carries away excess liquid, waste, and toxins. After the refuse is returned to the bloodstream by the lymph, it is filtered through the kidneys, and then excreted.

Lymph Nodes

Lymph nodes are connected by a network of channels called *lymphatics*, which are about the same width as a broom straw. These lymphatics are found all over the body, except for the central nervous system. When several lymphatics join together, they form what is called a *node*. Lymph nodes occur here and there in clusters throughout the body. They are not lymph *glands*, even though some people call them that, because they do not secrete hormones, and glands do. The function of these nodes is to act as filters.

You have clusters of lymph nodes under your arms, in your groin, behind your ears, behind your knees, and at various other places here and there throughout your body. There are also chains and clusters of nodes along your spine and in your abdominal cavity. Lymph tissue forms your tonsils and adenoids. These areas release *lymphocytes*. They are integral parts of your immune system.

Lymphocytes

Lymphocytes secrete the mood-altering brain peptide, endorphin, as well as ACTH (a main stress hormone). The lymph is a storage place for lymphocytes and *macrophages*. "Macrophage" means "big eater," and that is exactly what macrophages are. They are the cleanup detail, huge cells that roam your body, engulfing and devouring invading organisms, damaged cells, and other debris.

Lymph nodes act as mechanical filter traps, which is one reason they swell in size when you have an infection. The nodes are busy trapping germs. Any liquid that enters the lymph system must pass through at least one of these nodes before it enters the circulatory system. Lymph nodes also trap cancerous cells, which is why they are often biopsied to see whether a cancer is spreading. Tissues in the lymph nodes produce antibodies, which defend you from repeat attacks by alien invaders called *allergens*.

Lymph and the Immune System

The spleen is also part of the lymphatic system. It can be thought of as a superlarge lymph node wrapped in a tough capsule. This organ is located in the upper left abdominal cavity, behind your ribs and under your diaphragm. The spleen contains a large number of macrophages and, in the spleen, their job is to "eat up" the old, worn-out red blood cells.

Another very important part of the lymph system is the thymus gland. It is located between the upper part of the lungs, behind the sternum (breastbone), in the center of the chest and lower part of the neck. We are still learning about this complex gland and its part in the immune system. There are many good books about the immune system, and I encourage you to read one.

Interstitial Edema

Remember that the lymph, unlike the blood, requires outside forces to help move it on its way. Anything that interferes with these forces, such as lack of exercise, paradoxical (and shallow) breathing, muscle tightness and loss of range of motion, and even constipation will contribute to stagnation of the lymph fluid. All that excess liquid, waste, and toxins can become trapped in the sluggish lymph. Swelling, or edema, results. If your lymph is constricted, excess fluid can backup in the interstitial spaces, causing interstitial edema, or *lymphedema*. Lymphedema can cause pain, discomfort, and sensory dysfunctions, which may further restrict your movements.

Interstitial edema is common in FMS, and may be part of a bodywide swelling called *fluid retention syndrome*.[2] It may be due to the excess serum hyaluronic acid, which is found in FMS patients.[3] This biochemical is part of the ground substance that absorbs water (see chapter 15). High levels of hyaluronic acid have been documented in areas of interstitial swelling.[4] Physicians may often miss interstitial edema, because the excess fluid is spread out in the interstitial spaces.

J. B. Eisinger, M.D. (see chapter 15) has found that common edema is often linked to low thyroid, but interstitial edema is common in FMS and is probably also linked to it.[5]

Sam Yue, M.D. (see chapter 15) also found that many of his patients with FMS have lymphedema. In spite of rigid diets and diuretics, these patients gain weight and have periodic swelling of their extremities. He believes that proteins may leak out of the gut into the extracellular space (see chapter 23), but are unable to exit through the lymphatic system. This causes overall, diffuse swelling with what is called "nonpitting edema." The terms "lymphedema" and "interstitial edema" are often used interchangeably. Nonpitting edema may have many causes, but it is usually due to metabolic dysfunction. Abdominal lymphedema is quite common. Doctor Yue has found guaifenesin helpful for this.[6]

Women with FMS often report fluid retention and swelling. When doctors respond instinctively and prescribe a diuretic, or "water pill," the FMS can worsen. These preparations mobilize fluid by promoting muscle actions that induce more pain.

Neuromuscular electrical stimulation (NMES) can help control edema.[7] Some types of massage also help.[8] My primary care physician, Carolyn Taylor-Olson, M.D., suggested a low-tech solution that can help control edema. She recommends wrapping the swollen area in plastic wrap. That induces sweating, which reduces the interstitial fluid. Be sure to wash the sweat off the surface of your skin, as it may contain irritants.

Vodder bodywork targets the lymph system (see chapter 19). My therapist, Lindsay Crossman, wrote the following paragraphs about Vodder bodywork just for this book:

Vodder Manual Lymph Drainage Massage is a highly specialized form of massage that uses very gentle rhythmic circular motion with alternate pressure and release movements in the direction of the lymph flow. This helps keep the lymph flowing.

We start at the neck and direct pressure down toward the area where the neck meets the shoulders. The massage stroke starts away from the center of the body and works in toward the center. Massage of the limbs starts close to the torso and works outward. The pressure is gentle and the rhythm is slow.

Manual Lymph Drainage Massage facilitates a change from the sympathetic nervous system (sometimes referred to as the "fight-or-flight response") to the parasympathetic nervous system (the "rest and digest response") by triggering specific reflexes. I tell my clients that the slow, repetitive motion bores their sympathetic nervous system and puts it to sleep. It is significant to note that neither one system nor the other is more important. What is important is a balance between the two. In our world of ever-increasing stimuli, we frequently become out of balance. Much of our energy goes into dealing with stresses and other stimuli (sympathetic nervous system) at the expense of the parasympathetic functions.

Manual Lymph Drainage Massage also helps to alleviate pain. The gentle rhythmic stroking can inhibit the pain impulses to the brain, distracting the client from the pain. Manual Lymph Drainage encourages the movement of fluid. Before it enters the vessels—while it is still in the tissues—it is called interstitial fluid. Once it enters the vessels, it is called lymph fluid. If the flow is reduced, say, because of muscle spasms or constricted fascia, you can develop edema and stagnation. This condition may cause trigger points to develop. Furthermore, the lymph fluid also carries important nutrients, vitamins, hormones, and plasma proteins used as vital building substances and nutrition for the cells. There are two official schools that teach this Vodder Manual Lymph Drainage method, one in Walchsee, Austria and one in Victoria, British Columbia, Canada (see Resources).

Endnotes

1. Bjorntorp, P., G. Holm, and R. Rosamund. 2000. The metabolic syndrome—a neuroendocrine disorder? *Br J Nutr* 83 Suppl 1:S49-57.

2. Deodhar, A. A., R. A. Fisher, C. V. Blacker, and A. D. Woolf. 1994. Fluid retention syndrome and fibromyalgia. *Br J Rheumatol* 33(6):576-582.

3. Yaron, I., D. Buskila, I. Shirazi, I. Neumann, O. Elkayam, D. Parran, et al. 1997. Elevated levels of hyaluronic acid in the sera of women with fibromyalgia. *J Rheumatol* 24(11):2221-2224.

4. Liu, N. F., and L. R. Zhang. 1998. Changes of tissue fluid hyaluronan (hyaluronic acid) in peripheral lymphedema. *Lymphology* 31:173-179.

5. Personal communication. March 6, 2000.

6. Personal communication. July 17, 1999.

7. Lake, D. A. 1992. Neuromuscular electrical stimulation: an overview and its application in the treatment of sports injuries. *Sports Med* 13(5):320-336.

8. Danneskiold-Samsoe, B., E. Christiansen, and R. B. Andersen. 1986. Myofascial pain and the role of myoglobin. *Scand J Rheumatol* 15:174-178.

CHAPTER 6

Coexisting Conditions: Not Diagnoses of Exclusion

Any coexisting condition may also be a perpetuating factor. Anything that you can do to improve a coexisting condition may help your fibromyalgia (FMS) or chronic myofascial pain (CMP). For example, if you find a way to improve the quality of your sleep, your general health may improve considerably. Fibromyalgia and myofascial trigger points (TrPs) are great mimics of other medical conditions. Because the myofascia is everywhere and touches on or interacts with so many other parts of the body, it may cause diagnostic confusion. Someone may seem to have many different medical problems, but all of these problems could turn out to be part of FMS and CMP. Of course, that isn't always the case. Fibromyalgia and CMP often appear in conjunction with another disorder and then intensify the symptoms of that disorder. We may tend to shrug off our symptoms and blame everything on FMS and CMP, but this can be dangerous. If in doubt, check it out.

Common Coexisting Conditions

The following sections describe some of the most common medical conditions that may coexist with FMS and CMP. If you have a confirmed diagnosis of FMS and/or CMP, have not been responding to treatment, and have eliminated perpetuating factors (see chapter 7), you should have a thorough medical evaluation to establish whether you have any of these coexisting conditions.

Arthritis

There are over one hundred different forms of arthritis. The word "arthritis" means inflammation of a joint. Joints are simply the places where bones join together and "articulate." There are many structures that contribute to this articulation: tendons, ligaments, and cartilage, for example. If you have myofascial TrPs, as they contract your muscles, the bones can be pulled slightly out of alignment, causing wear and tear on the bony surfaces and stress and strain on the soft tissues around them. This results in *osteoarthritis*. Although osteoarthritis is almost always present in older people, the condition can occur at any age, especially after a joint injury. Note that *age alone does not cause inflammation*.

The inflammation of osteoarthritis is caused by misalignment of the joints. It signifies musculoskeletal dysfunction. It is known that people with abnormal joint alignment, previous significant joint injury or surgery, joint instability, above-average body weight, or inadequate muscle strength probably have increased risk of osteoarthritis.[1] "Inactivating the related myofascial TrPs and the *elimination of their perpetuating factors* appear to be important parts of early therapy to delay or abort the progression of some kinds of osteoarthritis."[2]

Rheumatoid arthritis (RA) is an autoimmune condition. With this illness your own body does not recognize some of its cells and attacks them, causing debilitating inflammations. Rheumatoid arthritis is a chronic, systemic (biochemical) inflammatory condition that results in crippling deformities of the bone. It almost always causes myofascial TrPs. Although the RA will continue to act as a TrP perpetuator because there is no cure for it and it is progressive, periodic TrP treatments can greatly lessen the pain load.

Polymyalgia rheumatica usually strikes women over sixty, causing marked pain and stiffness in the neck, shoulder, and hips. It is progressive, and causes a raised sedimentation rate on blood testing. It can have a dangerous complication called temporal arteritis, which is an inflammation of the temporal artery.

Ankylosing spondylitis is an autoimmune, progressive, and degenerative arthritis. Symptoms are recurrent back pain, sciatica, morning stiffness, fatigue and anemia. It is most common in young men.

It is vitally important for you to understand that *neither FMS nor CMP are types of arthritis.* Arthritis is inflammatory. FMS and CMP are not. Myofascial TrPs may *cause* conditions that set up osteoarthritis, in the same way that a fall may cause a joint injury. Neither the TrP nor the fall are arthritic conditions themselves. For more information on all types of arthritis, contact your local chapter of the Arthritis Foundation.

Attention Deficit Disorder

Attention Deficit Disorder (ADD) is a neurological syndrome. The classic symptoms include impulsivity, distractibility, and hyperactivity or excess energy. About 15 million Americans have it, and most of them are unaware that they do. People with ADD don't focus very well and may find it difficult to follow directions. They have trouble attending to one task at a time, and may have rapidly shifting moods. They can daydream a lot and often love high-stimulus situations with a great deal of action and novelty. They get upset when interrupted or when making transitions. There are deficits in attention and effort, impulsivity, problems in regulating level of arousal, and the need for immediate reinforcement. People with ADD often need external structure, limits, and controls.

Carpal Tunnel Syndrome

Carpal Tunnel Syndrome (CTS) is caused by pressure on the median nerve. This can occur anyplace along the nerve, not just in the wrist. Remember, a syndrome is a set of signs and symptoms—a description of a condition or set of conditions. Look for the cause. It might be nerve entrapment by myofascial TrPs.[3] Nerves are held in place by myofascia. If the myofascia is stiff and tight, causing pain, it does not require surgery but specific TrP therapy. If you are discussing possible surgery for CTS, make sure your doctor checks first for TrPs. Surgery for CTS has an increased likelihood of unsatisfactory results if you have myofascial pain or fibromyalgia.[4]

One researcher found that myofascial release, combined with the patient's self-stretching, reduced pain and numbness, and improved electromyographic results. An aggressive, conservative approach lessens the need for surgery in mild to moderate cases.[5] Another study stated that in more than ninety cases of cumulative trauma disorders, proper myofascial release technique, along with specific exercises, resulted in relief of symptoms and restoration of function.[6]

Chronic Fatigue Immune Dysfunction Syndrome

This is a condition in need of a name change. "Chronic Fatigue Immune Dysfunction Syndrome" (CFIDS) is too easily mistaken for generalized "chronic fatigue," which can occur from many sources such as constant overwork. CFIDS is not the same as FMS. Evidence for a triggering viral infection is lacking in the majority of patients with FMS, but is present in CFIDS.[7] CFIDS is characterized by a history of extreme exhaustion lasting at least six months, as well as by biochemical abnormalities. This exhaustion can be brought on by the slightest effort. Usually, aches and fever, sore throat, and an inability to concentrate are part of CFIDS. CFIDS seems also to be made up of subsets. Coexisting conditions must be identified and treated before CFIDS can be diagnosed, because unlike FMS and CMP, *it is a diagnosis of exclusion.* Any condition that cannot be confirmed by laboratory tests, such as FMS, does *not* exclude a patient from the diagnosis of CFIDS.[8]

Complex Regional Pain Syndrome

Complex Regional Pain Syndrome (CRPS) used to be called reflex sympathetic dystrophy (RSD). This condition is characterized by an overactive sympathetic nervous system, often from nerve damage caused by trauma or stroke. This results in an irregular blood supply to the affected area (hand, foot, knee, hip, shoulder, etc.), resulting in severe pain that often burns, swells, and causes changes in skin color and gooseflesh. The combination of FMS and CMP is often misdiagnosed as CRPS. In one study, myofascial pain was diagnosed in 82 percent of cases of CRPS.[9] Treating the TrPs may help ease the microcirculation problem.

Depression

There are several kinds of depression. Some symptoms of depression include feeling very sad most of the time, an inability to experience pleasure, lethargy, confusion, poor memory, sleep problems, and appetite changes. Also, it is natural to grieve when you have a chronic pain problem, but those feelings are not the same as a clinical depression.

Esophageal Reflux

Reflux means that something is flowing backwards, which is exactly what happens in this condition. At first, it is acid fumes that escape backwards through the valve between the esophagus to the stomach. These fumes can irritate the delicate esophageal lining, causing heartburn, sore throat, and TrPs. This irritation can set up a headache and disturb sleep. Then, the stomach fluids themselves start to leak into the esophageal area. If you lean over, or strain at a bowel movement, or put more pressure on the stomach in any way, the stomach acids can burn your esophagus and throat. Bending over or lying down can cause vomiting. Check your diet and check your TrPs. This condition should not be taken lightly. There is a strong and probably causal relation between reflux and esophageal adenocarcinoma.[10]

Gulf War Syndrome

Some studies have indicated that patients with Gulf War Syndrome also have some symptoms that overlap those of FMS, Chronic Fatigue Immune Deficiency Syndrome, and/or Multiple Chemical Sensitivity.[11] Many symptoms of Gulf War Syndrome may also be due to coexisting myofascial TrPs.

HIV

Both FMS and CMP may occur in HIV patients and may add considerably to the pain load. One study showed probable or definite FMS in 41 percent of HIV patients with musculoskeletal pain and in 11 percent of all HIV patients.[12] I have not seen any studies on HIV and TrPs, but I have never seen a person with HIV who did not have them. Treat the coexisting FMS and/or CMP.

Hypermobility Syndrome

Hypermobility Syndrome is characterized by joint relaxation that allows muscles to stretch beyond their normal range of motion. Exercise must be aimed at strengthening, not lengthening, the muscle, unless there are coexisting TrPs. Hypermobility perpetuates TrPs. Connective tissue hypermobility can be a contributing factor in hernia, uterine and/or rectal prolapse, mitral valve prolapse, or spontaneous pneumothorax. In children, joint hyperlaxity is an important (and often unrecognized) source of rheumatic symptoms.[13] (Joint hypermobility also may play a prominent role in FMS pain.)[14]

Hypometabolism

Hypometabolism and hypothyroid are different conditions. Hypothyroid is a low or low-normal thyroid level that makes people more susceptible to the development of TrPs. Hypometabolism is a condition of low usable thyroid activity that occurs due to thyroid metabolic dysfunction (see chapter 15).

Interstitial Cystitis

Interstitial cystitis (IC) is a chronic inflammatory condition of unknown origin. It is not the same as irritable bladder. It involves the muscles and the mucosa of the bladder and is primarily found in women. Periodic urinary incontinence may develop, with scarring of the urinary tract. Mast cells, which are a type of blood cell associated with histamine release, are present in large quantities at the nerve cells in the urinary systems of patients with IC. It is often helpful to avoid acid liquids, as they tend to irritate the condition.

The muscles in these areas gradually lose their tone, especially if TrPs are involved. Trigger points cause weakness and dysfunction before they cause pain. This dysfunction often becomes evident when periodic urinary incontinence develops. The mucosal linings of the urinary tract appear inflamed and scarred and there may be bleeding. The bladder wall may have thickened, although the mucosal lining is fragile. The mechanisms of hypersensitivity in IC may be the same as in FMS.[15]

Irritable Bowel Syndrome

People with FMS and CMP often have Irritable Bowel Syndrome (IBS) With this condition, muscles in the gut contract and relax at the wrong time, leading to a number of unpleasant symptoms. These symptoms include varying diarrhea and dry constipation. You may have a crampy urge to go but find that you cannot. You may also experience irregular contractions of the large intestines, bloating from gas, and hypersensitivity. Normally, the nerve endings in the gut transmit feelings only of fullness or stretching. With IBS, you can have pain as well.

Irritable Bowel Syndrome can disrupt your life. You may be afraid to go out because of your unpredictable symptoms. It can interfere with your travel plans and your ability to work. Usually the symptoms of IBS result from a combination of several factors. Poor nutrition, trigger points, medication and food sensitivities, yeast overgrowth, menstruation, and stress may aggravate IBS. Attention to diet, exercise, and stress reduction can help. Talk with your pharmacist about your medications. Some medications can cause side effects that can be similar to or contribute to IBS.

Irritable bowel syndrome does not cause inflammatory changes. It is not the same as ulcerative colitis. Stress worsens but does not cause IBS. IBS causes no bleeding, fever, significant weight loss, or severe, persistent pain. If you do have these symptoms, see your doctor right away.

Lupus

Lupus is a chronic, progressive autoimmune syndrome. There are two types of lupus:

1. Lupus myositis, or discoid lupus, is a disorder confined to the skin, and is not a generalized connective tissue condition. There is a scaling red, pink, or brown rash, often in the shape of a butterfly over the face, although it is not limited to that area. This rash is very photosensitive. In addition to the plaques, which are not always confined to the face, there can be scaling; the hair follicles can become plugged; and spiderlike telangiectasia can develop. This is a localized inflammation of the skin, sometimes seen with involvement of oral mucosa.

2. Systemic lupus erythematosus occurs in connective tissue. This kind of lupus can be fatal. It can also cause the butterfly rash and skin symptoms, but all of the connective tissue can be involved, not just the skin. There may be involvement with *any* or *many* organ systems, producing a host of symptoms. Symptoms may fluctuate. Fatigue, sun sensitivity, Raynaud's phenomenon, swollen joints, stiffness, muscle aches, swollen glands, low-grade temperature, hair loss, nausea and vomiting, and lack of appetite can all occur. Patients with lupus are at risk of developing secondary FMS.[16]

Lyme Disease

Lyme disease is caused by a bacterium called *Borrelia burgdorferi*, which is carried by certain types of ticks. Lyme disease often starts with a circular rash around the tick bite, and flulike symptoms. It must be treated promptly with antibiotics. It can trigger FMS. Sometimes this triggering of FMS can occur even if the Lyme disease is treated with prompt and adequate antibiotics.[17] However, even for FMS patients with positive Lyme antibody serology results, if the only symptoms are nonspecific muscle aches or fatigue, the risks and expense of antibiotic therapy may exceed the benefits.[18]

Migraine Headaches

Migraine headaches may have many causes and many triggers. Migraines are common in both FMS and CMP (see chapter 8).

Multiple Chemical Sensitivities (MCS)

Some people may become sensitized to one chemical after only a single exposure. Others become sensitized to that chemical only after repeated exposures. But in either case other environmental irritants, previously tolerated, begin to provoke allergic or sensitivity reactions. The signs and symptoms are many and varied. They include fatigue, headaches, muscle aches, coughing, watery eyes, and tremors. MCS is often present in people with FMS, which can make taking medication difficult.[19] Some studies indicate that MCS is due to neural sensitization of a nature similar to FMS.[20]

Multiple Sclerosis

Multiple sclerosis (MS) is caused by the breakdown of certain central nervous system tissues that occur in multiple, random sites. Myelin is the fatty sheath surrounding some of the nerves. In MS, this sheath is damaged and neurotransmitter information is diminished or lost, and areas of sclerosis (hardening) result. There are tests for MS. Multiple sclerosis does not lead to FMS, and FMS does not lead to MS.

Neuralgia-Inducing Cavitational Necrosis

Patients with these jawbone cavities will have a history of tooth extraction perhaps years before their pain complaints begin. Trigger areas are found inside the mouth. When these areas are compressed with finger pressure, they reproduce specific pain patterns, in spite of normal X-rays. Even though there can be considerable soft tissue destruction, the X-rays are normal until late in the condition. Only after significant removal or destruction of bone has occurred will X-ray changes be detected.[21] The initial instigating factor is a lack of blood supply to the area, which then begins to die. Direct trauma or TrPs can cause this. Sleep dysfunction is almost always present, caused by pain. On average, the patient endures pain for six years before getting a diagnosis. Antibiotics may ease the pain, but the abnormal tissues must be surgically removed for dramatic pain reduction.[22]

Neurally Mediated Hypotension

Neurally mediated hypotension (NMH) is low blood pressure caused by the central nervous system. *Neurally mediated syncope* and *syncope due to autonomic failure* are characterized by a temporary loss of consciousness due to a reduction of blood flow to the brain.[23] Dizziness or fainting can occur after a hot shower, a dip in a hot tub, or anything else that dilates the blood vessels. Standing for long periods can cause fainting. It can happen after eating a very full meal, or even while in a crowd.

Between episodes, patients with NMH can have orthostatic intolerance. This is dizziness if you stand up after a period of sitting or lying down. Prolonged fatigue lasting for days after moderate activity can be part of this condition. There is a strong association between FMS and NMH.[24]

Post-Polio Syndrome

Post-Polio Syndrome (PPS) affects some polio survivors, and can affect any area of the body. It may be triggered by stress-producing events, such as trauma, grief, or surgery. Symptoms may include difficulty breathing, muscle weakness, intolerance to cold, fatigue, twitching and spasms, sleep dysfunction, and difficulty swallowing. PPS can also cause progressive muscle wasting and recurrent paralysis. This can lead to life-threatening respiratory paralysis. As the primary polio infection may have appeared to be a flulike illness, some people were never initially diagnosed.

Posttraumatic Stress Syndrome

Flashbacks are part of Post-Traumatic Stress Syndrome (PTSS). In a flashback, you relive the initial trauma. General numbing of emotions is also a part of this condition. It may be accompanied by hyperarousal, hypervigilance, startle reactions, and/or difficulty falling asleep and staying asleep. This coexisting condition may influence how well you cope with FMS and how well you respond to treatments.[25] One study found 21 percent of patients with PTSS had unsuspected FMS, and indicated that previously reported diffuse pain in PTSS could be coexisting FMS.[26]

Raynaud's Phenomenon

Raynaud's phenomenon is a condition characterized by loss of blood circulation to fingers, toes, and ears in an exaggerated response to temperature drops or stress. Lack of blood in the extremities causes your skin to turn white. If the blood reaches the capillaries but is poorly oxygenated, your skin turns blue. When oxygenated blood returns to the affected areas, the skin turns red. Numbness, tingling, and burning may be present at these times. A subgroup of patients with FMS may have dysfunctional neurotransmitter receptors contributing to their exaggerated reaction to cold.[27]

Relief from Raynaud's is linked to improved circulation. Vibrational and repetitive movements, constrictions, and pressures should be avoided. Nifedipine is a medication commonly used to help improve the peripheral blood supply, but other medications such as relaxin are currently under investigation.[28] Therapy should include the release of myofascial entrapment of blood and lymph vessels in the area. Avoid triggering stimuli, such as nicotine, cold, and stress.

Reactive Hypoglycemia

Hypoglycemia is generally defined as a deficiency of sugar in the blood. There is a type of reactive hypoglycemia that is specific to low blood sugar that occurs in response to a high carbohydrate intake. Your blood sugar rises, affecting adrenaline levels, and then plummets. This may occur with insulin resistance (IR), when your body becomes resistant to the effects of insulin and your glucose level fails to be balanced by it. Many women have hypoglycemia just prior to their menstrual period. Stress can also trigger hypoglycemia. See chapters 7 and 23 for an in-depth look at reactive hypoglycemia.

Restless Leg Syndrome

If you have Restless Leg Syndrome (RLS), you feel abnormal, very deep sensations in your legs. These include but are not limited to itching, pulling, heaviness, cramping, hypersensitivity, aching, crawling, and tingling, as well as pain. These feelings are so uncomfortable that you must move, which brings temporary relief. Some allergy medications, seizure medications, and others can cause RLS. It can occur at any age, even in children. It is most common in the elderly, however, and is not always confined to the legs. These feelings may occur in the arms, trunk, or genitals. Most patients with RLS have a form of sleep dysfunction, and the symptoms may be progressive. Pergolide[29] or Ropinirol[30] may relieve RLS.

Seasonal Affective Disorder

People with seasonal affective disorder (SAD) feel very depressed in the winter and feel much better during the summer. In severe cases, they can fluctuate from severe depression during the darkest months of the year to manic episodes during the long summer days. Winter depression arrives in late autumn or early winter, accompanied by worsening fatigue and carbohydrate cravings. If you get the light you need in the morning during winter days, it often helps this condition. There is also a small percentage of patients who become depressed in the summer and who feel better or even become manic in the winter.[31]

Temporomandibular Dysfunction

Many people with FMS have temporomandibular dysfunction (TMD) symptoms.[32] These can range from clicking and snapping of the jaw to pain and severe bite dysfunction. Often, ringing and/or itching of the ears accompany this. TMD is often caused by TrPs. It is difficult for the dentist untrained in trigger point work to deal with TMD caused by TrPs, since the contraction of muscles due to TrPs can change drastically. You need to have the TrPs treated first, with dental work done in conjunction with the TrP work.

Vulvodynia

Vulvar pain, also called vulvodynia, is pain in the external female sexual tissues. (See chapters 8 and 11.)

Yeast Infections

Chronic yeast infections throughout the body often occur with FMS. Yeasts can perpetuate FMS and CMP, as can all infections. When you have an infection like this, much of the body's immune defenses are tied up fighting the infection, and that means there are fewer resources available to deal with FMS and CMP.

Yeast overgrowth can be responsible for at least part of the bloating, fibrofog, abdominal upsets, and muscle aches in patients with FMS and CMP. Treatment with a systemic antiyeast agent such as Diflucan, which crosses the blood-brain barrier, can result in dramatic long-term symptom improvement. It can also result in short-term symptom increase.

The latter situation is due to the yeast die-off phenomenon. The dead and dying yeast can create all sorts of havoc, in the form of toxins and waste. Patients with long-term systemic yeast problems usually have developed yeast antibodies, and often are also allergic or sensitive to molds. This allergy or sensitivity will also perpetuate FMS and CMP.

If yeasts seem to love your body, avoid antibiotics unless totally necessary. Antibiotics kill off the good critters (see chapter 23) that keep the yeast in check. Other perpetuating factors for chronic yeast problems are a diet high in simple carbohydrates, insulin resistance, the use of steroids, antacids, and medications such as Zantac, Pepcid, and Axid, These may lead to leaky gut/intestinal membrane hyperpermeability (see chapter 23).

Often foods high in yeast, such as citrus fruits, peanut butter, and cashews cause bloating or roof-of-the-mouth itch. Talk to your doctor about a blood test for anti-candida antibodies IgG, IgA, and IgM. This test doesn't measure the candida yeast, but it looks for antibodies that would form in response to it. This will give a good indication of whether you should consider taking allergy shots for mold.

Endnotes

1. Buckwalter, J. A., and N. E. Lane. 1997. Athletics and osteoarthritis. *Am J Sports Med* 25(6):873-881.

2. Simons, D. G., J. G. Travell, and L. S. Simons. 1999. *Travell and Simons' Myofascial Pain and Dysfunction: The Trigger Point Manual*, Vol. I. Second edition. Baltimore: Williams and Wilkins p. 792.

3. *Ibid.*, p. 688.

4. Straub, T. A. 1999. Endoscopic carpal tunnel release: a prospective analysis of factors associated with unsatisfactory results. *Arthroscopy* 15(3):269-274.

5. Sucher, B. M. 1993. Myofascial release of carpal tunnel syndrome. *J Am Osteopath Assoc* 93(1):92-94.

6. Leahy, M., and L. E. Mock III. 1992. Myofascial release technique and mechanical compromise of peripheral nerves of the upper extremity. *Chiro Sports Med* 6(4):139-140.

7. Matsumoto, Y. 1999. [Fibromyalgia syndrome]. *Nippon Ronsho* 57(2):364-369. [Japanese]

8. Fukuda, K., S. E. Straus, I. Hickie, M. Sharpe, J. G. Dobbins, A. Komaroff, and the ICFSSG. 1994. The chronic fatigue syndrome: a comprehensive approach to its definition and study. *Ann Int Med* 121(12)953-959.

9. Imamura, S. T., T. Y. Lin, M. J. Yriyrits, S. S. Fischer, R. J. Azze, L. A. Rosgano, et al. 1997. The importance of myofascial pain syndrome in reflex sympathetic dystrophy. *Phys Med Rehab Clinics of North Am* 8(1):207-211.

10. Lagergren, J., R. Bergstrom, A. Lindgren, and O. Nyren. 1999. Symptomatic gastroesophageal reflux as a risk factor for esophageal adenocarcinoma. *N Eng J Med* 340(11):825-831.

11. Kipen, H. M., W. Hallman, H. Kang, N. Fiedler, and B. H. Natelson. 1999. Prevalence of chronic fatigue and chemical sensitivities in Gulf Registry Veterans. *Arch Environ Health* 54(5):313-318.

12. Simms, R. W., C. A. Zerbini, N. Ferrante, J. Anthony, D. T. Felson, and D. E. Craven. 1992. Fibromyalgia syndrome in patients infected with human immunodeficiency virus. The Boston City Hospital Clinical AIDS Team. *Am J Med* 92(4):368-374.

13. Gedalia, A., J. Press, M. Klein, and D. Buskila. 1993. Joint hypermobility and fibromyalgia in schoolchildren. *Ann Rheum Dis* 52(7):494-496.

14. Acasuso-Diaz, M., and E. Collantes-Estevez. 1998. Joint hypermobility in patients with fibromyalgia syndrome. *Arthritis Care Res* 11(1):39-42.

15. Clauw, D. J., M. Schmidt, D. Radulovic, A. Singer, P. Katz, and J. Bresettte. 1997. The relationship between fibromyalgia and interstitial cystitis. *J Psychiatr Res* 31(1):125-131.

16. Grafe, A., U. Wollina, B. Tebbe, H. Sprott, C. Uhlemann, and G. Hein. 1999. Fibromyalgia in lupus erythematosus. *Acta Derm Venereol* 79(1):62-64.

17. Steere, A. C. 1995. Musculoskeletal manifestations of Lyme disease. *Am J Med* 98(4A):44S-48S; discussion 48S-51S.

18. Lightfoot, Jr., R. W., B. J. Luft, D. W. Rahn, A. C. Steere, L. H. Sigal, D. C. Zoschke, et al. 1993. Empiric parenteral antibiotic treatment of patients with fibromyalgia and fatigue and a positive serologic result for Lyme disease: a cost-effectiveness analysis. *Ann Intern Med* 119(6):503-509.

19. No author. 1999. Multiple chemical sensitivity: a 1999 consensus. *Arch Environ Health* 54(3):147-149

20. Bell, I. R., C. M. Baldwin, and G. E. Schwartz. 1998. Illness from low levels of environmental chemicals: relevance to chronic fatigue syndrome and fibromyalgia. *Am J Med* 105(3A):74S-82S.

21. Brown, C. R. 1996. Pain management: NICO. *The Implant Report* 8(9):916.

22. Shankland, II, W. E. 1995. Crainofascial pain syndromes that mimic temperomandibular joint disorders. *Ann Acad Med Singapore* 24(1):83-112.

23. Kaufmann, H. 1997. Neurally mediated syncope and syncope due to autonomic failure: differences and similarities. *J Clin Neurophysiol* 14(3):183-196.

24. Bou-Holaigah, I., H. Calkins, J. A. Flynn, C. Tunin, H. C. Chang, J. S. Kan, et al. 1997. Provocation of hypotension and pain during upright tilt table testing in adults with fibromyalgia. *Clin Exp Rheumatol* 15(3):239-246.

25. Sherman, J. J., D. C. Turk, and A. Okifuji. 2000. Prevalence and impact of posttraumatic stress disorder-like symptoms on patients with fibromyalgia syndrome. *Clin J Pain* 16(2):127-134.

26. Amir, M., Z. Kaplan, L. Neumann, R. Sharabani, N. Shani, and D. Buskila. 1997. Posttraumatic stress disorder, tenderness and fibromyalgia. *J Psychosom Res* 42(6):607-613.

27. Bennett, R. M., S. R. Clark, S. M. Campbell, S. B. Ingram, C. S. Burckhardt, D. L. Nelson, et al. 1991. Symptoms of Raynaud's syndrome in patients with fibromyalgia. *Arthritis Rheum* 34(3):264-269.

28. Ho, M., and J. J. Belch. 1998. Raynaud's phenomenon: state of the art in 1998. *Scand J Rheumatol* 27(5):319-322.

29. Staedt, J., H. Hunerjager, E. Ruther, and G. Stoppe. 1998. Pergolide: treatment of choice in restless legs syndrome (RLS) and nocturnal myoclonus syndrome (NMS). Longterm follow up on pergolide. *J Neural Transm* 105(2-3):265-268.

30. Estivill, E., and V. de la Fuente. 1999. [No title available]. *Rev Neurol* 28(10):962-963. [Spanish]

31. Wehr, T. A., D. A. Sack, and N. E. Rosenthal. 1987. Seasonal affective disorder with summer depression and winter hypomania. *Am J Psychiatry* 144(12):1602-1603.

32. Pennacchio, E. A., J. Borg-Stein, and D. A. Keith. 1998. The incidence of pain in the muscles of mastication in patients with fibromyalgia. *J Mass Dent Soc* 47(3):8-12.

CHAPTER 7

Initiating, Aggravating, and Perpetuating Factors

Perpetuating factors are those conditions or stressors that cause a myofascial trigger point (TrP) to remain in place, in spite of efforts to break it up. Perpetuating factors may occur alone or with others. They may be behavioral, such as posture, or biochemical, such as nutritional inadequacy. They also may be mechanical, such as poorly fitting shoes. Some of these perpetuating factors are also aggravating and initiating factors.

Travell and Simons say that the most important chapter in their text is the one on perpetuating factors.[1] This is true for my books as well.

The key to functioning better, with as minimal a symptom load as possible, is to identify as many of your perpetuating factors as possible and deal with them as thoroughly as you possibly can. Chronic pain is a key perpetuating factor; it has an entire chapter devoted to it (see chapter 9).

Frequently, one perpetuating factor will initiate or aggravate a TrP, and another will perpetuate it. For example, a fall could activate a TrP, and repetitive action at work could perpetuate it. Travell and Simons have documented this for myofascial TrPs. I have found that identifying and addressing perpetuating factors is appropriate for fibromyalgia (FMS), as well.

No Quick Fix

Every week I get mail from people telling me that they have found *the* cause of FMS and/or *the* cure. I don't get mail like that as often about chronic myofascial pain (CMP), possibly because many of the people now working with myofascial pain received their training from Travell and Simons and understand that it is *multifactorial*. That means many things can cause it, many things can aggravate it, and many things can improve it. The same is true for FMS. Whenever people tell me that they feel they are no longer improving in spite of receiving appropriate therapy, that usually means there are one or more perpetuating factors with which they are not dealing.

You can't change the past. and you can't change your genetic makeup. But there are many aspects of your life that can be changed, modified, or even eliminated. Changing conditions that might be adversely affecting the quality of your life can often have a huge impact on your ability to function, as well as on your quality of life.

Like a stone in your shoe, you must first identify the problem and accept that it is there before you can take steps to change or correct it. As you learned in the previous chapter, there are many possible coexisting conditions. All of these can be perpetuating factors. Cancer and other internal illnesses can produce and perpetuate TrPs. Other common conditions that can act as perpetuating factors include Crohn's disease, painful menstrual periods, ovulation, and even uncorrected vision problems. It is important to take care of these conditions as much as is possible; by doing so you will limit their ability to worsen FMS and CMP.

Perpetuating Factors

When you are seeking your perpetuating factors, you need not hunt alone. You should provide your medical team with specific data concerning your daily routines, including sleep positions, work conditions, and family dynamics. If you have a sleeping partner, consult him or her. Ask your health team for assistance in observing your body. They can tell you what to look for. Your doctor must be knowledgeable in ferreting out perpetuating factors, so that the right tests can be ordered.

Paradoxical Breathing

This is one of the most common perpetuating factors of both FMS and CMP and, in terms of time and money, it is the least costly to fix. The other perpetuating factors discussed in this chapter follow alphabetical order. But paradoxical breathing is so common and so important that it is discussed first to make sure that you don't miss it. This type of breathing may be perpetuated by FMS and by specific TrPs (see chapter 8). That is, if you have FMS or specific TrPs, you may have begun to breathe this way as a response to either condition. However, paradoxical breathing is something that you can change without expending anything but attention and effort.

Paradoxical breathing occurs when your belly flattens as you breathe in and expands when you breathe out. This is the reverse of the way healthy breathing takes place. If you are breathing in this shallow manner, you are probably not getting enough oxygen. Monitor your breathing throughout the day. Learn to be attentive to how you breathe until you get into the habit of breathing correctly.

Adhesions

"Adhesion" means, simply, materials stuck together. Adhesions often set up the conditions for TrPs and often accompany scars. The scars may be like the tip of an iceberg with much more extensive myofascial scarring and adhesion beneath them. Adhesions may be caused by surgery, infection, and conditions like endometriosis or physical trauma. Organs can adhere to other tissue, and even your bowels can be obstructed by adhesions. Surgical treatment often results in the reformation of the adhesions. Some types of bodywork can be very effective in breaking up adhesions regardless of their cause (see chapter 19).

Chiari Malformation: Cause and Effect?

There has been a recent flurry of media attention on the Chiari (pronounced khee–are–ee) malformation and also on cervical spinal stenosis. *Chiari malformation*, or Chiari Syndrome, occurs when part of the brain, called the cerebellar tonsils, extends downward a few extra millimeters and puts pressure on the brain stem and spinal cord.

Cervical spinal stenosis is a narrowing of the cervical canal. The spinal cord lies within the cervical canal, and a congenital narrowing or bony growth inside the canal can cause excess pressure on the brain. Cervical spinal stenosis and Chiari malformation are not the same as FMS or Chronic Fatigue Immune Dysfunction Syndrome (CFIDS). The surgery proposed for cervical spinal stenosis or Chiari malformation is an incision at the base of the scull to remove some bone to give the brain more room. Some doctors believe that some patients may have been misdiagnosed as having FMS or CFIDS when, in fact, they have cervical spinal stenosis or Chiari malformation.

On the night of March 10, 2000, there was a national television show *(20/20)* on ABC with Barbara Walters, who interviewed some of the doctors who perform this surgery. When questioned, one of these doctors stated that FMS had no known treatment! Neurosurgeon Dr. Michael Rosner of Charlotte, North Carolina mentioned that a trauma, and even heavy coughing, could trigger narrowing of the spinal canal. (So can any procedure that hyperextends your neck, such as some neck surgery.) The medical literature shows that reductions of 1.5 mm or less in the diameter of the spinal canal can come from simple *changes in posture*, such as a rotation in the pelvis.[2] What can one expect when there may be several areas of the spine rotated in CMP?

Tight muscles or abnormal posture may cause functional narrowing of the canal, and these can be caused by TrPs. Logic tells me that myofascial release of the dural tube, and adequate TrP releases of the scalenes and levator scapulae, should be accomplished and other perpetuating factors addressed before surgery is even contemplated. Always seek the least invasive procedures possible first. Of course, if magnetic resonance imaging (MRI) discloses a big cyst (another condition entirely) or a *large* bony growth causing cervical stenosis and pressure on the brain, surgery may be the only solution.

I have urged surgeons who are performing this operation to investigate the myofascial possibilities, and give noninvasive myofascial techniques and craniosacral techniques a try, but have never gotten a reply. Think about it. If a bout of heavy coughing can bring on this narrowing, isn't it more likely to be caused by a myofascial TrP than by a bony outgrowth? The temptation is to go for the "quick fix." Unless you have been misdiagnosed and don't have FMS or CFIDS, this isn't the place for one.

Environmental Factors

Pollution: The newspapers and the scientific journals are full of alarming accounts about the number of chemicals now in our environment capable of producing illness. Chemical pollutants can now be found in every person's body. The systems most affected by these compounds include the immune, neurological, and endocrine systems. These chemicals resemble or interfere with hormones, neurotransmitters, growth factors, and other informational substances.[3] We spend increasing amounts of time and effort, as well as finances, to detoxify our bodies while our environment becomes ever more suspect. It is vitally important that each of us become aware of ongoing environmental pollution, so that we can act to stop it. We must do what we can to improve the health of our environment if we wish to improve the health of our bodies and minds.

Allergic Conditions: Illnesses such as asthma and hay fever are perpetuators of TrPs and FMS. The neurotransmitter histamine seems to be implicated as a culprit in both conditions. FMS may worsen during times of high allergic load. "Myofascial TrPs are aggravated by high histamine levels and active allergies."[4] Fibromyalgia's allergic response may occur without the typical immunoglobin E presence, but other immunoglobins may be involved, and other allergic manifestations such as mast cells and eosinophils may appear (see chapter 8). Food allergies are common and potent in FMS, and skin testing is very unreliable. In some of us, our muscles seem to be the shock organ for the allergies. In other words, if you are stressed by allergies, they can make themselves known by muscular symptoms; for example, by swelling of the muscles and/or muscle aches.

Sensory Changes: These changes include the change to and from daylight saving time and weather changes like barometric and temperature pressure fluctuations, dampness, humidity, and drafts. A hyperactive nervous system can increase any kind of hypersensitivity. If this is the case for you, dress defensively in cool environments, and be especially careful of drafts; cold plus wind equals TrPs. Some days, rain hitting your window may feel as if it is pounding against each of your cells. Heat and high humidity can also be a perpetuator of pain, especially when the pain is augmented by swelling. Body warmth is important. When your muscles are cool, they contract to generate heat, and the added tension aggravates TrPs.

Ill-Fitting, Poorly Designed Furniture: Janet Travell, in her Spray and Stretch video series (see Resources), tells us that chairs were originally designed as thrones to raise a king above his subjects. They were not designed for comfort. This is doubly true for those of us with short upper arms and/or short lower legs. These anatomical features are other perpetuating factors whose effects can be intensified by ill-fitting furniture. Many bathtubs, sinks, and cabinetry are not designed for use by human beings. I often wonder what the designers look like.

I believe that the chair as we know it today symbolizes one of the many triumphs of packaging over performance. Basically, chairs are built the same approximate size for everyone, ignoring the fact that people come in all shapes and sizes. The chair is one of the chief regulators of posture, and poor posture is one of the chief perpetuators of TrPs.

Your body is designed for your weight to be carried by your bones, not your flesh. Your "sit bones" should be carrying about 60 percent of your weight when you are seated, with the other 40 percent transferred to your heels.[5] This is why your heels need to be flat on the floor, or on a footrest. There should be some space between the chair seat and the lower edge of the back of the chair, so that your buttocks can fit and your back is supported. Many chairs have lumbar supports that extend so far forward that people cannot get to sit at the back of the seat.

Some of the absolutely worst chairs are found in automobiles and airplanes. Traveling can really add extra stress to your body and mind, especially when you are driving. You are relatively immobile, many of your muscles are in shortened positions, and your circulation is often greatly impaired in the lower body. We are trapped in these instruments of torture when we are most immobile and most vulnerable. No wonder it can take us forever to recover from a trip.

It is important to move as much as possible, stretching every twenty minutes when you are in a car on an automobile trip. You can alternately tense and relax separate muscles as well, which helps to keep your blood supply and lymph flowing properly. It may be helpful to lean one area of your body at a time on a tennis ball. Keep moving the ball around. Working the ball around under your thigh may help the circulation in this area. Squatting is a helpful movement as it stretches your spine, opens your hip joints and lower back, and activates and flexes your ankles and feet. Bending at the waist is not a good thing, because your waist was not designed to be a hinge joint. You need to flex your knees, ankles, and hip joints. The hip is where you are supposed to bend.

Prolonged Sitting: So much effort has been spent on enabling us to reach many things while remaining sitting in one place, without understanding that this is not a good thing for our minds and bodies. If your work keeps you relatively immobile or in one posture for a long period of time, you may develop TrPs. Find a way to vary your position. Move. Raise your hands, wiggle. Stretch your feet and flex them up and down. Take microbreaks. Be sure that your workspace is ergonomically designed. This does not always mean spending a lot of money. For example, my myotherapist checked out my workplace before I started on this edition. I had most things fairly well situated, but we raised the computer screen by placing some large books underneath the monitor. I vary my chairs, and the keyboard height is nearly at my lap, thanks to a homemade stand.

Your work surface must be at the proper level for *you* to function in a healthy manner. Changes in the workstation alone may not be sufficient. Your own body shape and ways of moving must be recognized, addressed, and corrected by a combination of r ditioning, technique retraining, education, and counseling.[6]

Long fingernails can perpetuate TrPs when you use a computer ╮ nails trimmed. You should strike the keyboard with the points of your will be too much stress on too many muscle groups. Improper lighting a. your workspace can also perpetuate TrPs. Your reading material or copying mat placed at the height of your eyes, not lying flat to one side of your computer.

Crossing your legs when you sit is also a perpetuating factor because it constricts blo flow. This can be a problem for people with TrPs who often cross their legs to achieve better balance and support. The use of a gently sloping triangular footrest, to keep the foot in an ankle-down and toes-high position, is a great benefit. A large three-ring binder works well as a footrest.

The Norwegian Balans chair, designed by Peter Opsvik, also called the kneeling chair, can be helpful for a change of position. This chair has the effect of dropping your thighs and opening the angle of the thighs in relation to your spine, while still allowing you to work at traditional tables and desks. It changes the areas of compression. Instead of pressing on your hips and thighs, it presses on the front of your lower legs. However, this can activate other TrPs, so this chair may not work for you. I used a combination of an adjusted chair, a kneeling chair, and a large ball (see Resources) as I worked on this edition. This combination allowed me to work longer hours than I could have otherwise.

Immobility: Stiffness due to both FMS and CMP is most apparent after a period of immobility. Casts, even walking casts, can produce TrPs. Prolonged bed rest adversely affects people with FMS and CMP. Make sure your bed is a good one for *you*. We all have different requirements, and many of us need a large number of support pillows of different sizes and designs to get us through the night. How do you feel when you get up after sleeping? Which muscles are stressed the most? How were they positioned while you slept?

Foot Structure

Some common varieties of foot structure create additional hazards for the person with CMP. People with fallen arches often try specially made shoe orthotics without success. The undersurface of the foot near the middle continues to be painful, and the expensive inserts lie in the closet, unused. The TrPs perpetuating the flat feet need to be treated, and the foot problems corrected, often with properly applied mole foam and flexible arch supports.

Dudley J. Morton described several common variations on the normal foot structure. One type of Morton's foot is hypermobility of the first *metatarsal*. The metatarsals are the joints between the arch of the foot and the toes, not the toes themselves. The second variation is the foot with a short big toe metatarsal and longer second toe metatarsal. It often has a wide web between the second and third toes. When your first metatarsal is relatively short, it puts proportionately more stress on the second one because it hits the ground first. This tends to cause your foot to roll in an abnormal pattern, which may cause calluses to form. The outside heel of your shoe and the inside of the sole above the great toe show greater wear. Your foot may toe outward slightly and/or your knees may tend to pull, rotate, or collapse inward.

Morton's foot can result in a muscle imbalance and stress situation for the whole leg. (See figure 7-1.) The calf and foot muscles are directly affected. Other TrPs are perpetuated due to the attempts these muscles make to compensate for the calf and foot dysfunction. There is a common callus pattern with this condition that aids diagnosis. (See figure 7-2.)

Morton's foot can cause pain in your low back, thigh, knee, leg, and the top of your foot, and may include numbness and tingling. It can cause weak ankles that frequently turn or sprain, and difficulty ice-skating, roller blading, or skiing, due to stiff, unbending soles. This can

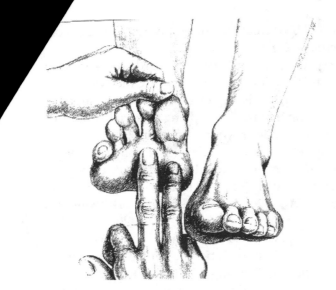

Figure 7-1: Morton's foot

produce asymmetry in the lower limb by muscular torsion, causing a TrP cascade, which causes the upper body posture to compensate, resulting in an upper body cascade as well. Morton's foot becomes evident when you bend your toes upwards. You can see if the second metatarsal is longer. A shoe that is too small, or is too tight-fitting over the toes and arch, or has high heels aggravates Morton's foot problems. People with this foot need a flexible sole for their shoes.

Morton's Neuroma: Morton's foot is totally unrelated to another foot condition, Morton's neuroma, which is named for *Thomas* Morton. In this condition, the metatarsals move a lot and can trap the nerve between them. The constant pressure on the nerve causes a thickening fibrosis. This fibrosis changes into scar tissue, causing more pressure. You feel as if you have a stone in your shoe all the time. Then you develop shooting pains from your foot. Finally, you have great pain constantly, may have to use a wheelchair, and surgery is necessary to remove the neuroma.

You can prevent the neuroma from worsening if you catch it early enough and find proper shoe supports, but they must fit your feet. The supports and your feet must fit properly into your shoes. In the typical FMS/CMP foot, I've observed that neuromas often occur between the second and third metatarsal heads.

The FMS/CMP Foot: There appears to be no technical term for what I call the FMS/CMP foot (called the "FMS/MPS" foot in the first edition, when myofascial pain was still a syndrome). This foot has a broad front, a narrow heel ("duck foot"), and a high arch. This arch can fall very suddenly, resulting in a functionally flat foot, which may be reversed if treated promptly with the proper TrP work and foot supports.

In the FMS/CMP foot there is usually a large space between the big toe and the second toe. There is also a typical callus pattern. This callus may wear a hole in your socks about the size of a dime right under the second metatarsal, in the middle of the ball of your foot. The big toe is often slanted towards the little toe.

Janet Travell researched shoes because they were damaging her patients. Pointed toes and any kind of heel are not good. The shoe should be flat. The sole of the shoe must be flexible at the metatarsal bend. There must be adequate room for the toes, and the heels must fit snugly. The shoe heel should be firm and fit well, to avoid sliding. Sliding irritates the Achilles tendon and can cause heel calluses. If the heel does not fit properly, the foot will roll, causing heavy callus formation on the sides and back of the heels. A thick foam or felt pad inside the shoe can prevent the rolling, calluses, and subsequent Achilles tendon irritation. The arch of your foot needs good support as well.

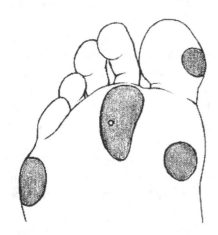

Figure 7-2: Morton's foot callus pattern

My trigger point myotherapist, Justine Jeffrey, helped me to explain Morton's foot in lay language. She wrote the following excerpt:

> The correction for Morton's foot involves some work on your part, the investment in a few supplies, and a full-length mirror. You will need *Molefoam®*—not moleskin—and Spenco 3/4 *soft* arch supports. It is important not to use full shoe arch supports because when the second metatarsal is corrected, the toes may feel cramped in the shoe. It is not uncommon for the measure of the first and second metatarsal to vary from foot to foot. In some people, only one foot is affected; or one foot may be a classic Morton's foot while the other is a classic fallen arch FMS/CMP foot.
>
> The sole of every shoe reacts differently with respect to the wear pattern caused by these problems. Each shoe you wear should be corrected individually and checked periodically, since the correction will wear down differently. No two pairs of shoes are alike, and your arches are not always in the same place on each foot. Keep trying till you find what works for you, focusing on Spenco 3/4 *soft* arch supports and *Molefoam* as your primary resources.
>
> First, stand in front of the mirror with no shoes on, with your feet about 1½ feet apart. Buckle your knees. Don't squat or try to control the way your knees move. Observe whether your knees knock together or, because your muscles have overcorrected through the years, split apart. Your goal is to have them positioned straight-ahead.
>
> Cut several 1-inch squares of *molefoam*. Place a square under the pad under the ball of the foot behind the great toe, adding squares of molefoam. Continue testing by repeating the process, buckling your knees until they buckle straight ahead instead of inward. Test placement of molefoam by lifting your heel until you are standing on the ball of your foot. The molefoam should be directly beneath the ball under your big toe. Lift the other toes off the ground just to make sure you have the pad cut small enough so that it will be placed only under the big toe. You may end up with one pad under one foot and three under the other. Now you know how much correction you typically need in your shoes. Add only one pad of molefoam to your shoe/s per week regardless of how many you may need. A drastic change may cause pain as your body adjusts to the change.
>
> Determine the placement of the molefoam in the shoe by using a combination of three techniques. First, fold your shoe where it bends, as if you were standing on your toes. The ball of your big toe typically goes to the very inside edge. Then, check the outside of your shoes to see if there is a bend pattern in the same place.

> I came upon a neat diagram, which showed how to lace your shoes for proper support. One way was for people who had narrow heels, one was for people who had a wide ball of the foot, and one was for people who had high arches. I wrote David Simons about it, asking what I should do if I had all three conditions. The subsequent discussions included Janet Travell and resulted in my discovery of yet another perpetuating factor—the FMS/CMP foot.

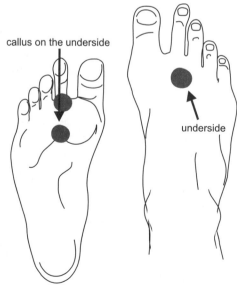

callus on the underside

underside

Figure 7-3: Typical FMS/CMP foot and callus pattern

Finally, and most important, see if you can feel an indentation or valley inside your shoe, formed by the ball of the big toe. If you have Morton's toe, most likely you will notice that the valley under your big toe is significantly deeper than the others. Place the molefoam square right in the valley. Be sure that the molefoam touches or even rides up a bit on the inside/central edge of the shoe or it is likely to slide just under the second metatarsal and undo all of your good work. Make sure it is exactly in the valley, not climbing up toward your big toe or toward the arch of the shoe.

Insert the 3/4 Spenco *soft* arch support. It will cover at least the beginning of your molefoam square, and possibly the entire square. Put on your shoes and stand in front of the mirror and collapse your knees. When you have the proper number of squares under the metatarsal, they will collapse straight forward.

When you shop for shoes, take along enough moleskin squares to duplicate what you will need to wear in your shoes. You need to ensure that not only your feet but also the corrective moleskin will fit comfortably in your shoes. If you have taught your knees to buckle outward to avoid knock knees, you may want to start with just the molefoam or just the arch supports. You will also have to unlearn the behavior of tightening your gluteus muscles and hamstrings to pull your knees outward.

Inappropriate Care

The quality and timing of acute pain treatment may be crucial.[7] Appropriate care may decrease sick leave and prevent chronic conditions from developing, saving costs. Prompt diagnosis and appropriate treatment of myofascial pain often results in relief for the patient.[8] Too often, patients have been given incorrect diagnoses or their complaints have been dismissed altogether. The lack of adequate care and support usually further worsens the symptoms, as TrPs spread and the central nervous system is further sensitized. If TrPs go unrecognized, patients may be subjected to strengthening regimens such as work hardening and weight training, and this inappropriate care may, of itself, cause disability (see chapter 19). One common failing is stretching or otherwise treating one side of your body and not the other. Often, the nonsymptomatic side, if there is one, is full of latent TrPs. Swinging or rotating your head around (the head-rolling exercise) can seriously overload the muscles and worsen TrPs.[9]

Infections and Infestations

The activity of TrPs tends to increase during any systemic viral, bacterial, yeast, or protozoal illness. Vulnerability to TrPs may start a few days before the symptoms from infection worsen, and may last for several weeks after the infection. Increased muscle soreness and stiffness may last several weeks following an acute viral infection, such as the flu. Many of the tender spots formed in the intercostal muscles after a herpes zoster infection are TrPs that respond to injection with immediate relief from pain.[10]

Viral disease is a common perpetuator, especially herpes simplex type 1. This virus may cause cold sores, canker sores, and mouth ulcers, or it may appear on the skin as areas of isolated vesicles filled with clear fluid.[11] Zovirax 5 percent ointment may ease this. Be sure to consult your doctor and correct any folic acid deficiency first.

Any bacterial or fungal infection, such as in an abscessed tooth, blocked sinuses, the pelvic area, or the urinary tract, can affect the severity of both FMS and CMP. An impacted wisdom tooth can perpetuate TrPs even when local infection is not present. It is also important to control any allergic component for sinus problems, and check for the possibility of a fungal infection in resistant sinus congestion. Research shows that fungal infections are present in a large percentage of patients with chronic rhinosinusitis.[12] Until you eradicate the TrPs, it may feel as though you still have an ongoing infection because they will perpetuate the symptoms.

Specific TrP therapy won't produce a lasting effect while a chronic infection is present in the upper respiratory system, the vagina, or if there is a parasitic infection like a tapeworm. Some infections, such as Lyme disease and hepatitis C, seem to initiate some cases of FMS.[13] There is a high prevalence of FMS in patients with hepatitis C virus, especially women. We are not sure yet what the association is, nor what it means.

Some people say that mycoplasmas *cause* FMS. There are people with mycoplasma infections who don't have FMS, and there are people with FMS who don't have mycoplasma infections. Any infection can contribute to the stressors that may cause FMS and CMP. There are a lot of dangers inherent in interpreting research. This is also true for the people who think that fluoride causes FMS. There is no one cause of FMS, and we need more research on the many possible contributory factors.

Lifestyle Choices

Certain behaviors, that is, particular things that you do, whether voluntarily or involuntarily, can be perpetuating factors. For example, grinding your teeth, clenching your jaw, late thumb sucking, chewing gum, breathing through your mouth, and the loss of your back teeth are some possible perpetuating factors for facial TrPs. The muscles you use for these activities are also the first to contract in situations of extreme emotional tension, desperation, and/or determination, so they are often afflicted with TrPs. If you are in the habit of frowning or squinting, you may have astigmatism or light sensitivity, which can be corrected.

Compression: Using a heavy shoulder bag can be very aggravating to TrPs, often starting a TrP cascade. You may be compressing other parts of your body by wearing a tight collar, necktie, bra, belt, or socks, or by habitually leaning in a certain way. This can be compounded if you tend to swell. For example, a bra that feels comfortable in the morning can become unbearably tight just hours later. Tight clothing can aggravate TrPs, causing constriction of blood vessels, which, in turn, can be worsened by the amplifying affect of FMS.

If you have large, pendulous breasts and they are causing TrPs that cannot be relieved in any other fashion, it may be advisable to discuss breast reduction surgery. Obesity may also be a factor in body compression.

The Good Sport Syndrome: The good sport syndrome is one that many readers will find familiar. Perhaps it's a family outing, or relatives are visiting and the house needs a supercleaning. Maybe your sister is moving and she needs help. You don't want to be thought of as a hypochondriac. You look just fine. So you pretend you *are* fine, and you act the "good sport." Then you pay. And pay. Pacing yourself properly is a hard skill to learn. But it is important that you learn how to respect your limits, and to teach others to respect them as well. The good sport syndrome may sometimes be coupled with the yo-yo effect.

Alternating periods of disabling pain and relative relief, called the *yo-yo effect*, are a sign that you are out of control. The yo-yo effect is operating when you overdo and then experience more pain. Then you are tempted to remain horizontal until you feel better again (and until your TrPs become latent). When you feel better, you overexert yourself again. Finally, your reactive muscle pain and tightness will force you to abandon all movement or exercise until you feel better, when, once again, you might overdo. This is a good sign that it's time to concentrate on pacing yourself.

Poor Posture: You may be contributing to poor posture by sleeping on two pillows, sleeping without adequate neck support (such as a well-fitting cervical pillow), protracted neck extension (watching a tennis match, or bird-watching), reading in bed with a light to one side, or rolling over in bed by lifting your head and leading with it. To check this, lie down on your bed. Now roll over paying attention to which muscles you use, and how you use them. Do you lift

> I have seen more people with active TrPs become disabled by repetitive motion exercises and inappropriate physical therapy than from anything else.

your head? Your head should remain flat when you turn. Otherwise you are placing stress on any TrPs you might have in your neck.

Poor posture can result from poorly adjusted reading glasses and improper focal length, or any such disability that continuously influences posture. This includes deafness in one ear, or an injury that restricts your range of motion. Anything that encourages you to tilt your body to one side can be a perpetuating factor. You must also avoid a round-shouldered posture, which happens when you roll your shoulders inward. This shortens the muscles in your chest and neck, perpetuating the TrP cascade. This may start by your picking up the habit of leaning on a table or desk in front of you. It often begins at school. How you hold your fingers is also important when you write. Try using a felt-tipped pen or special-grip pen and avoid pressing hard. Hold the pen flat, not vertically, and this may make it easier to write.

Muscle Abuse: Perhaps you overuse your muscles by pushing yourself too hard, or your boss pushes you too hard by requiring mandatory overtime, or you use muscles that you haven't warmed up properly. The failure to listen to your body is a form of abuse. Pain, fatigue, weakness, tingling, numbness, heaviness, clumsiness, stiffness, and lack of control are all signs that something is wrong. You get only one body in this life. Take care of it.

Repetitive Motion: This is one of the most common perpetuators of TrPs. For example, if you start an exercise program, such as weight training or work hardening, before you have gotten rid of your TrPs, the repetitive motion can be a perpetuating agent. Trigger points in the neck and shoulder muscles may restrict the movements of your arm at shoulder level. Hanging curtains, folding sheets, throwing a ball overhand, keeping an arm raised at school, ironing, or almost any repetitive motion in this area will perpetuate these TrPs and may activate others. Quick and jerky movements, pushing cold, tired muscles to overwork, working in or under a draft, or rushing through movements may perpetuate TrPs.

Smoking Cigarettes and Drinking Alcohol: Nicotine is a great stimulator. When you light that cigarette, you also light up your autonomic nervous system.[14] Since that system is already hyperstimulated in FMS, this is something you don't need. Smoking is a terrible abuse of your body. It is especially bad for people with FMS and CMP. Nicotine causes blood vessels to constrict and decreases blood flow. This adds to any existing microcirculation problems. Carbon monoxide in a smoker's blood binds to hemoglobin, which is the oxygen-carrying workhorse of the body. This then blocks the oxygen available to the muscles.

Some CMP patients have an idiosyncratic reaction to alcohol, experiencing myofascial pain the day after or soon after drinking.[15] Alcohol stresses the body; it uses up your valuable detoxification resources. Absorption of any toxic product makes the development of active TrPs more likely.

Mechanical Factors

Mechanical skeletal asymmetry and disproportion are like land mines, just waiting to go off. Think of the function and balance of the muscles. To provide balance, your body compensates for inequality. Often that compensation is viewed as the problem, rather than as the body's attempt at a solution.

Sometimes body asymmetry is revealed by facial asymmetry. If you put a small mirror in front of the middle of your face and check each side, how different are they? Trigger points may cause some of the difference on one side. Any long-standing loss of range of motion on one side of your body usually means that the other side is overworked.

It is important that apparent unequal leg length not be automatically treated with a heel lift. Legs apparently of unequal length may, in actuality, be unequal due to TrPs causing muscle torsion. Small children need to be checked before the inequality results in imbalance of gait and other kinds of compensatory muscle behavior. Note that if you use a shoe insert, you will often find that walking barefoot or in slippers results in a return of your symptoms.

If the smaller segment of your pelvis, the hemipelvis, is smaller on one side than the other, it tilts the bowl of the pelvis, often resulting in a compensating scoliosis.[16] Bones do what muscles tell them to do. This perpetuating factor can be relieved by the use of a butt lift. This is a small book of the right size that fits under the buttock needing the extra lift. Too often, the result—the scoliosis—is treated, without recognizing that it is the body's way of compensating for a structural irregularity. When a doctor sees developing scoliosis in children or young adults, s/he should ask, "Why?" If you can't sit comfortably without crossing your legs, you may have this problem. A compensatory tilt will develop in the upper body, resulting in TrPs in the neck muscles.

Head Forward Posture: This is one of the most common perpetuating factors. It is vital that any physical assessment you undergo does screening for head-forward posture. This posture is indicated by a measurement of less than 6 cm curvature of neck.[17] Your head should be balanced on the top of your spine. If it juts forward, it creates excessive strain on the neck muscles, which in turn create excessive strain on your other muscles. It throws your whole body out of alignment trying to compensate for the weight of your head, which is considerable. This posture affects your lung capacity, puts pressure on your discs, and affects the blood supply to your head. Whiplash injuries and broken necks are more common due to the head forward posture. If your head is already forward at the time of injury, your neck loses much of its ability to absorb the shock of impact.[18]

Body Asymmetry: To determine whether body asymmetry is an issue for you, take an inventory of your body, which is something we rarely do. To make this assessment, you need to stand naked in front of a mirror. From the front, your shoulder blades, shoulders, nipples, and the space between your arms and your ribs should match on your right and left sides. The points of your hips should match, as should your knees and ankles. From the back, your shoulders should be even and level. Your shoulder blades should match and not protrude. Your elbows and hip points should match, as should the backs of your knees, your ankles, and your heels. When you stand straight, your feet should touch each other from the big toe to the heel. If you stand with your back against the wall and with your heels about three inches away from the wall, your head should feel comfortable against the wall. If it feels unnatural, then it is likely that you have a problem.

If there is an internal rotation of your knees, shoulders, and/or hips, it creates a tightness of the musculature. This can create deformities and inequalities. Some types of hypermobility may be due to this type of rotation. Muscles resist correction and they resist change. Your diaphragm, the big flat muscle that separates the chest cavity from the abdominal cavity, also may be warped and stiff, affecting your breathing, although you may not be able to notice this deformation externally.

Each elbow should reach the outside top point of your hip bone. The corners of your mouth should be aligned with the corners of your eyes, and the sides should be symmetrical. If one shoulder is low, you may be tipping the other even lower to compensate.

If you wear glasses, you will know whether your ears are different heights. This can affect your vision, so be sure to mention it to your eye doctor.

If you have one leg longer than the other, your gluteal muscles will often respond by developing TrPs. The abnormal weight distribution usually causes pronation (toeing out). Check the alignment from the side view as well. See if you are tilted forward from the neck or from the hip. You will need a hand mirror to check your back view. Any sign of asymmetry is a sign of dysfunction.

My husband and I were at a Mensa gathering. It was during the winter Olympics, and I reached our room in time to see Elvis Stojko do his long skating program. My husband asked me how well he had done. I replied, "It was great. But gee, he has short upper arms!" I later told this story to Janet Travell, and she laughed. She knew she had gotten that lesson across.

Short Extremities: Proportionally short upper arms often cause you to lean one way or the other to reach arm supports. Your elbows can't reach most armrests, so you lean sideways. This causes stress to your shoulder elevator muscles and contracts muscles along one side. This condition seems especially prevalent in Native Americans, although it is not uncommon in other ethnic groups.

Proportionally shorter lower legs is a perpetuating factor. You may seem tall when you sit down, but your lower legs may be shorter in terms of your overall height. If this is the case, when you sit, you need a footrest to ensure that the circulation isn't cut off from your hamstrings. People of shorter stature also need to make this correction.

Ill-Fitting Shoes and Socks: A shoe with a tight upper layer and little room between the shoe and foot encourages the formation of TrPs. If you are using a shoe insert, take it to the store when you plan to buy shoes. Orthotics, which are specially made shoe inserts, are usually unnecessary unless there is a foot deformity. The need is for soft cushioning, not hard orthotics, which may perpetuate TrPs.[19] Shoes with extensive wear on the heels and soles may also perpetuate a foot problem. Shoes with rigid soles that allow only ankle movement and no room for toe movement can perpetuate TrPs in your legs and feet. We need shoes with flexible soles. Selecting the right sole is important for other reasons, too. Wearing shoes with smooth soles on a hard slippery surface can perpetuate TrPs because your muscles must be constantly on guard against falling. Chilling of the feet, as of any muscle, can also activate or perpetuate TrPs.

Note that it isn't unusual for people with FMS and CMP to retain indentations on their legs from their socks for a whole day or longer. Knee socks and stockings with elastic may have the same circulation-blocking effects.

Metabolic Factors

Many possible coexisting conditions such as sickle-cell trait or anemia may be perpetuating factors because a percentage of your blood is not functioning properly. That means your muscles get less oxygen and anything that interferes with the supply of oxygen to your muscles will perpetuate TrPs and add to the woes of FMS. Imbalance of estrogens or testosterone can also perpetuate both FMS and CMP (see chapter 11).

Vitamin and mineral inadequacy, insulin resistance, and other nutritional factors are extremely common perpetuating factors of FMS and CMP (see chapter 23). It is important for your medical team to know what foods you avoid, as well as what you do eat, and how your food is prepared. Vitamin insufficiency is a common perpetuating factor. "Some individuals have an unusually high requirement for specific vitamins."[20] In FMS, often there are low blood serum levels of essential amino acids, including tryptophan, which contributes to sleep regulation, pain control, and immune system function. The result can be lack of sleep, pain, or frequent infection. These are all perpetuating factors.

Patients with hypometabolism or hypothyroidism are more susceptible to TrPs. They often get only temporary relief from therapy.[21] Fibromyalgia patients often have need for thyroid supplementation (see chapter 15).

Intolerance to low-dose thyroid supplementation may be due to vitamin B1 deficiency. Supplement with thiamin and then try again. You should always ensure adequate thiamin (B1) levels before starting thyroid supplementation. Note that smoking impairs the action of thyroid hormone and will accentuate the symptoms of hypothyroidism.[22]

Lack of restorative sleep perpetuates both FMS and CMP. This may have metabolic as well as other causes (see chapter 10).

Obesity puts stress, both physical and emotional, on anybody. Unfortunately, as with many problems associated with FMS and CMP, there are built-in self-perpetuators, such as altered carbohydrate metabolism and chocolate craving (see chapter 23).

Microcirculation

A disturbed microcirculation, in combination with muscle activity, can cause localized muscle pain. When FMS developed in patients who had started with localized pain, one study found indications that muscular changes could initiate and maintain the sensitization of some nociceptive nerve cells. This is also a key finding in chronic regional muscle pain. However, this may not be true of FMS patients who did not start out with localized pain.[23]

Overwork

Those people who are competent at their tasks are often especially vulnerable to overwork.[24] They need to learn to use their talents wisely, where they are most needed, and delegate other tasks. This is very true in the fields of FMS and CMP where it often seems there are too few knowledgeable people to handle the urgent needs of a great many.

The tendency to overwork is my weakest point. The year 2000 has been one of survival mode for me. Even when I explain to some people that I am doing four medical journal articles, one clinical study, and writing a book this year they often still insist that I can "just do this one thing" for them. Their causes are worthy, but I am only one person. I have learned to say "No."

I have a message here for those managers who, when they want something done, give it to someone who is already doing the most he or she can do. That burns out the best people. Supervisors should intervene to assist these workers to take steps to protect themselves from a lifestyle that decreases career longevity and promotes psychological discontent.

Psychological Issues

Acute pain from a specific cause that diminishes in the course of natural healing is generally manageable psychologically. You know why you hurt (and so do your friends and family), you know what to do about it, and you know it will end. Recurrent or chronic pain, especially pain caused by an undiagnosed or invisible cause, has a destructive effect on your sense of self. If you have FMS and/or CMP, visit after visit to doctor after doctor may provide little or no relief. Every doctor may give you a different diagnosis. Because some of the symptoms of FMS may also be symptoms of depression, eventually some doctors might begin to urge a psychiatric evaluation, which further erodes your self-esteem. Your frustration mounts, and true depression and progressive disability may follow.

It is harmful when others, especially physicians and other health care professionals, imply that you are somehow to blame for your afflictions. It is also very stressful when otherwise well-meaning friends and relatives try to pass your symptoms off as nothing important.

"You're *young*, you shouldn't be using a cane!" "My feet hurt, too." " Just get up and move around more. You're just out of shape." "You're just clumsy. If you weren't so preoccupied with your health, you wouldn't knock things over all the time." "It's not as if you had something like cancer" (meaning something *real*). Such comments (and worse) become painfully familiar.

When people are told that they must learn to live with their FMS and CMP pain because it is due to arthritis or some other cause, it may cause them to restrict their physical activity in order to avoid pain. This immobility perpetuates TrPs, because their muscles shorten even more with disuse. In addition, patients are often put on heavy doses of aspirin, steroids, and other anti-inflammatory medications, which frequently add a whole new layer of symptoms and further stress.

The Depression Factor: It's unlikely that a doctor would tell a patient in agony with a severe rheumatoid arthritis flare to put on a happy face, ignore the pain, and get on with life. But such words are said to FMS and CMP patients every day, and these statements have enormous negative effect. There is nothing you can do about the poor treatment and cruel comments you may have received in the past. You do need to educate others, but you must learn not to take negative talk personally. You can help yourself by learning positive, life-affirming, peaceful ways to cope both with your illness and with the ignorance and disbelief of others (see chapter 20). It's important for you to focus on the present, to work on enhancing your own health, and to take over the management of your own health care. You can't change other people. But you can change your reactions to them.

Avoid generating negativity. Guilt, blame, hurt, anger, fear, and frustration are negative emotions. When they are hurled at you, that is abuse. You shouldn't take abuse from anyone. The world directs more than enough negativity your way. It is equally true that you must not abuse yourself. Don't generate more negativity. Anything you accomplish is deserving of respect and praise. "Love others as yourself" takes it as a given that you first love yourself. This may be a difficult lesson.

Psychological symptoms are often secondary to chronic pain, but they still need to be treated. The longer the duration and the greater the intensity of unrelieved pain, the greater the depression is likely to be. Relieving the depression allows you to take more responsibility for putting into action the various therapeutic processes you need to improve your life. Anxiety and tension tighten your muscles. One study showed that patients with myofascial disorders reported significantly worse pain, higher depression scores, more interpersonal conflict, and less support from others than did the patients with arthritis, yet they did not differ from the arthritis patients on personality traits.[25] This would indicate that the pain and the nature of the pain cause depression and conflict. A psychologically healthy person finds the functional restrictions imposed by a FMS and CMP terribly frustrating and unrewarding.

Too many insurance companies and doctors are focused on "secondary gain." This term includes everything you might gain by being ill. This includes extra attention, lessening of responsibilities, time off from work, etc. Most of us have gained little from being in chronic pain except the special insight that a chronic pain condition can bring. On the other hand, our losses may be staggering. It is important for insurance companies and doctors to focus on how effective your life coping skills were before the onset of FMS and CMP. Do you try to function or do you only talk about it? What was your level of function before the event that started the pain? A higher level of function is not realistic. As your TrPs and FMS symptoms are relieved, are you resuming activities and functioning better?

Sexual/Physical Abuse: There is a subset of patients with FMS who have a history of sexual/physical abuse.[26] Researchers have found that childhood traumatic events are significantly related to chronic pain states.[27] Any kind of psychological stressor can be a perpetuating factor, and sustained or severe psychological trauma can be initiating factors. Even working under pressure or frustration can cause you to tense your muscles and to develop TrPs.

You can be defeated by your own attitude. When you have chronic pain, you can get caught up in a cycle of denial and negativity. You may feel worn down, dealing with the constant grind of a chronic invisible pain condition. Life may seem terribly unfair. Sometimes it is. That is not the issue. What are you going to do about it? *That* is what you need to focus on. Life is about change.

Don't Compare Yourself with Others: You don't know what their stressors are, nor what they deal with day by day. You may think you have it rough, and you may, but so do many of us. Those of us who have elaborate support systems built them, piece by piece. Each of us is different, and the comparison does not matter if it gets you down. Catch yourself when you start focusing on how bad your life is. You are victimizing yourself with that attitude, and adding another perpetuating factor to your list. At this point in time, there are more options and information available to people with FMS and CMP than ever before. Doctors are receiving proper training. Researchers are finding pieces of the puzzle. What matters most in your attitude is you, and what you have to work with, and what you need to do to change things for the better.

Psychological Testing: Presently, the MMPI I and II (Minnesota Multiphasic Personality Indicator) are still the best tests we have for assessing personality, but they don't take into consideration the fact that many of the answers may be affected by or determined by physical illness. There is no opportunity to explain the "why" of an answer. Computers score most of the tests. If you get the raw data scores and check out the "indicative" questions, and then make allowances for those answers that were affected by your physical symptoms, your personality profile may be entirely different. For example, you may avoid parties. This can reflect fatigue level or sensory overload, rather than lack of sociability. Your mental health counselor must be made aware of this, and you may want to schedule a session specifically to talk about test answers before a personality profile is created. This will provide your counselor, and you, with a more accurate result.

Reactive Hypoglycemia (RHG) and Insulin Resistance

There is a certain type of hypoglycemia, or low blood sugar, that accompanies many cases of FMS and CMP. This is not the same as the fasting hypoglycemia that shows up on the glucose tolerance test. Reactive hypoglycemia usually occurs two to three hours after a high carbohydrate meal, overstimulating insulin release, which then triggers an adrenaline response. This can cause symptoms such as tremors, rapid heart rate, and sweating. Anxiety also stimulates adrenaline, as does caffeine and nicotine. Reactive hypoglycemia may lead to insulin resistance (IR).

After your body has turned the food you eat into glucose and the glucose has moved through the walls of your gastrointestinal system, it can travel freely to some areas, but other areas are restricted. Your body needs an agent to take the glucose to the mitochondria so it can be turned into energy, just as a visitor to a power plant needs an escort. Insulin receptors open the doors of the mitochondria and allow the glucose to enter and to be processed into adenosine triphosphate (ATP).

Adenosine triphosphate is the fuel that runs your body. When you have IR, the mitochondria no longer recognize the security pass, and the glucose is denied entrance. This could be due either to changes in the shape of the insulin receptor or to changes in the way your cells respond to insulin itself.

Insulin is also the agent that causes excess glucose to deposit as belly fat. Obesity can be one sign of insulin resistance, but thin people can have IR, too. Insulin resistance may not show up on glucose tolerance tests, but you can test for serum insulin response to an oral glucose load.

This will pick up IR. Insulin also controls salt and water retention, and IR may be involved in a combination of rising blood pressure and galloping cholesterol. People with IR often display clinical abnormalities other than impaired glucose tolerance, including central obesity, hypertension, and abnormal coagulation.[28] Reactive hypoglycemia and IR not only perpetuate FMS and CMP, they can institute a metabolic cascade on their own, leading to, among other things, type II diabetes. These conditions, until fairly recently, were not taken as seriously as they should be by some in the medical community. This is changing. The research on these conditions is vigorous.

Hypoglycemia can produce a significant deterioration in performance on any of the visual information processing tasks.[29] That means it can add to the mental confusion of "fibrofog." Cognitive, perceptual, and motor deficits are part of the symptoms found in hypoglycemic conditions.[30] It is logical to check people with chronic pain for signs of insulin resistance, since sleep disturbances may adversely affect glucose tolerance.[31] Note that even moderate exercise is associated with improved insulin sensitivity in healthy individuals.[32] *You* can control your exercise levels.

In one study, traits characterizing the IR syndrome were found to be clustered to a significant degree among Native Americans.[33] I have observed that at least some tribes of the Native American population have many people with FMS and CMP, and many of those individuals have reactive hypoglycemia and insulin resistance as perpetuating factors.

Trauma

Whiplash: Any assessment following whiplash injury must include examination for TrPs. Myofascial pain from TrPs is present in a hundred percent of cases of chronic whiplash pain, including those with facet joint injury and pain arising from the joint itself.[34] Generalized central hyperexcitability is common in patients with chronic whiplash syndrome.[35] There are increased rates of FMS following neck spine injury.[36] Concussion may go unrecognized, because when cortical activity is interrupted, as it is during a concussion, a retrograde amnesia often develops. You don't remember the head impact and you may not remember loss of consciousness.

What does it take to injure the central nervous system? We don't know. We do know that it doesn't take a motor vehicle accident to cause a whiplash effect. How many times have you been subjected to what my myotherapist calls a "brain bash"? These are the incidental head traumas we receive every day—hitting your head on a cupboard door or a car hood, or falling and hitting your head against the corner of the coffee table; all of these incidents may take their toll, contributing to head and neck injury.

Postural Rotation and Asymmetry: These conditions may be caused by problems at birth or before birth.[37] There is a theory that symmetrical pressure on the vertebrae can cause later structural asymmetry such as scoliosis. We don't know how often kinematic ischemic suboccipital syndrome (KISS) occurs during the birth process. Ordinarily, the ligaments in your upper neck have the same strength as radial tire bands. In KISS, there is decreased elasticity in the suboccipital muscles. If the dentate ligament is rotated, this can affect the brainstem and the dorsal spinal cerebellar pathway. The cerebellum controls posture, proprioceptors, gait control, agility, balance, and coordination.[38] People in one study who had experienced a whiplash injury demonstrated proprioceptor problems.[39] Once proprioceptor function is compromised, which may happen both from myofascial TrPs and possibly from FMS, more falls and other traumas may result.

We also know that many neurotransmitters, including norepinephrine, serotonin, dopamine, and acetylcholine are affected by brain injury.[40]

Traffic Accidents: There is a thought-provoking article that many people may not know about. It is an interesting study on traffic accidents.[41] It was done to determine if a correlation existed between the external forces of injury and the muscles responding to those forces. The study was looking for evidence of weakness and resulting muscle shortening, or TrPs. There is such evidence. This study indicated that these TrPs can persist indefinitely. Only one accident occurred at a speed greater than 40 mph. The patients were categorized by the direction of impact, and whether the victim was a passenger or driver. They were even able to list the muscles and the frequency of occurrence of TrPs, in regard to the direction of impact and position of the victim at the time of impact. I offer the following quotes:

> Objective testing indicates the injured underreport rather than exaggerate their physical complaints and limitations.[42]

> Patients tend to underreport their functional limitations and pain. One needs to question the process of labeling the patient who does not respond to ordinary treatment in a timely fashion, whose insurance has been expended, who in general is frustrating those who are doing exhaustive studies, are biased toward surgery as a general solution, or who "fake, bake and shake."[43]

> Reports that read, "No Neurological Disorder," or "No Orthopedic Disorder" are quite common with those who examine muscle overload patients for Workers' Compensation or Personal Injury Litigation. This study suggests that the role of an independent medical examiner might be one that focuses upon muscle overload.[44]

If you have been involved in an automobile accident, make sure you have the presence of both FMS and CMP assessed by competent practitioners. From what we know, early intervention will prevent an injury-induced metabolic cascade, and treatment with agents that activate cerebral metabolism may mitigate chronic symptoms.[45]

Repetitive Motion: This is a specific type of trauma. It is important to vary your motions as much as possible. You may even need to relearn how to move. Often we need to go through an unlearning of bad habits and then a mental as well as a physical retraining effort.

Surgery: Surgery is a carefully orchestrated and planned trauma. Surgeons may be untrained in dealing with FMS and CMP, although anesthesiologists are becoming increasingly more aware of both conditions. During prolonged surgeries while being kept in stationary and sometimes odd postures, muscles may undergo passive overstretching. These muscles will develop TrPs that, if untreated, will persist as chronic pains. Myofascial pain should be considered for any patient who develops pain in one or more muscles following surgery with general anesthesia.[46] For more information, see "What Your Surgeon Should Know" in *The Fibromyalgia Advocate*.[47] General anesthesia must be coupled with local analgesia during surgery to prevent TrPs, and combined with meticulous postsurgical pain control[48] to prevent development of TrPs. Painful TrPs in surgical scars are common and can be relieved by trigger point injection[49] and specific myofascial scar release therapy.

Vertebrae Fusion: I have heard of countless cases where vertebrae have been surgically fused because of degeneration, only to have the discs above and/or below degenerate, requiring more spinal fusion. If the muscles are contractured and TrPs are pulling the bones out of alignment causing the eventual disc degeneration, they must be treated. Dealing with the disc or the vertebrae does nothing to reduce the strain from the muscles. We know that TrPs are more likely to occur in certain muscles in the presence of cervical disc lesions at specific levels.[50] You must deal with the TrPs, or the surgery will simply cause more strain, resulting in more contracture and future problems. (See chapter 8.)

Mitigating Trauma: There are many other kinds of trauma. Some may seem small but they can be devastating. For every trauma there is a way to mitigate the impact. For example, injection of irritating substances into a latent TrP site can activate it. This includes tetanus toxoid, flu shots, B vitamins, and penicillin. But this activation can be avoided by peppering the injection site with procaine immediately after the injection.[51]

What You, the Patient, Can Do

As you learn more about your body in this book, you will find that there are steps you can take to eliminate or lessen the effects of perpetuating factors. Because TrPs are probably at the heart of much of your pain, it's important that you always try to prevent more TrPs from developing. You can do so in the following ways:

- Treat injuries aggressively. • Seek crisis intervention when appropriate. • Build proper and sufficient exercise and sleep into your program. • Use your body properly. • Control psychological trauma and stress load. • Make lifestyle modifications.

This chapter may seem overwhelming, and it does not even include all the possible perpetuating factors. How do you handle them? One at a time. Make a list of the perpetuating factors you may have and want to investigate. The key is to take better care of yourself.

Endnotes

1. Personal communication.

2. Harrison, D. E., R. Cailliet, D. D. Harrison, S. J. Troyanovich, and S. O. Harrison. 1999. A review of biomechanics of the central nervous system—Part I: spinal canal deformations resulting from changes in posture. *J Manipulative Physiol Ther* 22(4):227-234.

3. Colborn, T., M. J. Smolen, and R. Rolland. 1998. Environmental neurotoxic effects: the search for new protocols in functional teratology. *Toxicol Ind Health* 14(1-2):9-23.

4. Simons, D. G., J. G. Travell, and L. S. Simons. 1999. *Travell and Simons' Myofascial Pain and Dysfunction: The Trigger Point Manual.* Second edition. Baltimore: Williams and Wilkins, p. 105.

5. Cranz, G. 1998. *The Chair: Rethinking Culture, Body and Design.* New York: W. W. Norton and Co.

6. Pascarelli, E. F., and J. J. Kella. 1993. Soft-tissue injuries related to the use of the computer keyboard. A clinical study of 53 severely injured persons. *J Occup Med* 35(5):522-532.

7. Linton, S. J., A. L. Hellsing, and D. Andersson. 1993. A controlled study of the effects of an early intervention on acute musculoskeletal pain problems. *Pain* 54(3):353-359.

8. Bruce, E. 1995. Myofascial pain syndrome: early recognition and comprehensive management. *AAOHN J* 43(9):469-474.

9. Simons, Travell, and Simons. 1999. *Op. cit.,* p. 443.

10. Chen, S. M., J. T. Chen, T. S. Kuan, and C. Z. Hong. 1998. Myofascial trigger points in intercostal muscles secondary to herpes zoster infection of the intercostal nerve. *Arch Phys Med Rehabil* 79(3):336-338.

11. Simons, Travell, and Simons. 1999. *Op. cit.,* p. 223.

12. Ponikau, J. U., D. A. Sherris, E. B. Kern, H. A. Homburger, E. Frigas, T. A. Gaffey, et al. 1999. The diagnosis and incidence of allergic fungal sinusitis. *Mayo Clin Proc* 74(9):877-884.

13. Rivera, J., A. de Diego, M. Trinchet, and A. Garcia Monforte. 1997. Fibromyalgia-associated hepatitis C virus infection. *Br J Rheumatol* 36(9):981-985.

14. Gershon, M. D. 1998. *The Second Brain.* New York: HarperCollins.

15. Simons, Travell, and Simons. 1999. *Op. cit.,* p. 226.

16. Egoscue, P., and R. Gittines. 1998. *Pain Relief.* New York: Bantam.

17. Simons, Travell, and Simons. 1999. *Op. cit.,* p. 262.

18. Egoscue and Gittenes. 1998. *Op. cit.*

19. Travell, J. G., and D. G. Simons. 1992. *Myofascial Pain and Dysfunction: The Trigger Point Manual*, Vol. II. *The Lower Body*. Baltimore: Williams and Wilkins.

20. Simons, D. G., J. G. Travell, and L. S. Simons. 1999. *Op. cit.*, p. 107.

21. *Ibid.*, p. 213.

22. Simons, Travell, and Simons. 1999. *Op. cit.*, p. 218.

23. Henriksson, K. G. 1999. Is fibromyalgia a distinct clinical entity? Pain mechanisms in fibromyalgia syndrome. A myologist's view. *Baillieres Best Pract Res Clin Rheumatol* 13(3):455-461.

24. Davidhizar, R. 1991. Liabilities of competence. *Adv Clin Care* 6(1):44-46.

25. Faucett, J. A., and J. D. Levine. 1991. The contributions of interpersonal conflict to chronic pain in the presence or absence of organic pathology. *Pain* 44(1):35-43.

26. Alexander, R. W., L. A. Bradley, G. S. Alarcon, M. Triana-Alexander, L. A. Aaron, K. R. Alberts, et al. 1998. Sexual and physical abuse in women with fibromyalgia: association with outpatients' health care utilization and pain medication usage. *Arthritis Care Res* 11(2):102-115.

27. Goldberg, R. T., W. N. Pachas, and D. Keith. 1999. Relationship between traumatic events in childhood and chronic pain. *Disabil Rehabil* 21(1):23-30.

28. Sowers, J. R., and B. Draznin. 1998. Insulin, cation metabolism and insulin resistance. *J Basic Clin Physiol Pharmacol* 9(2-4):223-233.

29. McCrimmon, R. J., I. J. Deary, B. J. P. Huntly, K. J. MacLeod, and B. M. Frier. 1996. Visual information processing during controlled hypoglycaemia in humans. *Brain* 119(4):1277-1287.

30. Piotrowski, C. 1997. Hypoglycemia as a mitigating factor in vehicular accidents. *Perceptual Motor Skills* 84 (3 pt 2): 1241-1242.

31. Scheen, A. J., M. M. Byrne, L. Plat, R. Leproult, and E. Van Cauter. 1996. Relationships between sleep quality and glucose regulation in normal humans. *Am J Physiol* 271(2 pt 1): E261-E270.

32. Mayer-Davis, E. J., R. D'Agostino, Jr., A. J. Karter, S. M. Haffner, M. J. Rewers, M. Saad, et al. 1998. Intensity and amount of physical activity in relation to insulin sensitivity: the Insulin Resistance Atherosclerosis Study. *JAMA* 279(9):669-674.

33. Greenlund, K. J., R. Valdez, M. L. Casper, S. Rith-Najarian, and J. B. Croft. 1999. Prevalence and correlates of the insulin resistance syndrome among Native Americans. *Diabetes Care* 22:441-447.

34. Gerwin, R. D., and J. Dommerholt. 2000. Unpublished data.

35. Koelback Johnson, M., T. Graven-Nielsen, A. Schou Olesen, and L. Arendt-Nielsen. 1999. Generalized muscular hyperalgesia in chronic whiplash syndrome. *Pain* 83(2):229-234.

36. Buskila, D., L. Neumann, G. Vaisberg, D. Alkalay, and F. Wolfe. 1997. Increased rates of fibromyalgia following cervical spine injury. A controlled study of 161 cases of traumatic injury. *Arthritis Rheum* 40(3):446-452.

37. Biederman, H. 1992. Kinematic imbalances due to suboccipital strain in newborns. *J Manual Med* 6:151-156.

38. Rockwell, J. 1995. The 1995 Convention of the National Association of Myofascial Trigger Point Therapists: Parker Chiropractic College, Dallas, Texas. September 17–19.

39. Loudon, J. K., M. Ruhl, and E. Field. 1997. Ability to reproduce head position after whiplash injury. *Spine*. 22(8):865-868.

40. Anderson, K., and J. M. Silver. 1998. Modulation of anger and aggression. *Semin Clin Neuropsychiatry* 3(3):232-242.

41. Baker, B. A. 1986. The muscle trigger: evidence of overload injury. *JONOMAS* 7(1):35-44

42. *Ibid.*, p. 39.

43. *Ibid.*, p. 40.

44. *Ibid.*, p. 40.

45. Mamelak, M. 2000. The motor vehicle collision injury syndrome. *Neuropsychiatry Neuropsychol Behav Neurol* 13(2):125-135.

46. Prasanna, A. 1993. Myofascial pain as postoperative complication. *J Pain Sympt Manage* (7):450-451.

47. Starlanyl, D. 1998. *The Fibromyalgia Advocate: Getting the Support You Need to Cope with Fibromyalgia and Myofascial Pain Syndrome*. Oakland, CA: New Harbinger Publications.

48. Simons, Travell, and Simons. 1999. *Op. cit.*, p. 57.

49. Defalque, R. J. 1982. Painful trigger points in surgical scars. *Anesth Analg* 61(6):518-520.

50. Hsueh, T. C., S. Yu, T. S. Kuan, and C.-Z. Hong. 1998. Association of active myofascial trigger points and cervical disc lesions. *J Formos Med Assoc* 97(3):174-180.

51. Simons, Travell, and Simons. 1999. *Op. cit.*, p. 692.

CHAPTER 8

Signs and Symptoms

In one episode of the television series *Babylon 5*, the ambassador from Centauri tells his aide, ". . . this, this is being nibbled to death by, eh, what are those Earth creatures called? Feathers . . . long bills . . . webbed feet. Go quack." "Cats," is the answer. The ambassador repeats, "Like being nibbled to death by cats!" He identified his symptoms, but could not identify the cause, and the person he consulted was misinformed. Sounds familiar, doesn't it? This is frequently the problem for patients (and care providers) when myofascial trigger points (TrPs) and fibromyalgia (FMS) are involved. This chapter will help to change that.

To make this long chapter more manageable, it has been divided into four sections. The dividing lines may seem a little fuzzy, because they are. Everything in the body is connected and dividing lines are often arbitrary. Learning how to use the information in this chapter will give you a greater measure of control over your life. Some of the information is still in the theoretical stage, and we have indicated that. We are blazing trails. Don't let the specific muscles' Latin names baffle you. They can help your doctor to make a correct diagnosis. They will also help your bodyworker. I use nonmedical terms as often as possible, but I try to be specific enough so that you can locate the TrPs. For a more complete set of diagrams, see the video, "Chronic Myofascial Pain Syndrome: A Guide to the Trigger Points." (See Appendix B under Starlanyl.)

The diagrams in this chapter are not part of FMS. They are part of *myofascial pain and TrPs*. Myofascial TrPs respond to specific treatment if the perpetuating factors are addressed. One of the first challenges Dr. Simons gave me was to separate FMS symptoms from those caused by TrPs. I remember how overwhelmed I felt at the time. You may have to read this chapter in bits and pieces to avoid sensory overload! Some doctors look at the symptom list for FMS and say, "At some time in their lives, everyone has had allergies, postnasal drip, swollen glands, runny nose, sore throat, stiff neck, morning stiffness . . ." and so forth. These doctors are missing the point entirely.

Healthy people may have one or two of the symptoms. If someone has *many* of these symptoms and they are chronic or repeating, there is a pattern. Some of the symptoms, like mottled skin, are here because other people can see they are real. Some are here because they may be clues to FMS and/or to chronic myofascial pain (CMP). Some of your symptoms may be due to myofascial pain, not to fibromyalgia. *This means that there is something you can do about these symptoms that may alleviate them.*

Most of the diagrams in this chapter are from the medical texts *Myofascial Pain and Dysfunction: The Trigger Point Manuals*, reproduced here with the permission of their authors and publisher. They are not intended to replace the complete set in the texts. If you recognize these diagrams, give thanks to Janet Travell and David Simons for mapping them out and for founding myofascial medicine.

In the diagrams, the "X" does not mark the *only* spot in which a TrP can occur, only the most *common* sites. Trigger point sites in a given muscle may occur anywhere and in any layer of the muscle. Each muscle may hold multiple TrPs. Diagnosis is challenging when FMS and CMP occur together. Trigger points can even overlay FMS tender points.

Section I: No Bones About It

1. **Did you have growing pains and chronic aches as a child?** Many people with FMS and/or CMP believe that their problems started recently. When questioned, however, they often remember "growing pains."[1]

2. **Do you attract blackflies and mosquitoes?** There seem to be something about the FMS biochemistry that attracts these insects. The bites swell into huge, hard lumps that take forever to go away and often leave scars. This symptom seems to be diminished by guaifenesin or T3 therapy (see chapter 21). Keep cool and unscented, wash off areas of sweat frequently, and wear white clothing. Excess hyaluronic acid may be one of the reasons that mosquitoes love us (see chapter 15). The lactic acid in sweat also acts as an attractant.

3. **Do you bump into things frequently?** *Proprioception* is the name of the sense that allows you to know where you are in relation to the space around you, and where each part of your body is, in relation to the other parts. People with FMS sometimes have indications of a movement disorder and sensory disturbances.[2] If you can't sense where you are in relation to the world around you, your movement is instinctively inhibited. Proprioception gives you clues about your posture and balance. It requires integration of touch and pressure sensations from your skin, muscles, and tendons; visual and motor information from your brain; and balance feedback from your inner ear.

    You may have problems discerning the location of your teeth in relation to surrounding structures. If so, you may bite your tongue or cheek. A soft ridge may form along your cheek, parallel to the line where your teeth come together, due to frequent trauma from your teeth. This may be due to TrPs in the chewing muscles, especially the pterygoids.[3] I also suspect the buccinator TrP. This TrP is found in the muscle that is attached at the corners of your mouth. TrPs aren't shy. Once you find them and press them, they let you know that you've hit the right spot. Ouch!

4. **Do you have allergies and sensitivities?** Allergies seem to be part of the FMS bag of tricks. Histamine, a familiar name to allergy sufferers, is a neurotransmitter. In the posterior hypothalamus, a gland that is dysregulated in FMS, there are histamine-containing nerve cells. These may bathe the hypothalamus and other parts of the brain with excess amounts of this irritant. It's common for patients with myofascial pain and allergies to have increased histamine response to bodywork.[4] More research needs to be done on this.

    Mast cells live in the connective tissue and are hypersensitized by allergens. They also produce histamine. I have observed that many people who experience an increased immune response during allergy season, or are ill or in flare, respond well to antihistamine therapy to decrease their pain level. Other people cannot tolerate any antihistamines and develop a rapid heart rate.

> At the Focus on Pain Seminar in 2000, someone noticed that my *Trigger Point Manual* was indexed with many tabs.
> "Gee," she said, "you must be compulsive."
> "No", I explained, "I *use* the book."

Avoid antihistamine combinations that include epinephrine or norepinephrine. People with FMS don't always react normally to skin tests due to their altered biochemical responses. Often many of our "allergies" are actually sensitivities without an immune component, or they have a mechanism that does not utilize Immuglobin E (IgE), the typical allergy marker.

5. **Do you have a changing or hoarse voice?** Asthma, sinus difficulties, postnasal drip, and allergies can create TrPs around the area of the trachea and larynx due to *bronchospasm*. This can create changes in your voice, or even voice loss. It can be aggravated or perpetuated by acid reflux. As I worked on this edition, to save my fingers I purchased a vocal interface for my computer. I didn't take into account the fact that my fingers *and* my throat have TrPs. I had to let my fingers do the walking, and sometimes they limp.

For years I lost my singing voice. I could no longer trust my voice to carry a tune or to project. Work on my head, neck, and chest TrPs brought my voice back. Your throat has a lot of little muscles and any of them may get TrPs. You may need an anatomy book to locate the following TrPs, which can occur in any part of the muscles. **Warning:** Some long and unfamiliar Latinate names are coming. Don't panic. If you have the related symptoms, just write down the muscle names and send your doctor and bodyworker to their (hopefully well-worn) copies of the *Trigger Point Manual.*

The digastric muscle (Fig. 8-1) can be involved with voice difficulties. Other anterior neck muscles can refer pain to your laryngeal region, the front of your neck and mouth. Often, both mouth breathing and paradoxical breathing perpetuate these TrPs. Active TrPs in any laryngeal muscles may produce a hoarse voice. Activation of TrPs in the suprahyoid muscles, infrahyoid muscles, and the deeper anterior vertebral muscles (the longus colli in particular), can result from a whiplash injury, sore throat, or postnasal drip.

Intermittent cold may help these TrPs. Deep anterior neck muscles can refer pain to the laryngeal region, anterior neck, and mouth and affect your voice. They require special consideration from your bodyworker. The mylohyoid muscle can refer pain to your tongue. Head and neck pain can come from the stylohyoid muscle. Trigger points in the cricoarytenoid muscle cause pain when you talk, as well as causing a sore throat.[5] I have observed a constricted feeling in the neck is common with omohyoid involvement. Trigger points in the omohyoid muscle can elevate your first rib. It will stand out prominently when your head is tilted to the other side. These TrPs can prevent a full stretch of the trapezius and scalene muscles and must be released before these muscles can be released. Trigger points in the stylohyoid muscle may

The discoloration on my skin first began to be noticeable on my forearms. They became brown in rectangular patches. The color faded slightly with the winter and then darkened again in the sunlight. After a few years, the blotches turned an angry red and itched when they were exposed to the sun, although sunblock did prevent this symptom from occurring. I visited a dermatologist, who had no answers, except to rule out infection.

The clue for me came when I inadvertently left some salt gel residue from a muscle electrostimulator electrode on my forearm. I soon developed a brown mottled semicircle on my arm. It became obvious to me that the electrolytes—the "salts"—in the gel had reacted with something in the sunlight to cause the brownish mark on my arm. Observing my movements in the garden, I noticed that I often wiped my forehead on my arms. The photo-reaction of the gel salts with sunlight and the salts in my sweat and, perhaps, unusual FMS biochemical components produced the mottling. I still have the mottling on my arms two years later, but, since I began wearing headbands while gardening and frequently washing off any sweat accumulation, the mottling has not increased.

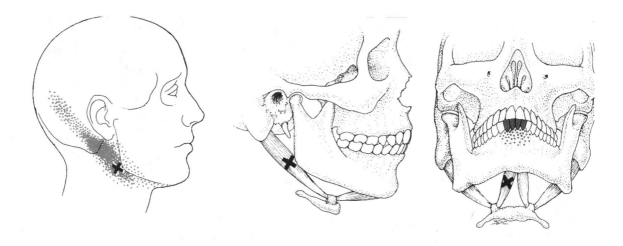

Figure 8-1: Trigger points in the right digastric; stippled and dark parts show areas of referred pain.

entrap the carotid artery and affect blood flow. Trigger points in the longus capitis and/or longus colli muscles can cause difficulty swallowing, as well as the feeling of having a lump in the throat. Spasm of the longus colli muscle can cause dry mouth, a sore throat, a persistent tickle in throat, or the feeling of a lump in your throat when you swallow.

If TrPs exist in any of these muscles, check for tight tissue in the jaw, pectoral, and abdominal regions. Treat these with TrP releases (see chapter 3), postural training, and passive stretch exercises. Correct your breathing, jaw grinding and clenching, and bite.

6. **Do you have dry, itchy skin or frequent skin irritation?** Fibromyalgia skin biopsies reveal significantly higher values of Immunoglobin G (IgG) deposits in the skin and vessel walls and a higher reactivity for one type of collagen. These patients also have more mast cells, which often indicates allergy.[6] A type of nerve fiber called C-fibers prompts the histamine-type itch. This may respond to Benedryl crème, and ice may help temporarily. Keep your skin moist with lotion to minimize discomfort. The antidepressant, doxepin, which has an antihistamine component, may improve itching. There is a Japanese topical mast cell inhibitor cream, Tranilast, that you may be able to get from a compounding pharmacist (see chapter 24), but presently it is not marketed in the United States.

C-fibers may also be responsible for some burning sensations. Opioids relieve pain but not itch and may themselves cause severe itching. Widespread *cutaneous* TrPs have been called the "skinache syndrome." After one subcutaneous injection of lidocaine, 68 percent of ninety-four patients had their symptoms relieved.[7] People with FMS sometimes have what I call "fragile skin syndrome." If you have this, even turning clothes inside out while doing laundry can peel the skin from your cuticles until it bleeds. Filing 3 x 5 cards can do the same, as can tucking in sheets, or any other action that rubs downward across the front of the fingers. Bleeding hangnails are also common.

7. **Do you have mottled, blotchy skin?** The skin mottling seen in FMS may be due to the reaction of hyaluronic acid and other acid salts in your sweat to sunlight and/or heat. Many of us have more mottling in places where the sweat tends to pool, such as the base of the neck.

8. **Do you have swelling/edema?** Fluid retention syndrome, or idiopathic edema, occurs almost exclusively in women. It can produce a variety of symptoms ranging from headache and blurring of vision to abdominal pains and diarrhea. The most common symptoms are bloating,

fatigue, and generalized weakness.[8] The added fluid in your body often causes heat intolerance. Suspect interstitial edema, and check for symptoms of insulin resistance.

Edema may start with the release of sensitizing substances, such as histamine, bradykinin, or prostaglandins during times of trauma.[9] This trauma includes repetitive use. These substances cause your pain receptors to fire. Sometimes these nociceptors keep firing, even after the sensitizing substances are gone. This causes local edema, which may begin to compress blood and lymph vessels. All this contributes to local microcirculation problems, which, in turn, cause the release of more sensitizing substances. This type of edema may be helped by a high protein diet.

9. **Do you crave carbohydrates or sweets?** Such craving may be caused by reactive hypoglycemia (see chapters 7 and 23). Try eating a balanced diet and avoid excess carbohydrates.

10. **Do you have nails with vertical ridges that break off and/or curve under?** Nail ridges or beads, fragile nails, and/or nails that curve under are common in FMS. The nails curve downward at the tips, turning under. This "clubbing," also called "beaking," may be inherited. This may be associated with chronic lack of oxygen, chronic infections, or adrenal problems. When the body is under stress, as it is in any chronic pain state, it cuts down on the nutrients it sends to less important areas, such as the fingernails. Hair loss may also be related, because hair tissue is similar to fingernail tissue. There may even be detachment of the nail bed from the overlying plate. This condition, called "onycholyis," may be a sign of an endocrine disease.[10]

11. **Do you have overgrowing connective tissue? Do you scar easily and abnormally?** Ingrown hairs, adhesions, easy scarring, cuticles that thicken and split resulting in sore hangnails, cysts and fibroids, pierced ears that overgrow, scrapes or mosquito bites that turn into burnlike scarring—all of these symptoms may be related. I've observed that people with FMS frequently have overgrowing connective tissue, fibroid tumors, and possible encapsulation of certain types of tissues. Scars that form may be of an unusual nature. They can resemble burns. The dark brown "burn mark" finally peels away, sometimes in layers, leaving a scar. I have no idea why this happens. Yet.

12. **Do you have fibrocystic breasts?** Although this symptom is generally linked to FMS, I believe it may be due to lymphatic congestion and fascial constriction of the ducts of the breasts.

13. **Do you have "galloping cholesterol"?** I know of people with steadily rising cholesterol and triglycerides. They are often put on statin drugs like Zocor for lowering cholesterol, and may get to temporary lower levels, but they don't get steady control. High triglycerides that are not a reflection of your diet may be linked to released wastes from myofascial work (see chapter 2). The high cholesterol and triglycerides also may be linked to thyroid metabolic problems and I believe they are also linked to insulin resistance. We need some studies on this.

14. **Do you experience unusual reactions to medications?** Considering the neuroendocrine changes possible in FMS,[11] the possibility of leaky gut syndrome (see chapter 23) or multiple chemical sensitivity (see chapter 6), it should not be surprising that many of us may react in unusual and unpredictable ways to some medications. Sometimes just a small portion of the normal dose of a medication will have very strong effects. Others may take large doses of the same medication and feel no effect, or the opposite of the expected effect.

15. **Do you have thick secretions?** With FMS you may experience thick secretions. The mucus from your nose can be so sticky it gets on your eyeglasses and is hard to remove. You may

find it difficult to cleanse yourself after a bowel movement, and require lots of toilet paper and moist towelettes (and you probably never told your doctor about *that* symptom!). Your eyes may be crusty from sleep when you wake. I even had this symptom as an infant. My eyelashes were very long and would get stuck together as I slept.

16. **Do you have a disturbed sweating mechanism?** One of my readers wrote and asked about this symptom. The reader had experienced an unpleasant body odor and dark sweat during flare, and her 14-karat gold rings turned her fingers black where they touched. If she started drinking a lot of grapefruit juice as soon as she noticed the dark areas developing on her fingers, she could drastically reduce the intensity of the flare. Any ideas on this, biochemists? It is likely that the body is trying to eliminate toxins and built-up metabolic waste products in the sweat. Your sweat and your urine may smell very bad at such times of waste disposal. This may be your body's way of doing a chemical detox, and it is a signal to take it easy for a while, drink a lot of fresh water, eat healthy food, and exercise gently. Wash off your sweat as soon as possible. Your body is getting rid of it for a reason. Some medications also cause abnormal sweating. Ask your pharmacist about that possibility.

17. **Do you have dermographia (writing with a fingernail on your skin leaves red welts)?** This and other *neurogenic* (nervous system–provoked) skin responses increase in patients with chronic rheumatic pain.[12] This is part of a reaction to the neurotransmitter histamine at TrPs and other trauma sites. This can occur with any kind of bodywork, mild touch, heat, stress, or chemical contact. Some people with both FMS and CMP also experience a profound change in their ability to tolerate heat and cold, as well as an increase in the sensitivity that results when the upper layer of skin is pinched, lifting it off the underlying tissues. These people respond to touch with reflexive muscle guarding. This can make some forms of bodywork counterproductive.

18. **Do you have an extreme susceptibility to infection?** This symptom can occur in a cycle of immune system dysfunction. You may experience a time when you don't catch colds or other types of germs that may be going around, and your immune system seems to be on hyperalert. Your allergies may run wild. Other times, your immune system has no success attacking infections at all. At those times, you have to put antibiotic ointment on every scratch to prevent it from becoming infected. Both allergies and an inefficient immune response can be signs of immune system dysfunction (see chapter 5).

19. **Do you have delayed reactions to overactivity?** With FMS, when you overdo things, the reaction hits hardest the next day or even the day after that. This may set up the yo-yo effect (see chapter 7), and is a sign you need to work on pacing yourself better.

20. **Do you get the shakes when you are hungry?** If they subside as soon as you eat, see the sections on reactive hypoglycemia in chapters 7 and 23.

21. **Do you bruise easily? Do your bruises take a while to appear and a long time to fade?** There are probably several mechanisms contributing to this phenomenon, some which we have not yet identified. Many of us have been on aspirin, NSAIDs (nonsteroidal anti-inflammatory drugs), or other medications, which may be partially responsible. These symptoms may be caused by constrictions in the myofascia, other microcirculation dysfunction, or capillary fragility.

22. **Do you have hair loss?** Loss of hair may take place with FMS. It can come out by handfuls, clogging drains and leaving a trail on your pillow that looks like the abominable snowman slept there. This may be an indication of thyroid dysfunction. Some patients find that thyroid supplementation helps this condition (see chapter 15), and others have been helped by

guaifenesin. Some people have reported that adding more protein to their diet helped their hair loss.

23. **Do you have jumpy muscles?** If your muscles "jump" when you are just about to fall asleep, and you feel as though you have fallen into the bed from a height, this is a "sleep start." You haven't been levitating. This can startle you, causing an adrenaline surge and chasing away your hard-won near-sleep (see chapter 9).

24. **Do your hands hurt when you put them into cold water?** This may be a sign of impaired circulation, as it is in cases of Raynaud's phenomenon (see chapter 6), as well as enhanced FMS sensitivity. Modify your tasks to avoid cold water. For example, wash your lettuce in lukewarm water. It can "crisp" in the refrigerator.

25. **Have you experienced a recent weight gain or loss?** If you have experienced a recent weight gain, it may, in part, be due to the medications you have been taking. Elavil (amitriptyline), for example, has a tendency to give folks the "munchies." Interstitial edema may be part of a rapid weight gain, as may excess histamine.

     Then there is carbohydrate craving (see reactive hypoglycemia in chapters 6 and 23). Excess eating may be activated by a need to chew. Jaw tightening and grinding (bruxism) is a common symptom in both FMS and CMP. This can be almost like a "restless leg syndrome" of the jaw. You may not even be aware of the quantity of food you are eating, until you try writing down everything that you put in your mouth for a week. Eating just before going to bed seems to put on weight more easily. A subset of people with FMS lose weight and have to struggle to regain it. This may be due, in part, to Leaky Gut food sensitivity in FMS (see chapter 23).

26. **Are you hypersensitive to light?** Even if you aren't a Hollywood star, you may not be able to go anywhere unless you wear dark glasses. In FMS, some part of this sensitivity may be caused by a connection between light sensitivity and the hypothalamus. Many people with FMS and CMP often have problems driving at night. The lights of oncoming cars really distress us. This may be due to altered reactivity of the eye's pupils. This is under neurotransmitter control. Beta-carotene may help somewhat.

27. **Does the noise of fluorescent lights irritate you?** This sound can be disruptive to your coherence of thought. You may get a massive headache or become irritable because of noises that others rarely notice. The flickering of fluorescent lights as the bulbs wear out can be hazardous to your peace of mind. Readers have reported varying responses ranging from mild irritation and disquiet to near seizure and petit-mal-type fugue states. There is a subset of FMS patients with a seizure disorder or seizurelike effect. This may be similar to "video-game epilepsy," which is not unique to FMS, although FMS sensations are often amplified. One study found 50 percent of photosensitive patients are also sensitive to a 50-Hz television flicker.[13] Some FMS patients with this sensitivity may do well on Neurontin.

28. **Do some patterns (stripes, checks) make you dizzy?** Some people have reported becoming dizzy to the point of falling, caused by looking at certain patterns of light and dark. You may need to avoid fabric stores, conveyer belts, airport carousels, and escalators. I can use escalators if I don't look at the striped steps. The patterns of light and dark cast by the trees at the side of the road can affect you, depending on the lighting. Even certain floor patterns can cause dizziness. Some of this can be caused by eye muscle TrP proprioception disturbances.[14] There may be a proprioceptive component to FMS.[15]

29. **Do you have electromagnetic sensitivity?** Do you become wired by electrical storms? That is, do you become edgy, tense, unable to sleep? Are you up all night when the moon is full?

Can you sometimes sense the feelings of others? This is what I call electromagnetic (EM) sensitivity. Some people with FMS may be hypersensitive to EM transmissions, especially when they are in flare.

Some people with FMS have told me that their presence stops watches and computers. They say that phones and VCRs are also affected. Usually, they have been afraid to mention this to their doctors. They may not have connected this effect either with FMS or CMP. One doctor called me from New York to talk about this. One of his patients could walk under streetlights and turn them off. He had observed this personally.

It seems likely that many people with FMS and CMP may be electromagnetically sensitive due to a combination of enhanced autonomic nervous system activity, central nervous system sensitization, and souped-up receptors. Remember, FMS amplifies sensations. The skin over TrPs is high in electrical conductance—it is measurably abnormal.[16] It has also been documented that EM fields can affect heart rate.[17] We need more research on this.

30. **Do you experience numbness or tingling?** Electrolytic imbalances due to interstitial edema may contribute to this. For nerves to conduct sensations, charged particles (ions) of potassium, chloride, and sodium, called electrolytes, must pass back and forth across the nerve's outer sheath. When a nerve is compressed, this transfer is slowed or stopped. When the pressure is released, the sudden movement causes pain and tingling. Numbness and tingling in referred pain zones are common symptoms of some TrPs, caused by nerve entrapment by the myofascia.

Section II: The Head Bone's Connected to the Neck Bone

1. **Do you have motor coordination problems and clumsiness?** If you have motor coordination problems, the sternocleidomastoid (SCM) group of muscles could be part of your problem (Fig. 8-2). You may frequently bump into doorjambs, walls, and other stationary objects, and knock things over. All of us with FMS and CMP go tripping through life cleaning up one mess after another. We learn to keep our sense of humor activated and a good supply of paper towels handy.

> My theory is that with muscle tightening, normal fluid passages become constricted, and fluid backs up in the sinuses, so we get a constant post-nasal drip all night long, although the membranes of the nose may feel very dry and even may bleed on occasion.

Proprioceptor dysfunction may be associated with *any* TrP, but it is especially linked to SCM TrPs. These TrPs can cause any (or all) of the following problems: dizziness, imbalance, neck soreness, a swollen glands feeling, runny nose, maxillary sinus congestion, tension headaches, eye problems (tearing, bug-eyes, blurred or double vision, inability to raise the upper eyelid, dimming of perceived light intensity), spatial disorientation, postural dizziness, vertigo, sudden falls while bending, unintentional veering while walking, staggered walk, impaired sleep, nerve entrapment, and disturbed weight perception. This last symptom can result in spilling food and drink, and in throwing an object across the room when you are just trying to pick it up. Be careful how you move in bed. When you turn over, roll your body with your head remaining flat on the bed, and use your arms to help. Don't lift your head and lead with it as you roll, or you can cause or aggravate neck TrPs.

2. **Do you have sinus stuffiness that "travels" at night?** The nighttime stuffiness moves to whichever side of your head is on your

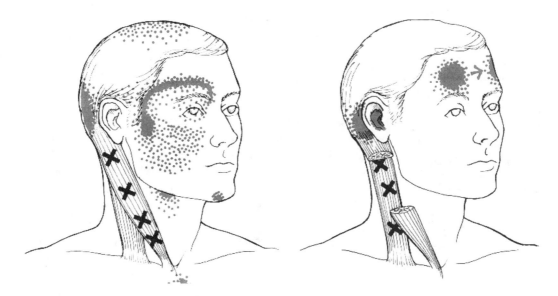

Figure 8-2: Sternocleidomastoid (SCM) trigger points

pillow if you are lying on your side. Gravity drains the congestion to the lower side. This condition goes along with postnasal drip and, often, a constantly runny nose. This is worsened by the head-forward posture (see chapter 7) and congestion of normal fluid passages caused by TrPs. Check for a TrP slightly above the outer edge of your upper lip and toward your ear. This TrP is in a cutaneous facial muscle, the zygomaticus major, and it can add to sinus pain. It may also cause a restriction of several inches of your jaw opening.

I have found that the use of a small massager in the sinus areas helps to loosen thick mucus and promotes a sneeze. You can cleanse your throat and nasopharyngeal area using very warm salt water as a nose wash. Try this before you go to bed to minimize sinus and nasophrangeal stuffiness without medication. If you suspect the area is raw, don't use much salt or too high a temperature. (Use about a half-cup of water, and add one gentle shake of salt.) Lean your head as far back as you can. Use a dropper with a small amount of the salt-water mixture. Insert the dropper into your nostril, with your head bent as far back as it can go. First rinse the lining of your nose with the dropper pressed against the top of the inside of the nostril. Then spit out the water and blow your nose gently. Repeat the process in the other nostril. Then repeat each side, with the dropper pressed against the bottom of the inside of the nostrils. You can irrigate many areas this way

Gargling with salt water may also help clear away the thick secretions and prevent further irritation. If you do this procedure every night before going to bed, you may find your nose and throat become less sensitive to the salt and the temperature. *Don't use the massager or salt-water nose drops if you suspect an infection, as you do not want to take a chance on spreading the germs.*

3. **Do you frequently have a runny nose?** Many FMS and CMP patients experience a runny nose without an obvious cause. The side with the worst head and neck rigidity is often the side you sleep on most and it is subjected to more of the drip ... drip ... drip ... on the back of the throat, all night. Using the salt-water irrigation and massager may help. Pay attention to what foods might provoke this reaction as well. Sugar is a frequent culprit. One reader suggested using Viva towels as handkerchiefs. They are soft and large, and may be washed in a machine. *Soft* cloth handkerchiefs are also helpful.

> When I go clothes shopping, I don't even look at anything unless it has pockets for handkerchiefs. I use cotton ones—the old-fashioned kind. They are easier on the nose and the pocketbook—if you can find them.

4. **Do you have a chronic, dry cough?** This may be due to a TrP at the lower end of the sternal (breastbone) division of the SCM (Fig. 8-3). It can also be caused by esophageal reflux (see chapter 6), or TrPs in the longus colli muscle.

5. **Do you have ear pain?** Medial pterygoid TrPs can cause deep ear pain or stuffiness of the ear. The sternal portion TrPs of the sternocleidomastoid muscle group can also cause deep ear pain (Fig. 8-2). Medial pterygoid TrPs also refer pain to the tongue, pharynx, and hard palate, below and behind your temporomandibular joint, and deep into your ear. This referred pain may include the area behind the jaw and in front of your ear, and/or the floor of your nose and throat. If these symptoms are caused by medial pterygoid TrPs, the pain is increased whenever you try to open your mouth wide, whenever you chew food, or whenever you clench your teeth. You may also experience soreness inside your throat and painful swallowing.

These TrPs are activated by the forward-head posture. Other activators or perpetuators are clenching or grinding your jaw, gum chewing, anxiety, and emotional tension. They can also be activated by an infection in the region. The TrPs are more often the cause, rather than the effect, of dental abnormalities.[18]

The medial pterygoid TrPs may entrap part of the lingual nerve, causing a bitter metallic taste. These TrPs can often be worked on from inside the mouth, behind the last molar. A TrP in the back of the tongue can cause pain in the throat deep behind the angle of the jaw.

6. **Do you experience ringing in the ears?** Tinnitus (pronounced tin-uh-tuss) may have many causes. Deep masseter TrPs may cause you to hear a ringing or low roaring (Fig. 8-4). The sound may vary. For example, you may experience a crackling noise. These TrPs can cause itchy ears. The itch, which can drive you to distraction, can be relieved by acupressure on the TrP and sometimes by cold compresses on the TrP.

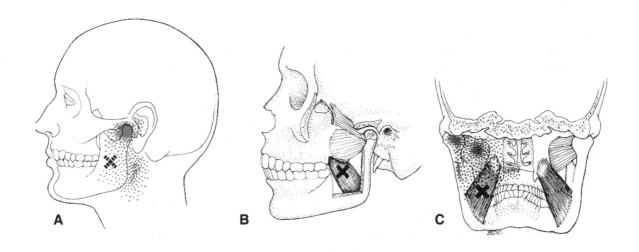

A   B   C

Figure 8-3: Trigger points in the medial pterygoid; (A) stippled parts show external areas of referred pain; (B) location of the TrP is on the inner side of the mandible; (C) looking forward, showing internal areas of pain.

There may be an FMS link to tinnitus, even when you can change the loudness of the sounds by moving the muscles of your face. Researchers have associated this symptom with *neural plasticity*[19] (see chapter 9). Tinnitus may intrude to such a degree that you can't live a normal life. It may contribute to insomnia, inability to concentrate, depression, and even suicide. Some researchers have found intravenous lidocaine can bring relief.[20]

7. **Do you have fluctuating blood pressure?** There are several possible mechanisms involved fluctuating blood pressure. Some are mechanical. There are blood vessel swellings in your neck, called *carotid sinuses*. These sinuses are lined with pressure receptors that help to control the blood pressure by constricting and dilating the blood vessels. Trigger points could affect them. Trigger points can also cause entrap-

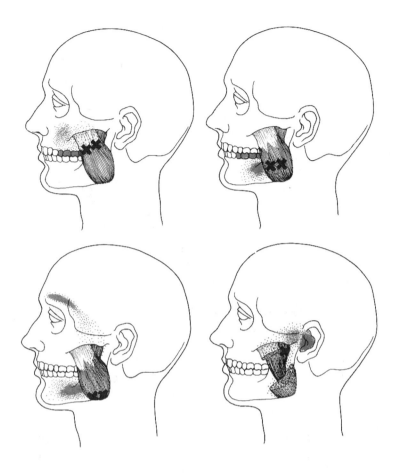

Figure 8-4: Trigger points located in various parts of the masseter

ment of blood and lymph vessels. This can affect blood pressure. High blood pressure can also aggravate scalene TrPs, causing a mutual aggravation spiral. Fibromyalgia can be involved because the central nervous system affects blood pressure by regulating the dilation of blood vessels with informational substances.[21]

8. **Do you have dry eyes, nose, and mouth?** The symptoms of dry eyes, nose, and mouth are called sicca syndrome. With either or both FMS and CMP, your mucous membranes can become excessively dry, including the lining of the vagina and the gastrointestinal tract.

9. **Do you have problems with swallowing and chewing?** Trouble with swallowing may develop due to the presence of digastric TrPs (Fig. 8-1.) This leads to head and neck pain and a "swollen glands" feeling. Researchers confirmed that their patients with facial pain and abnormal swallowing had digastric hyperactivity *in every case*.[22] It hurts to work digastric TrPs! Start with warm moist packs on your throat for a few minutes. Then put your elbows on the table, and rest your thumbs on either side of your jaw, under your chin. You are trying to get a release of the myofascia, by "milking" away excess fluid. Use a gentle backward motion from the base of your chin, stroking or pressing up to the base of your ear. Start gently and listen to your body. It will tell you how much pressure to use. Gentle bodywork may help you to deal with these TrPs.

Internal medial pterygoid TrPs (Fig. 8-3) may cause problems swallowing, and you may also experience the following symptoms: pain when chewing, jaw clicking,

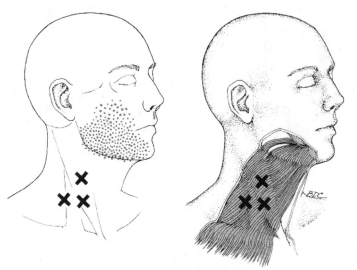

Figure 8-5: Trigger points in the platysma. The stippled area shows the prickling pain in the skin over the jaw.

temporomandibular dysfunction (TMD), sore throat, excessive saliva, and sinus pain, drooling during sleep, or choking on saliva.

10. **Do you have a prickling "electric" face?** This is most often due to platysma TrPs. The platysma is a flat, thin, cutaneous facial muscle lying over your throat area (Fig. 8-5). These TrPs refer the prickling pain across skin covering your jaw.

11. **Do you have red and/or tearing eyes?** The SCM muscle can cause your eyes to become red and to tear. Talk with your eye doctor about the possibility of using artificial tears to soothe your irritated eyes. You may want to try a formula that can be safely stored in the refrigerator so that you can also enjoy the mechanical effect of cold that helps to constrict swollen red vessels in your eye.

12. Do your jaws pop or click? This is often caused by masseter TrPs (Fig. 8-4), although the trapezius and temporalis TrPs can be involved, too (Figs. 8-6 and 8-7), leading to a complex, overlapping pain pattern that may be confusing.

13. **Do you grind and clench your jaw?** This may occur at night, even though you don't know it. Your muscles will remember. When your brain doesn't know what to do in response to mixed or erratic signals it receives from poorly regulated neurotransmitters and dysfunctional receptors, it doesn't know how to respond. Its default setting is to clench the teeth. The masseter TrP may be involved (Fig. 8-4) and stress is a frequent contributor. Chewing something before bed, and using hot moist packs on your jaw (both sides) may help your brain to "chill out" and relax these muscles.

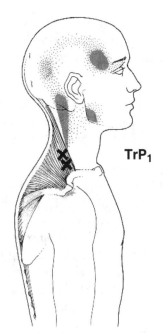

TrP₁

Figure 8-6: Trigger points in the upper trapezius

14. **Do have unexplained toothaches?** If you have toothaches that cannot be explained by dental problems, the digastric, masseter, and temporalis (Figs. 8-1, 8-4, and 8-7, respectively) TrPs may cause them. A TrP-induced toothache is usually intermittent. During a long dental procedure, which often activates these TrPs, take periodic rests to exercise and relieve the stress on your jaw muscles. These TrPs are sensitive to heat and cold and touch, as well as causing pain. If you have these TrPs, show the patterns to your dentist and teach him or her about TrPs.

15. **Do you have eye pain?** Cutaneous (skin) facial TrPs can cause pain in your ears, eyes, nose, and teeth. These TrPs

are shallow and can occur anywhere on the face. Try some finger pressure work on your face, but be gentle.

16. **Do you have double vision, blurry vision, or changing vision?** Trigger points can form in the muscles that hold your eyes in place. Fatigue makes things worse. The culprits may be TrPs in the extrinsic eye muscles (Fig. 8-8), or the SCM, trapezius, temporalis, or cutaneous facial muscles (Figs. 8-2, 8-6, and 8-7, respectively). See chapter 19 for eye exercises. Trigger points in the splenius cervices muscles can cause blurring of near vision, as well as pain in the side of the head to the eye on same side, and in the eye orbit (Fig. 8-9).

17. **Do words jump off the page, or disappear when you stare at them?** The orbicularis oculi cutaneous facial TrPs (Fig. 8-10) will cause this. They also refer pain to your nose and cheek and above your eye. Putting clear plastic over the page to decrease print contrast may help with jumping words.

18. **Do you have frequent headaches?** Most "tension-type headaches" are caused by TrPs.[23] If tension, allergy, hormones, or other stressors have initiated or activated the TrPs, you need to find them to get rid of them.

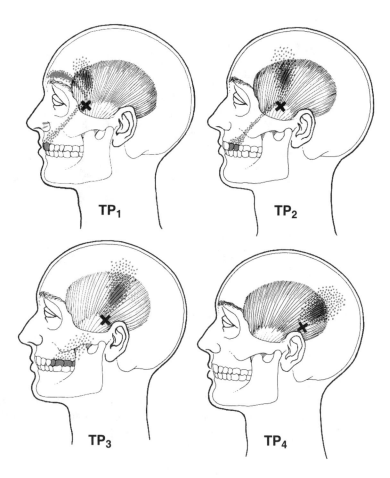

Figure 8-7: Trigger points in the temporalis; stippled and dark parts show referred pain patterns.

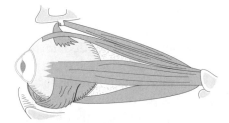

Figure 8-8: Trigger points can occur in any of these extrinsic eye muscles.

Any TrP that can cause a sore throat can also add to headache pain. You can frequently lessen the headache by putting cold compresses on your throat or the back of your neck.

Many upper body TrPs may contribute to headaches. Find the pattern that most resembles your headache pain pattern, and check the TrP area on your body. Head and neck pain may also be referred from the nasal and sinus cavities and from the teeth as well.[24] Posterior cervical TrPs (Fig. 8-11) may entrap the occipital nerve. This can cause numbness, or a tingling, burning pain in a band around your head. Other posterior cervical TrPs can refer pain to the back of your neck down to the shoulder blade, and in the back of your skull on the side with the TrPs. If you read or work at a desk with your neck bent over for a long time, these TrPs may become aggravated.

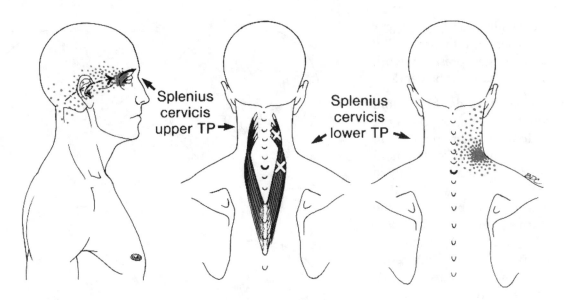

Figure 8-9: Trigger points in the upper and lower splenius cervici

19. **Do you experience migraines?** Thanks to the advanced imaging devices now available, researchers have mapped migraines as they spread across the top of the brain and down the brainstem where the pain receptors are located. The migraine, as it spreads, can activate subcortical centers that may be involved in pain reception.[25] The migraine itself is a neuroelectric and metabolic event. The excitability of the cell membranes of the brain determine how likely a migraine is to occur.

Some of the pain of a migraine may be caused by inflammation of the *meninges*. They are membranelike coverings of the brain and spinal cord. Ah-ha! A myofascial connection. Surely you knew that was coming in somewhere. Dr. Marco Pappagallo and his research team, using SPECT (single photon emission computerized tomography) images, found that menningeal blood vessels become hyperpermeable during migraines.[26] Hyperpermeable means that that these blood vessels are very easily penetrated. These areas of hyperpermeability corresponded to the areas of pain. Animal studies indicate that the trigeminal nerve, the main nerve from the brain to your head and face, causes the initial inflammation. Yes, migraines are noninfectious, neurogenic meningitis.

Depakote or Neurontin may be very helpful to decrease central nervous sensitivity. Carisoprodol may also help some people. Hormonally induced headaches sometimes seem helped by the use of a low-dose Climera hormone patch.

Many migraines are caused by myofascial TrPs.[27] Trigger points in the digastric (Fig. 8-1), sternocleidmastoid (Fig. 8-2), cutaneous facial (not shown), temporalis (Fig. 8-7), trapezius (Fig. 8-6), splenii (Fig. 8-13), and posterior cervical muscles (Fig. 8-11) are all possible migraine-inducers. The migraine connection may be another way in which FMS

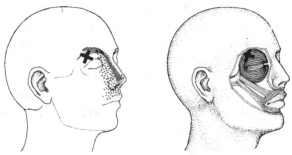

Figure 8-10: Trigger points in the orbicularis oculi

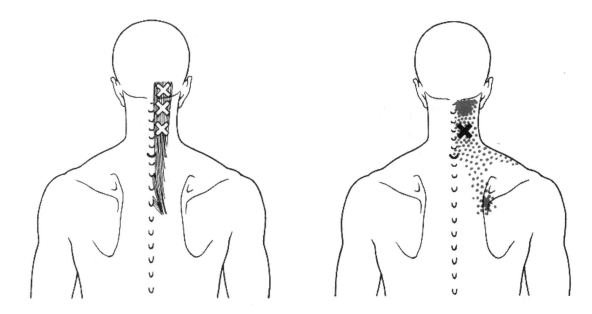

Figure 8-11: Trigger points in the posterior cervicals

(hyperpermeability and hypersensitivity) can combine with chronic myofascial pain trigger points to cause more than double the trouble.

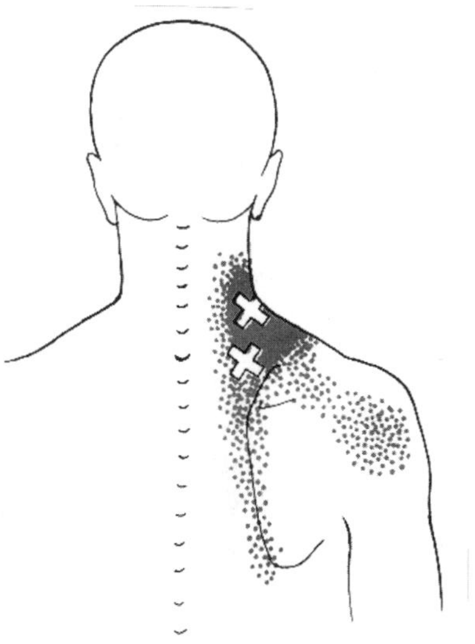

20. **Do you have a stiff neck?** Levator scapulae TrPs (Fig. 8-12) are a common cause of stiff neck, although this can be caused or perpetuated by upper trapezius TrPs and posterior cervical TrPs (Figs. 8-6 and 8-11). Levator scapulae TrPs may be activated by a cold sore, tilting your head to one side regularly, or even watching a tennis match. Trigger points in this muscle may aggravate vertebral changes caused by a narrowing of the cervical dural tube. (See Chiari malformation in chapter 6.) Avoid holding a phone receiver in the crook of your neck while talking.

21. **Do you experience dizziness when you turn your head or move?** Here's that sternocleidmastoid trigger point again (Fig. 8-2). These TrPs cause so much misery, mostly because they are allowed to. Doctors must become familiar with their proprioceptor effects. Otherwise, the doctors may suspect neurological or psychiatric dysfunction.

Figure 8-12: Referred pain pattern of trigger points in the right levator scapulae

Trigger points in this group of muscles can make heading into traffic while driving miserable; you try to look both ways while holding your head in your hands to avoid dizziness. Or you can be stooping over to change the cat litter and, when you stand up, you can tumble right over backwards. If you have these TrPs, it is important to keep your neck warm and away from drafts. If the TrPs are active, it is a wise precaution to use a soft, triple-folded hand towel pinned loosely around your neck as a splint or chin rest before you drive or ride over bumpy roads.

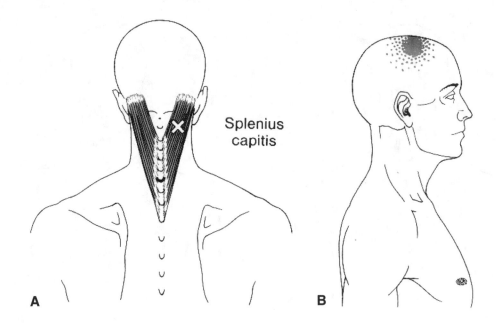

Figure 8-13: (A) Trigger point in the splenius capitus; (B) referred pain on the crown of the head

22. **Do you have a sore spot on the top of your head?** This is often caused by the splenius capitis TrP (Fig. 8-13). Just the motion of the wind on your hair can hurt the crown of your head. It may be painful to brush your hair. This pain can also be referred from TrPs in the sternal portion of the sternocleidomastoid muscle group.

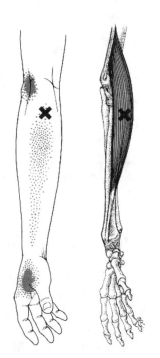

Figure 8-14: Trigger point in the right brachioradialis

Section III: The Shoulder Bone's Connected to the Backbone

1. **Do you feel pain or discomfort if you wear a heavy coat or carry a shoulder bag?**
   This is often caused by the upper trapezius TrP (Fig. 8-6). The trapezius muscle can get many TrPs and each one has its own pain pattern or symptoms. One trapezius TrP can even cause a shivery feeling and gooseflesh to appear on your arms or legs. Try to keep your bag as light as possible. Fanny packs are also options.

2. **Do you have pain when you write, a changing signature, and/or illegible handwriting?** This can be due to many shoulder and arm TrPs. Figure out how you can cut down on paperwork. Do hand and finger stretches often while you work. Use ergonomic motions with a well-designed workspace. Thumb pain and tingling numbness may be due to brachialis muscle TrPs entrapping the radial nerve, as well as the adductor and opponens pollicis muscle TrPs (Fig. 8-15). Brachialis TrPs are often found in a vertical line along the front center of the biceps in your upper arm. Adductor and opponens pollicis

TrPs also can cause "trigger thumb," weeders' thumb, clumsiness, and handwriting that is both painful and illegible. Brachioradialis TrPs are most often responsible for writer's cramp, and for the weak grip that allows objects to slip out of your hand (Fig. 8-14).

Interosseous muscle TrPs (not shown) are located in the back of your hand, in a line between the end of your finger and wrist. They transmit pain along the side of the finger that is in line with them. The most intense pain is usually at the last joint. Pain, finger stiffness, and awkwardness are common with these TrPs, as is the formation of Heberden's nodes. These nodes are associated with osteoarthritis, but may be part of TrPs.[28] When these nodes first form, there is usually no true joint swelling, and they are tender. They harden with time. The interosseous TrP referral zone can include the back and palm of your hand. The pain pattern varies as to the location of the TrP. Tenderness may be referred to the joint. If you have these TrPs, you can't button buttons. Writing and grasping are also difficult. These TrPs may entrap digital nerves. Finger TrPs may be latent for years. Then their pain, restriction of motion, and stiffness is often ascribed to rheumatoid arthritis or to "old age." Avoid prolonged or repetitive pinching grasps. Change your

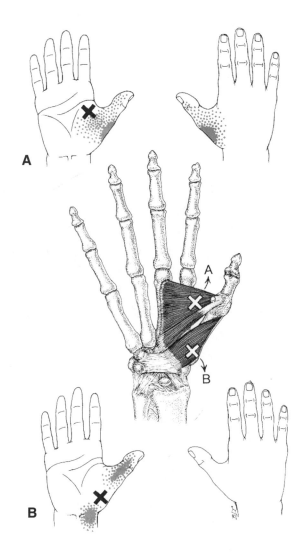

Figure 8-15: (A) Trigger point in the adductor pollicis; (B) trigger point in the opponens pollicis

daily activity patterns and interrupt sustained periods of contraction with exercises. Reduce the duration and force of your pincer grip activities. "Inactivating the related myofascial TrPs and the *elimination of their perpetuating factors* appear to be important parts of early therapy to delay or abort the progression of some kinds of osteoarthritis."[29]

3. **Do your fingers turn color with the cold?** If your fingers turn colors with cold or stress, you may have Raynaud's phenomenon (see chapter 6).

4. **Do you have esophageal reflux?** Trigger points in the upper external abdominal oblique muscle TrP may aggravate and perpetuate reflux. Check the area where your ribs meet your breastbone (Fig. 8-16).

5. **Do you experience shortness of breath?** This is often due to serratus anterior TrPs and is commonly associated with a "stitch in the side"(Fig. 8-17). This TrP can contribute substantially to the pain of a heart attack. It can also cause a catch in the lower inner side of the shoulder blade. The pectorals are often involved as well. Restricted chest expansion causes less air

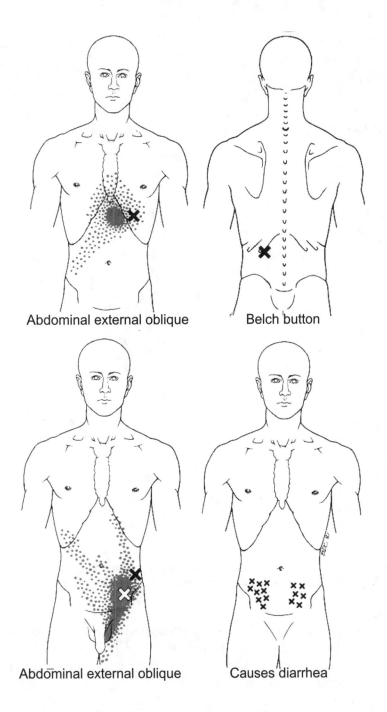

Abdominal external oblique

Belch button

Abdominal external oblique

Causes diarrhea

Figure 8-16: Trigger points for the external abdominal oblique muscles, "belch button," and some lower abdominal muscles; stippled and dark areas show pain pattern.

to be taken into your lungs because your breath is shallower. Intercostal (between the ribs) TrPs (not shown) primarily cause aching pain locally. Feel around your ribs for these TrPs. They are most often located on the front of your body, close to your side. The pain increases when you take a deep breath, cough, or sneeze. In the area near the breastbone, these TrPs may cause cardiac arrythmia.[30]

Trigger points in the dome, or center, of the diaphragm (not shown), refer pain to the upper border of the shoulder on the same side as the TrP. Trigger points along the edges of the diaphragm send pain to the edges of the ribs close by. These TrPs can cause the "stitch in the side," chest pain, or inability to take a full breath. The pain will be most intense as you breathe out after taking a deep breath. Diaphragm TrPs cause restricted rotation of your spine if you twist to look behind yourself. Chronic cough and paradoxical breathing will perpetuate these TrPs, as will head-forward, slumped-shouldered posture. Local impact trauma, chest surgery, herpes zoster, and rib fractures are possible initiating and perpetuating factors, as are tumors, and some exercises. Severe, episodic shortness of breath is often a part of FMS as well. Maximum lung pressures are low in FMS, which could indicate respiratory muscle dysfunction.[31]

6. **Do you have hypersensitive nipples and/or breast pain?** This is commonly due to TrPs in the pectoralis muscles (Fig. 8-18). Many of us have latent TrPs in the pectorals and sternalis muscles (Fig. 8-19). Doorway stretches help these TrPs (see chapter 19). There is a TrP on the right side between the fifth and sixth ribs about midway between the nipple and the outer edge of the

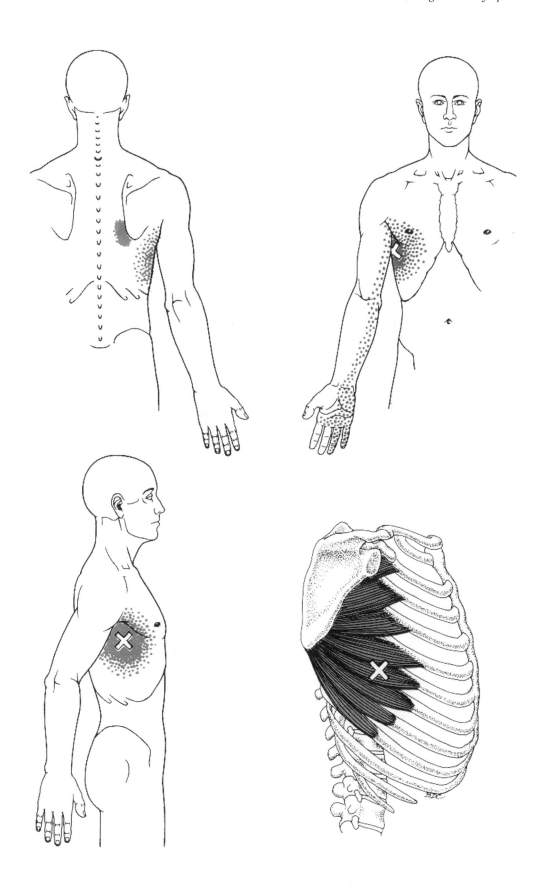

Figure 8-17: Trigger points in the serratus anterior; stippled areas show the referred pain patterns.

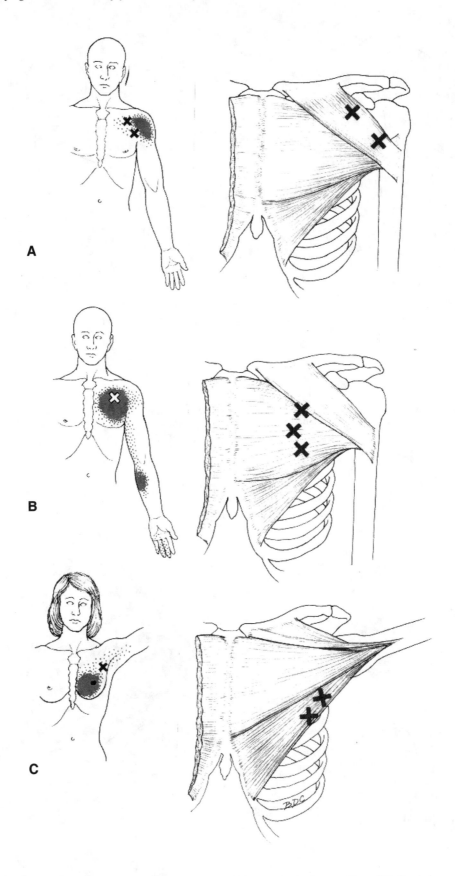

Figure 8-18: Trigger points in the left pectoralis major: (A) the clavicular section; (B) the intermediate sternal section; (C) the lateral free margin of the muscle

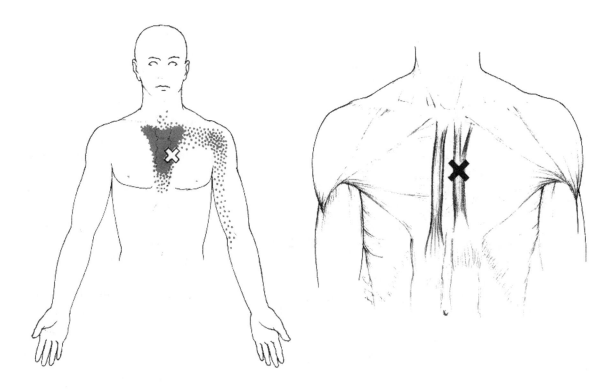

Figure 8-19: Trigger point in the left sternalis; stippled and dark areas show pain patterns.

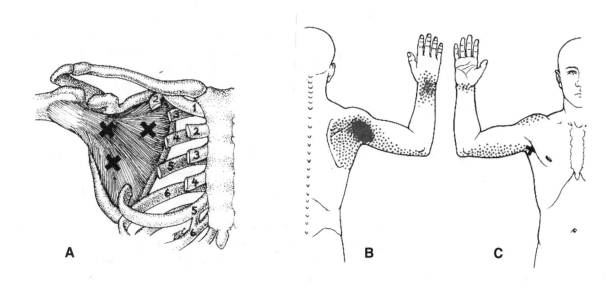

Figure 8-20: (A) The X's show trigger points in the right subscapularis. (B) and (C) show the trigger points and the referred pain zones emanating from those trigger points.

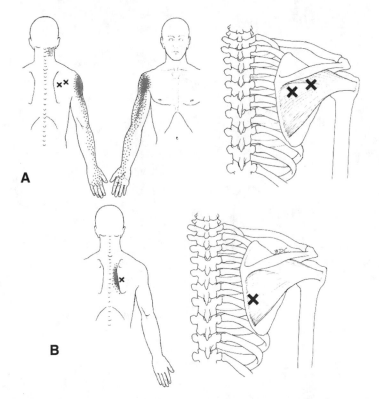

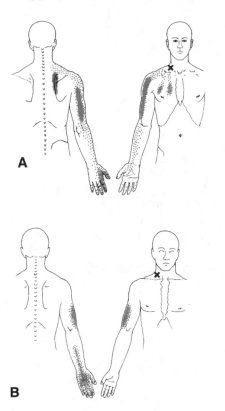

Figure 8-21: Trigger points in the right infraspinatus: (A) common location of trigger points; (B) a more unusual location for a trigger point

Figure 8-22: Location of trigger points in the right scalene: (A) scalenus anterior; (B) scalenus posterior

sternum that can be involved with cardiac arrythmias. Treating the TrP may rid you of the arrhythmia.

Pectoralis minor TrPs (not shown) are located most often in an area about midway between your collarbone and nipple, and midway between the edge of your breastbone and the outer edge of your upper arm. They send pain over the front of your chest and shoulder. Pain may run down the inner side of your arm, and include the last three fingers. Pain from a left side pectoralis minor TrP can mimic the pain of angina. These TrPs can entrap nerves, lymph, and blood vessels. Your wrist pulse may disappear as you move your arm. When you relieve the TrP, the pulse is restored.[32]

Numbness and odd sensations of the fourth and fifth fingers are common. You may feel peculiar sensations over some parts of your forearm and over the palm side of the first three and a half fingers, and you may have difficulty reaching forward and up, or reaching backward with your arm at shoulder level. I believe that these TrPs may be involved in some cases of Raynaud's. Paradoxical breathing perpetuates this TrP, as does poor posture. Check standing and sitting postures and movements. Don't sleep curled up on your side with your lower shoulder forced forward. Blood vessel entrapment by these TrPs does not produce the hand puffiness associated with scalene entrapment. Connective tissue TrPs may be located in scar tissue in the attachment area in the front of your shoulder and can cause referred tenderness, hot prickling pain, and/or lightning-like jabs to the pectoralis area. Myofascial therapy can relieve this.

7. **Do you have a "frozen shoulder"?** Subscapularis and other TrPs (Fig. 8-20) can cause a frozen shoulder.

These TrPs severely restrict rotation of your arm at shoulder level. Hanging curtains, folding sheets, throwing a ball overhand, or even holding an arm up at school to answer a question are perpetuators and can be very painful. Driving long distances aggravates this TrP, as does anything that causes your arms to remain in a shortened position. The doorway stretch (see chapter 19) helps.

8. **Do you have a painful, weak grasp that sometimes lets go?** This may be due to many TrPs, but the infraspinatus (Fig. 8-21), brachioradialis TrPs (Fig. 8-14) and scalenes (Fig. 8-22) are usually part of the picture. The pain felt when turning a doorknob or using a screwdriver can be intense with infraspinatus TrPs. You may have extreme hand weakness, and loss of control when drinking or pouring anything liquid. Keep some straws and paper towels handy, and work those TrPs with a tennis ball (see chapter 19). These TrPs can entrap blood vessels and nerves and may cause pain that can disturb your sleep. Scalene TrPs may also cause numbness, or tingling (usually in your little finger and the finger next to it), and hand swelling. The puffiness is especially noticeable when you first wake up. The scalene and sternocleidomastoid muscles may become "welded" together in a myofascial knot. It takes persistence and skill (and adequate pain control) to unravel this knot, which may become calcified with time.

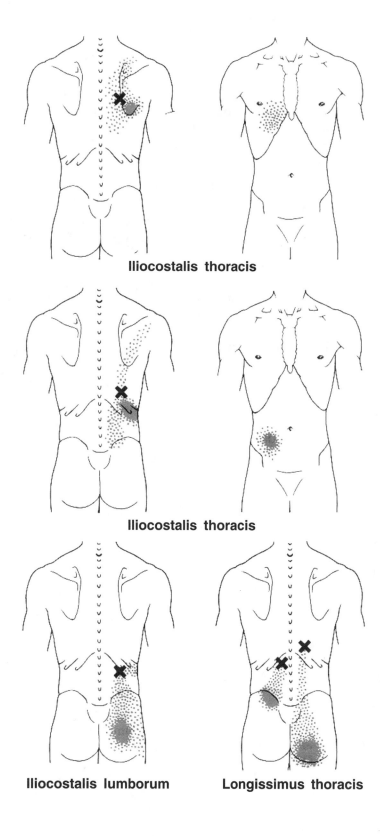

Iliocostalis thoracis

Iliocostalis thoracis

Iliocostalis lumborum   **Longissimus thoracis**

Figure 8-23: Trigger points in the superficial paraspinal muscles

9. **Do you have heart attack–like pains, rapid heartbeat, and/or a fluttery heartbeat?** These symptoms can be caused by pectoral and sternalis TrPs (Figs. 8-18 and 8-19). If you have angina or have had a heart attack, treating them can reduce your symptom level. Pain from sternalis TrPs may be relieved by a few well-directed sprays of vapo-coolant (see chapter 21).

10. **Do you have mid-back pain?** Many TrPs can cause mid-back pain. Some of the most common are in the superficial paraspinals (Fig. 8-23). These respond well to circular massage, myofascial release, and tennis ball acupressure (see chapter 19). Depending on where they are, they can cause chest pain similar to angina, pain in the gut, loin pain as in a kidney infection, and even cause retraction of the testicle. Trigger points in these muscles may cramp or "catch," restricting stretches.

11. **Do you have intestinal cramps or bloating?** Trigger points in your abdominal muscles may contribute to a lax, pendulous abdomen filled with gas. The TrPs inhibit further muscle contraction. These TrPs can cause burning, fullness, bloating, and swelling.

12. **Do you experience nausea?** TrPs in the deep paraspinal muscles (Fig. 8-24) can cause this. You can work these TrPs with the tennis ball or other ball (see chapter 19). Trigger points in these small muscles located along the spine can cause endless nerve entrapments and symptoms, depending on where they are. One type of deep paraspinals, the multifidi, TrPs refer pain to corners of your vertebrae. Low-back multifidi also transmit pain to the abdomen, and can perpetuate irritable bowel syndrome (IBS). At the base of the vertebrae they refer pain to the tailbone. All multifidi TrPs can cause nerve entrapment symptoms including supersensitivity and numbness or lessened sensitivity of the skin on your back.

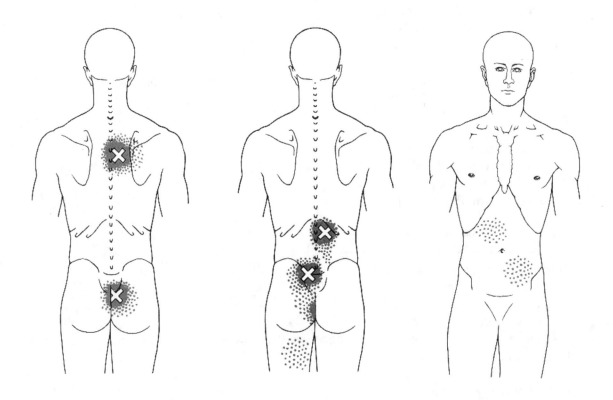

Figure 8-24: Trigger points in the deep paraspinals (multifidi); stippled and dark areas show pain patterns.

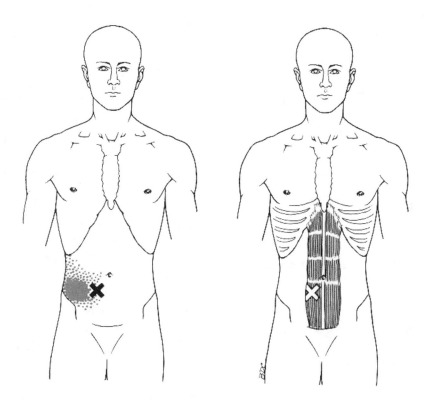

Figure 8-25: McBurney's point trigger point in the rectus abdominis muscle

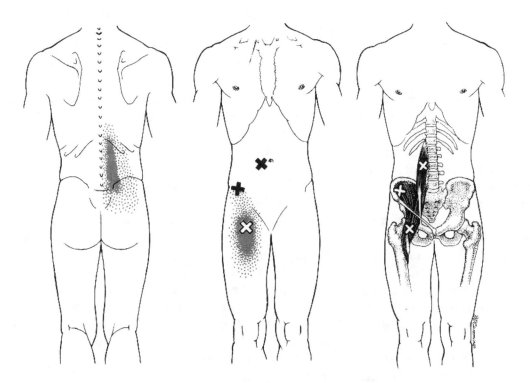

Figure 8-26: Trigger points along the iliopsoas and referred pain patterns

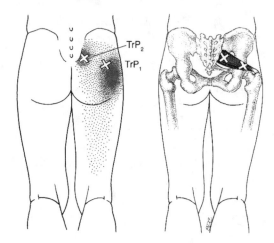

Figure 8-27: Trigger points in the right piriformis

13. **Do you experience appendicitis-like pains?** This can be caused by TrPs in the iliopsoas (Fig. 8-26), piriformis (Fig. 8-27), or some superficial paraspinal (Fig. 8-23) muscles. The rectus abdominis is the broad, flat muscle in the front of your body. It reaches from below your breastbone to the pelvic area. It is the stomach muscle on body builders that is responsible for that washboard shape. Trigger points can occur at any place in this muscle, but they tend to cluster on the upper end where the breastbone and the ribs meet, and on the lower end in the area of the pubis. There is one TrP that forms in the rectus abdominis (Fig. 8-25), which can cause pseudoappendicitis. It can also refer pain to the pelvis or to the penis. Pain caused by TrPs in the iliopsoas (Fig. 8-26) may seem like appendicitis, but it often includes pain that radiates down the front of the thigh and *up and down* either side of the low-back spine. This specific pain pattern helps you distinguish the TrP that is causing it.

14. **Do you have an irritable bladder and/or bowel?** This can be due to the pyramidalis (not shown), multifidi (Fig. 8-24), and abdominal TrPs (Fig. 8-16). The pyramidalis TrP is found in your lower abdomen, a little to the side of midline. It is at about the same height as the *lower* hipbone ridge. Trigger points in the upper rim of the pubis appear to add to the irritability and spasms of the genital- urinary tract. This may be part of the reason why so many of us have to urinate so often. With FMS and CMP, not only is the bladder hypersensitive, it may not hold as much. In addition, you may not be able to empty your bladder totally due to TrPs in the rectus abdominis, or in scars from abdominal surgery. Trigger points in upper left rectus abdominis can also cause superficial pain in the heart area. Trigger points in this muscle may be responsible for symptoms of gall bladder disease, pelvic disease, and peptic ulcer. Groin stretches and craniosacral and myofascial release work may help.

There are specific TrPs that may cause or intensify diarrhea, nausea, vomiting, food intolerance, colic, burping, and/or painful menstrual periods. (See Fig. 8-16 for the external oblique, lower quadrant oblique, belch button, and abdominal TrPs.) Vomiting can also be caused by TrPs in the upper rectus abdominis. Abdominal TrPs can develop in any muscle that is subjected to acute or chronic overload, or in muscles that are in the zone of referred pain from a diseased organ. Other activating or perpetuating factors include total body fatigue, overexercise, emotional tension, exposure to cold, infections, constipation, poor posture, and body asymmetry. These stresses are additive. *If these or any TrPs keep recurring, in spite of proper treatment, you must find the perpetuating factor.* That could be a hidden heart or abdominal problem, for example. Trigger point pain may cause *more severe* pain than visceral pain and may activate months or even years after a visceral trauma.[33]

Iliopsoas TrPs (Fig. 8-26) can worsen constipation, which, in turn, can perpetuate TrPs. Back pain caused by iliopsoas TrPs is very common in pregnancy. Symptoms of TrPs in the iliopsoas include pain in the front of the thigh and pain in the low back in an *up and down* pattern close to the vertebrae. Pain from these TrPs can extend as high as the shoulder blade. People with active or latent psoas TrPs tend to walk stooped over. Diarrhea and other side effects from flu or other infection may set up these TrPs. Until the TrPs are treated appropriately, the symptoms may continue when the infection is over.

15. **Do you have burning or foul smelling urine?** This may be an indication of the excretion of biochemical wastes and toxins. It can also occur with guaifenesin treatment (see chapter 21).

16. **Do you experience pain with intercourse?** This symptom may be caused by vaginal and pelvic floor TrPs (Fig. 8-28). Abdominal and low-back TrPs may be the cause of aching discomfort and cramps during intercourse. If you feel sharp pain, the culprit may be the piriformis TrP (Fig. 8-27). The piriformis and other short lateral muscles in this area activate the same referral pain pattern, often called the piriformis syndrome. In this syndrome, the myofascia can entrap many different nerves, blood, and lymph vessels. These TrPs are often part of a conglomerate of TrPs in the hip and pelvis. Piriformis syndrome also can include pain and unusual sensations radiating to your low back, groin, perineum, buttock, hip, and the back of your leg and foot. You may experience rectal pain during bowel movements. Even spreading the thighs apart can be painful. Piriformis TrPs also may result in tightening or immobility of the sacroiliac, which causes further dysfunction.

    Symptoms of these TrPs are aggravated both by sitting and by using the muscles involved. You can also experience swelling in the affected leg. Your foot can feel numb, and you may walk with a broad-based, staggering gait.

    These TrPs may be caused by acute muscle overload, such as may occur during a fall or lifting a heavy weight. Acute muscle overload may occur when you run, or by sitting immobile in a car. Chronic infections, chronic arthritis of hip, or Morton's foot can bring on these TrPs. Bodywork that uses an elbow in this area is *not* recommended, as the sciatic nerve could be compressed. If you sleep on your side, use a small pillow placed between your legs. When you sit, use a rocking chair and keep your body moving. Change position as often as you can while sitting in a car and stop to walk at intervals.

17. **Do you have urethral syndrome?** Urethral syndrome is a collection of symptoms characterized by urinary frequency and urgency or the inability to urinate fully. This is a description, not a diagnosis. Look for the *cause* so that you can get some relief. Trigger points that may cause or contribute to this include TrPs in the low abdominal wall, low rectus abdominis, pelvic floor muscles, piriformis, and high adductor magnus.

18. **Do you experience pelvic and/or rectal pain?** *This section is very important for men as well as women.* So much of this type of pain is misdiagnosed and people are left living with pain and other symptoms that could be remedied. Trigger points often cause pelvic pain and are responsive to therapy. Figure 8-28 is different from the other TrP diagrams in this book, in that it shows actual muscles rather than TrPs. You need to know the location of the different muscles to find those TrPs. Recognizing and treating these TrPs can help avoid unnecessary surgery for pelvic pain.[34]

    The TrPs that occur in the muscles of the pelvic floor refer pain to an area between your buttocks in an oval shape from the base of the sacroiliac triangle to the base of the tailbone. The obturator internus muscle TrP referred pain pattern is a little different, in that the area of pain between the buttocks is more rounded, and there is also a spillover pain that can occur in a V-shape down the back of your thigh. These TrPs may cause generalized symptoms such as painful intercourse in women, particularly during entry, as well as an aching pain between the anus and the vagina. In men, these TrPs cause aching pain in the area behind the scrotum, discomfort while sitting, and they may cause impotence. The piriformis (Fig. 8-27) may contribute to these symptoms. The combination of irritable bowel syndrome and pelvic floor TrPs causes a misery that is hard to diagnose and harder to endure.

Pelvic Floor Trigger Points

Specific muscles cause specific symptoms as well as the generalized ones mentioned above. It is important that you know which symptoms come from which muscles, even though the muscle names are unfamiliar multisyllables. These TrPs all cause poorly localized pain, which means that you may not be able to tell where the pain is coming from. Often the sacroiliac (SI) joint is jammed as well, and you need it to be mobile for proper pelvic functioning.

The *sphincter ani* is a band of circular muscle that constricts the anal opening. Trigger points here refer pain to the back of the pelvic floor and vagina. They may cause poorly localized anal aching, and painful bowel movements. Straining, coughing, laughing, or weight-lifting can aggravate these TrPs.

The *levator ani* (lee-vay-tor ay-nye) supports the pelvic floor and assists the anal and urethral sphincters that help control defecation and urination. Trigger points here refer pain to the perineum (the area between the rectum and genitals), to the vagina or penis, to the bone on top of the tailbone, to the tailbone itself, rectum, posterior pelvic floor, vagina, the base of the penis and scrotum, and low back. These TrPs are aggravated if you lie on your back or have a bowel movement. They can cause incontinence when you cough or sneeze. You may lose the ability to empty your bladder thoroughly. These TrPs often cause low back pain in pregnancy. They may be responsible for attacks of rectal pain after intercourse. This symptom may also be caused by TrPs in the sphincter ani, bulbospongiosus, or ichiocavernosus. *Any of these TrPs may be activated during a pelvic exam.* This may be avoided by the use of a topical anesthetic that is approved for mucous membranes.

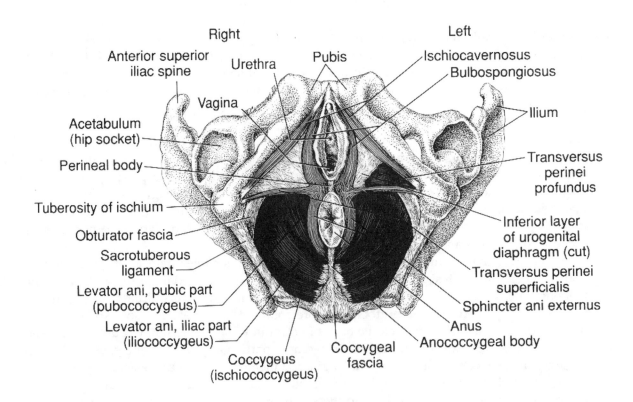

Figure 8-28: Female pelvic floor muscles as seen from below, with part of the deep fascia removed. Trigger points can occur in any parts of these muscles, and in reciprocal and related muscles in the male.

Coccygeus TrPs, in the tailbone muscle, refer pain to your tailbone, hip, and back. They are often responsible for low back pain late in a pregnancy.

Obturator internus TrPs cause pain to the vaginal area, around the anus, and tailbone. There may be an area of spillover pain to the back of your thigh. These TrPs can give you a sensation of fullness in the rectum.

Vaginal wall TrPs may refer pain to the lower abdomen and uterine area around the cervix. You may feel this pain as bladder spasms, dysmenorrhea, or cramps. There are many young girls lying in school nurses' offices with only aspirin and a hot water bottle, who wait in agony for their pain to subside. My heart aches for my own lost days and goes out in shared grief to them. These trigger points are *treatable!*

The *bulbospongiosus* is a muscle with a long name that you need to know. This muscle constricts the vagina, and is involved in erection of the clitoris (yes, women have erections, too!) and the penis. Trigger points in the ischiocavernosus muscle refer pain to the perineum and to nearby urogenital structures. These TrPs can contribute to pain during intercourse, particularly during entry, as well as causing an aching pain in the perineum. Contraction of the bulbospongiosus helps men to empty the urethra at the end of urination. Trigger points in the tissue behind the scrotum can cause discomfort when sitting erect and may cause impotence.

Often pain and pressure in the vaginal and perineal area respond well to internal work on the bulbospongiosus. This muscle is in a rim around the vaginal area. You can often feel the TrPs as lumps in this muscle. These TrPs may respond to finger pressure, but the use of a topical anesthetic is mandatory. Remind your doctor that FMS amplifies TrP pain and other symptoms.

Trigger points in scar tissue produced by any surgical incision are common, but they seem to be especially prevalent in the vaginal cuff following hysterectomy. The *vaginal cuff* is the area at the top of the vagina that would normally be attached to the neck of the uterus. Surgeons can lessen the chance of developing surgical scar TrPs by injecting the incision area of the cuff with a local anesthetic immediately before surgery. Of course, any outer layers of the initial incision should also be injected.

Scar tissue TrPs in the pelvic area can cause pain that is easily mistaken for ovarian cramps, menstrual cramps, and bladder spasms. Also common in this area are nonmyofascial TrPs in the fat layers under the skin, the fat pads overlying the sacroiliac region, and in fatty tumors called lipomas.

Trigger points in the back half of the pelvic floor refer pain that is hard to locate. It just hurts! If you have TrPs in this area, you feel the need to shift sitting position frequently. If you sit for a long time, getting up may cause pain and require extra effort.

Hemorrhoids, pelvic adhesions, fibroids, or cysts may initiate, aggravate, or perpetuate these symptoms. They will not, however, prevent successful TrP treatment. Pelvic floor TrPs respond to trigger point myotherapy, myofascial release, moist heat, massage, stretching, pulsed galvanic stimulation, and posture correction. Stripping massage is a painful but effective treatment,[35] although the pain may be prevented by the use of a topical anesthetic. It is important to resolve any coexisting condition, such as chronic inflammatory pelvic disease. Slumped posture is a major perpetuator. These TrPs also can be activated by pelvic or abdominal surgery, a severe fall, or an auto accident. They can pull the coccyx in toward your pelvis. Then, the doctor may incorrectly blame the pain on the tipped tailbone, rather than the TrPs that caused it. Once you get adequate bodywork, you may be surprised—and relieved—to know how much of the pain was caused by the TrPs rather than the initiating condition.

Vulvodynia is a condition of pain in the external female genitalia without infection or other pathology. It may be so severe that intercourse is impossible, and the ability to sit may be severely curtailed. Trigger points may cause much of this pain. Vaginal wall TrPs may contribute to vulvodynia. Vaginal TrP taut bands can often be felt during pelvic exam. The use of a topical anesthetic may inactivate them, but you need to educate your doctor about TrPs.

Vaginismus is another condition that may coexist with TrPs in the pelvic area, and compound your misery. If you have this condition, your vaginal area goes into spasm whenever entry is attempted. This can include pelvic exams. Relief may quickly follow internal work on the bulbospongiosus and other pelvic floor TrPs, but the use of a topical anesthetic is necessary.

All too often, *dyspareunia*, painful intercourse, is blamed on psychological reasons. Some patients with FMS may have had psychological sexual trauma in their past. Some have not. In either case, pelvic floor biofeedback and TrP work will often relieve pain that has been present for years. If you are such a person, your relief may be quickly followed by anger that your physicians did not know about TrPs before this. You may forgive him or her more quickly if you see they have signed up for one of Dr. Gerwin's courses on identifying and treating TrPs, or, at the very least, that he or she has purchased the Gerwin videos (see Appendix C). Ignorance is bliss for the doctor, not for the patient! Awareness demands action.

Many pelvic floor TrPs can be prevented or eased by using a large sports ball as a chair and bouncing on it occasionally with your legs to either side. This helps stretch the pelvic floor muscles. One TrP that can be stretched this way can contribute to all sorts of pelvic pain, and it is often missed. The adductor magnus is a muscle that runs along the inner *thigh*, and the TrP that can cause diffuse pain *inside* the pelvis is about three-quarters of the way back from the front of the inner thigh, right under the place where your leg joins your body. This area is hard to reach, but it responds well to groin stretches. Lunge stretches and sitting on the floor with the soles of your feet together, stretching your thighs, can ease these high adductor magnus TrPs. This pain referral zone can include the pubic bone, vagina, rectum, and bladder. In some patients with these TrPs, pain only occurs during intercourse. In others, it may mimic pelvic inflammatory disease or prostate trouble. Adductor magnus TrPs also can compress the femoral blood vessels.

19. **Do you have menstrual problems such as severe cramping, delayed periods, irregular periods, long periods with a great deal of bleeding, late periods, missed periods, membranous flow, and/or blood clots?**
   These symptoms often have many causes. Some may be due to an imbalance of the HPG axis[36] and to other hormone dysfunctions (see chapter 11). Rectus abdominis, pyramidalis, and other pelvic, abdominal and vaginal TrPs, as well as that high adductor magnus TrP, may cause or contribute to menstrual cramping.

20. **Do you have pain in your buttocks and tailbone after you sit for a while?** Check the gluteus maximus TrP 3 (Fig. 8-29) for tailbone pain, and also the coccygeus muscle in the pelvic floor. Interrupt any sitting every twenty minutes to stretch these muscles, and place a pillow between your knees when sleeping on your side.

21. **Do you have low back pain?** *"Low back pain in the population at large is not usually a surgical problem,* and the chances of there being significant pathology requiring surgical or other forms of intervention may be less than 1 percent of those affected. Low back pain per se is in the majority not a neurologic problem, an orthopedic problem, or a neurosurgical problem, so that consultation with these specialists, unless there are strong suspicions otherwise, has limited value. The overwhelming cost of low back pain to the economy can be decreased along with suffering and the adverse impact that pain has on all social strata."[37] If early attempts at symptom relief fail, a multidisciplinary pain clinic may help *if people at the clinic are aware of the diagnosis and treatment of myofascial TrPs.*
   The quadratus lumborum (QL) muscle TrPs are often at the root of low back pain, and they are too often overlooked. The QL is a hard muscle to describe, even with pictures,

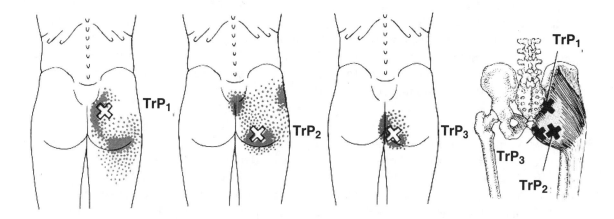

Figure 8-29: Trigger points in the gluteus maximus

because there are many layers. A good bodyworker can often tell which muscle is involved with a TrP by the direction of muscle fibers, but some QL muscle fibers are horizontal, some vertical, and some diagonal.

There are shallow and deep QL muscles along the spine. Deep TrPs are usually found fairly close to the edge of the vertebrae, right above the back crest of the hip and along a line above that. Superficial TrPs are found a few inches farther out, and the line extends longer. Your bodyworker or doctor can palpate these TrPs, but you need to be positioned correctly on your side, with a folded towel beneath the QL area on the lower side, so that the area between the bottom of your rib cage and the top of your hip is easier to examine.

In addition, your legs need to be positioned differently for each segment of the QL. The thoroughness of the QL examination will let you know how familiar your doctor or bodyworker is with the Travell and Simons texts. It is perfectly okay for them to do the exam with the textbook out for reference. In fact, it is the preferred way to do the exam until they become proficient. Trigger point palpation takes a lot of practice, and this TrP is at the root of much low back pain.

Quadratus lumborum TrPs are exceedingly important. They cause pain in circular areas of the buttocks, pain that curves around the upper arch of the hip, and pain along the bottom outside of the buttock and thigh. There is a spillover pattern in a curve on the abdomen from a little in front of the top of the hip to the bottom pelvic rim. These TrPs can cause pain when walking, when turning in bed, when getting up from a chair, and when coughing or sneezing. You can get a deep lightning bolt of pain to the front of the thigh from these TrPs. Pain may extend to the groin, testes, scrotum, or down the leg like sciatica pain.

The QL muscles on either side are designed to work together. If one side is shortened, the other side is lengthened. If there is any body asymmetry, or short upper arms, the QL muscles try to compensate. Trigger points in the QL can cause a *functional* scoliosis. The muscles get so contractured on one side, and lengthened on the other, that the bones are moved out of alignment. It is *very important* that this be taken care of as soon as possible before arthritic changes occur.

You may have a feeling of heaviness in your hips, cramping in your calves, and burning sensations in your legs and feet from these TrPs. Your bed and sleeping position can affect the QL very strongly. These TrPs can result in lost sleep, and can even cause loss of energy and endurance because of all the energy needed to suppress the pain. This pain is

". . . persistent, deep, aching pain at rest, often severe in any body position but excruciating in the unsupported upright position and in sitting or standing."[38] The QL, piriformis, iliopsoas, gluteus minimus, and other TrPs can form composite referral patterns that cause pain that can be nearly unendurable (especially with FMS amplification), and may be beyond the ability of most pain medications to help. Sometimes, a change of position and putting ice packs on the TrPs can help temporarily, but to get lasting relief, you need to tend to the TrPs and perpetuating factors.

Put pillows in between your legs if you sleep on your side, or under your knees if you sleep on your back. Use care in sitting and standing. Avoid bending forward and sideways to lift or pull. If you must climb stairs or use a ladder, move at a 45-degree angle to keep your back straight. Avoid pulling on your pants or socks and shoes while standing. Always lean or sit down. Never stand and lean over a low work surface. The pressure relief technique is helpful for these TrPs. While standing up, place your hands on your hips at waist level, and press in and down. This may allow you to walk long enough to get to your car and to your bodyworker's office.

22. **Do you have sacroiliac (SI) joint dysfunction?** Abnormal muscle tension from any cause can put this joint into an abnormal, displaced position. It can become frozen in place. For proper functioning, this joint must be able to move. These TrPs can start when you are bending forward while tilting your pelvis and twisting. This can happen during a golf swing or while shoveling snow; while stooping and reaching, after a slight fall, or during almost any movement in late pregnancy.

There are many TrPs that refer pain to the SI. The obturator externus and the gluteus maximus TrPs already mentioned are two. The gluteus medius (not shown) TrP 3 is another. This TrP is located in the midline of the side, just under the crest of the upper hipbone arch. It sends a big ball of pain right to the middle of your low back, just below your waist. Those multifidi in the area of the sacroiliac (SI) can send pain there, too. These small muscles are located right next to your vertebrae, and any multifidi can cause nerve entrapment, adding to the grief. In addition, there are some TrPs low on the rectus abdominis that can refer pain in a band crossing the hips at that level and including your SI. Yes, these sneaky little TrPs are in your *belly* and they cause pain in your *back*. Trigger points in the soleus muscle (Fig. 8-30) in your *calf* can refer pain to the edges of your sacroiliac. That's what referred pain is all about, and why your bodyworker and your doctor need to know these referral patterns.

Section IV: The Hip Bone's Connected to the Leg Bone

1. **Do you have pain radiating down your leg from your hip?** This throbbing ache can feel like a toothache festering in your hip. There are a lot of muscles in your hip, and it's hard

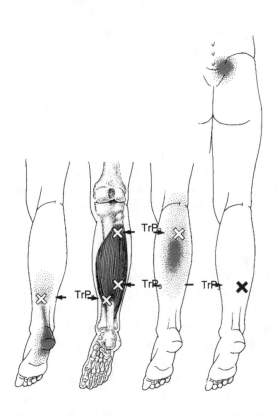

Figure 8-30: Trigger points in the soleus

to be sure you have found the precise culprit. Often the TrPs work as a team, egging each other on. Superficial paraspinal (Fig. 8-23), gluteus minimus (Fig. 8-31), hamstrings (Fig. 8-32), piriformis (Fig. 8-27), and iliopsoas (Fig. 8-31) TrPs may form a composite pain pattern that is called the "piriformis syndrome," and is often mis-diagnosed as sciatic pain. The piriformis TrPs are the ones responsible for the pain radiating down the leg. Usually, it is the most recently formed TrP that screams the loudest. Often, when that TrP is inactivated, a previous one clamors for attention. This can get frustrating, especially when the pain switches from one side to the next. Sound familiar? That means that you most likely have TrPs in both hips. Often, the TrPs in one hip are secondary TrPs that formed when the other side was "favored" because it hurt. The side that took up the slack of the TrP-weakened side then developed TrPs and hurt because of the extra work it was required to do. When one side is treated and feels better, the other one reminds you that it is not in the proper position. It hurts. Sometimes the pain shifts back and forth for a while with treatment, until the muscles regain their proper movements. This shifting should not be taken as a sign that the treatment isn't working. It's actually a good sign, because your muscles are moving once again, and aren't stuck.

Overextension can cause or aggravate TrPs. So can driving. Move around as much as you safely can. If you have these TrPs, avoid chilling your muscles, especially in the hip area. Become aware of your sleep positions, and talk to your bodyworker about them. Find out what may need to be modified. Any problem that can cause an alteration of your gait, even blisters on your feet, can cause or aggravate these TrPs. Tennis ball acupressure daily on the *side* of your hip, followed with moist heat, may help these TrPs. Start gently. It hurts.

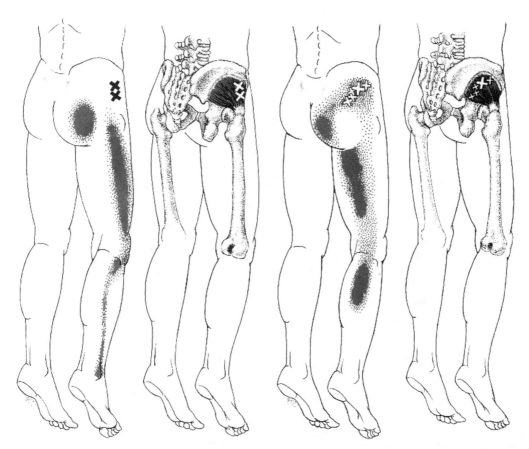

Figure 8-31: Trigger points in the gluteus minimus; stippled and dark areas show referred pain patterns.

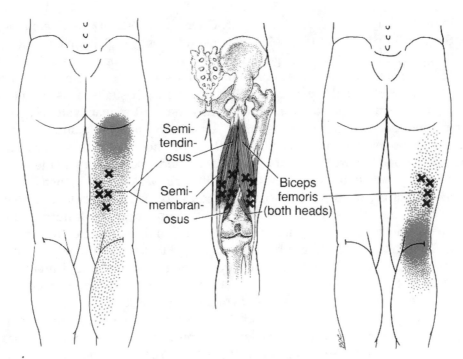

Figure 8-32: Trigger points in the hamstrings; stippled and dark areas show referred pain patterns.

2. **Do you have tight hamstrings?** Trigger points in the adductor magnus, rectus femoris (Fig. 8-33), iliopsoas (Fig. 8-26), and gastrocnemius (Fig. 8-34) are often involved with hamstring TrPs. Defusing the TrPs in this area is a very complex procedure. There is one layer of muscle after another, crossing over each other, often each muscle has layers of TrPs. The adductor muscles, located on the inside of your thigh, often have to be released before the hamstrings respond to therapy. Tightness of the hamstrings is common with low back pain. It's wise to start treatment of low back pain by releasing the hamstrings.

Tightness of muscle is not always spasm. Muscle tension is often misdiagnosed as spasm. We feel this as stiffness. I believe that it is often a significant cause of pain. There is a type of tension caused by excess electrical activity. Electromyograph (EMG) can measure this.

There is also tension caused by biochemical processes. This is not detected by normal tests because there is usually no electrical component. This is independent of muscle contraction and is caused by the amount of interstitial fluid being held by the state of the ground substance.[39]

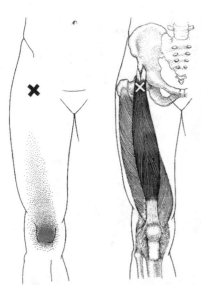

Figure 8-33: Trigger point in the rectus femoris

3. **Do you have weak ankles?** Peroneal TrPs (Fig. 8-35) are the most common ones that cause your ankle to buckle outward. The buckling may cause soft-tissue damage and falls. These TrPs can produce pain in the ankle and on the top of the foot and can cause you to trip over your own feet. They can come from the immobilization of a leg in a

cast, trauma, or from variations of foot structure such as Morton's foot. Inner ankle pain is usually due to peroneus brevis or tibialis TrPs.

4. **Do you get sharp, lightning-like pains up the front of your lower leg?** This pain occurs suddenly and travels like electricity up your lower leg, especially when you kneel. Sometimes it can be avoided if you make sure your toes stay curled under when you kneel, keeping the top of your foot off the floor. If the muscles are rigid, it can be difficult to palpate the tibialis anterior TrPs (Fig. 8-36).

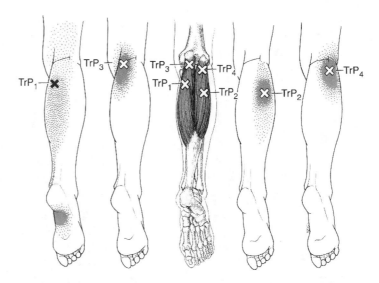

Figure 8-34: Trigger points in the gastrocnemius muscle; stippled and dark areas show referred pain patterns.

5. **Do you stumble over your own feet?** The tibialis anterior TrPs (Fig. 8-36) are often responsible for the disturbances of gait called "foot slap" and "foot drop." These terms describe the loss of "foot clearance" when you take a step. Your foot hits the ground instead of moving forward. Sometimes, so does the rest of you. Your brain may not know how high to lift your foot, or your muscles may not be giving your brain sufficient feedback so it doesn't know how many motor neurons it must activate to lift your foot high enough to clear the ground. Note that tibialis anterior TrPs can also cause big toe pain.

6. **Do you have upper/lower leg cramps?** Sartorius TrPs (Fig. 8-37) may cause upper leg cramps, and TrPs in the gastrocnemius and soleus muscles (Figs. 8-34 and 8-30) are usually the culprits in calf cramps. The QL may be a part of the leg cramps as well. Dehydration, electrolytic imbalance, heat stress, metabolic and other illnesses, as well as some medications can all cause leg cramps.

7. **Do you have nocturnal calf cramps?** Gastrocnemius TrPs are one common and treatable cause (Fig. 8-34). Therapy for myofascial TrPs is as effective as oral quinine during the treatment period, and the effects lasted longer.[40]

The soleus muscle (Fig. 8-30) assists the heart by returning blood from the lower legs. The way that this works is that large cavities in the deep veins beneath the soleus and the veins above the soleus collect venous blood. When you use this muscle, tough fascia helps pump it back from your legs. This soleus pump sleeps when you do, which

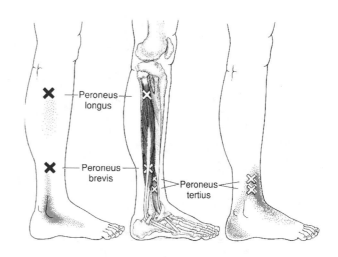

Figure 8-35: Trigger points in the peroneals

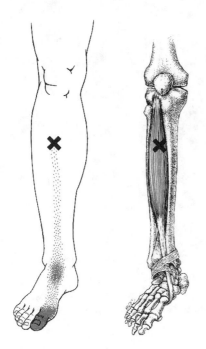

Figure 8-36: Trigger points in the tibialis anterior

adds to the pooling of blood in your lower legs, and to circulatory insufficiency in your calf muscles. This is one reason that calf cramps so often occur when we lie down, or when we first arise from sleep. There may be swelling of the foot and ankle with these TrPs. Soleus TrPs usually cause referred heel pain and tenderness and pain in the back of the calf, but one of these lower leg TrPs can even refer pain to your jaw!

Do not point your toes like a ballerina while you sleep; keep your feet at right angles to your legs to avoid or ease these TrPs. A rolled up blanket or beach towel under your upper sheet may help to keep your feet straight. When you make your bed, try tucking in the bottom end of the cover sheet very loosely, with folds, to allow room for your feet to stick up. Don't ever sacrifice function for packaging.

8. **Do you experience muscle cramps and twitches elsewhere?** Ordinary muscle cramps are caused by overstimulation of a muscle by nerves, unlike spasms, which are caused by a chemical imbalance in the muscle. You could have a metabolic disorder, a coexisting illness, or a vitamin or mineral imbalance. Your body is talking to you. Pay attention!

Check the TrP charts for a pain referral pattern that is in the area of the cramp or twitch. Then find the location of a TrP affecting that area. Check your body to see if a TrP is causing the symptom. Eye twitching may be due to many things,

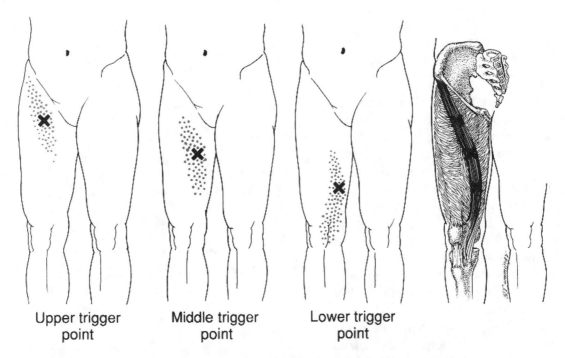

Upper trigger point   Middle trigger point   Lower trigger point

Figure 8-37: Trigger points in the sartorius; stippled areas show referred pain patterns.

but I think that this also may be affected by a TrP. I noticed that when my eye twitched, if I pressed on the hollow behind the outer corner of the eye, the twitch would often go away. One of my friends, Wesley Shankland, discovered a new muscle in that area since the first edition of this book went to press. He has been asked by the NIH to assist in describing it, so you won't find it in anatomy books yet. The "pre-anterior belly" of the temporalis muscle, now named the zygomandibularis, is a discrete, separate muscle. This gives you some idea of the complexity of the human body, if we are still discovering new muscles! This muscle was present at 100 percent of thirty-eight sites checked,[41] so it's been there all along. I believe that a TrP here can cause eye pain, pain behind the eye, anterior temporalis pain, and zygomatic pain. We need more research on it.

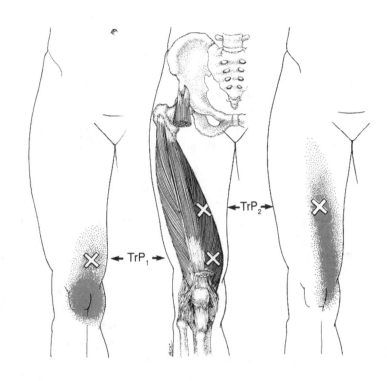

Figure 8-38: Trigger points in the vastus medialis

9. **Do you have a buckling knee?** This falling failing is often due to a combination of vastus medialis TrPs (Fig. 8-38) and adductor longus TrPs (Fig. 8-39). The adductor TrPs can form as a result of abdominal congestion and pelvic pain, often during a menstrual period or prostate trouble. Your knee aches, frequently on the inner side, and it may give out, especially when you are walking over rough ground. When treating these TrPs, it is important to treat the hamstrings. They are usually tight when this TrP is active. Avoid prolonged immobility. A buckling knee from a vastus medialis TrP may result when your thigh muscles are tightened by TrPs and can't do their job. The vastus medialis muscle then tries to take up the slack, until it can no longer cope (Fig. 8-38).

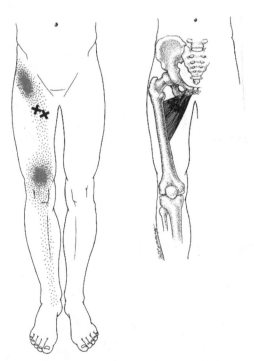

Figure 8-39: Trigger points in the adductor longis and brevis; stippled and dark areas show pain patterns.

10. **Do you have a buckling hip?** This is often caused by a combination of TrPs in the rectus femoris (Fig. 8-33) and the vastus intermedius (not shown). The vastus intermedius lies under the rectus femoris muscle. The buckling hip TrPs in the intermedius are usually about a handswidth below and slightly outward of the rectus femoris TrP shown in Figure 8-33.

11. **Do you have difficulty climbing stairs?** This can be due to TrPs in the sartorius (Fig. 8-37), rectus femoris (Fig. 8-33), and/or vastus medialis (Fig. 8-38) muscles. One way to avoid aggravating these TrPs is to climb steps with your feet and body held at a 45-degree angle to the steps. Don't face the steps; climb with your body at a diagonal. Superficial paraspinal TrPs can also cause this.

12. **Do you have foot pain?** This can come from a variety of causes. Heel pain is often caused by TrPs in the soleus (Fig. 8-30). Frequently, people are treated surgically for a heel spur, even though there may be a heel spur on the other heel, too, but it causes no symptoms. After the "painful" heel spur is removed, the pain often remains, because the TrP, which is the actual cause of the heel pain has not been treated. The TrP must be treated and the perpetuating factors remedied. Doctors must be trained to treat patients, not X-rays. There are many foot TrPs. Some TrPs in the lower leg also cause foot pain.

    Deep intrinsic foot TrPs can cause pain under your heel, intolerance to orthotics, a staggering walk, and thickened calluses. These TrPs can also cause a strange "fluffy" feeling of numbness, a sense of the skin swelling over the region of the metatarsal heads (these are the joints in the toes like the knuckles in the fingers), and a tingling of the great toe (Fig. 8-40). Active or latent TrPs in the dorsal interosseous muscles can be associated with hammertoe. Any foot deformity will perpetuate TrPs. Deformations of the toes may disappear after correction of TrPs.

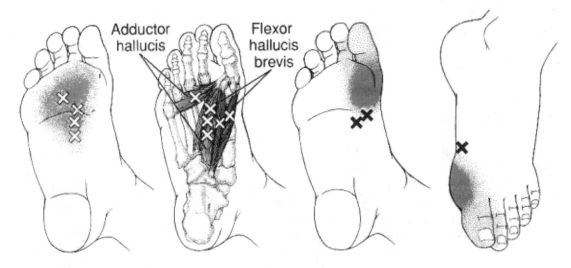

Figure 8-40: Trigger points in some of the deep intrinsic foot muscles

13. **Do you experience rolling waves of contractions or muscle mounding?** The rippling muscle syndrome occurs when impact or pressure on a muscle initiates a rolling wave of contraction that spreads across the muscle in both directions. Myoedema is a localized muscle contraction, or bunching up of muscle tissue, that occurs after impact on the muscle. Both of these conditions are due to exaggerated release of calcium in response to mechanical deformation.[42] I have seen (and experienced) myoedema in response to compression. Both of these conditions are due to exaggerated release of calcium in response to mechanical deformation.

14. **Do you experience strange sensations (of running water, ants crawling under your skin, etc.), hypersensitivity, and/or numbness on your outer thigh?** This is called *meralgia paresthetica*. It occurs because of a very large, superficial nerve on the outer thigh, called the lateral femoral cutaneous nerve. Several muscles can entrap this nerve as it leaves the pelvic area, including the iliopsoas (Fig. 8-26), sartorius (Fig. 8-37), and tensor fascia latae (not shown). Meralgia paresthetica is often associated with a lax, pendulous abdominal wall.

15. **Do you have a staggering walk and balance problems?** If caused by myofascial pain, these symptoms are usually caused by SCM (Fig. 8-2) and/or gluteus minimus (Fig. 8-31) TrPs. Flexible shoes with good support will help control some balancing problems, but perpetuating factors, such as Morton's foot, must be addressed.

16. **Do your first steps in the morning feel as if you are walking on nails or broken glass?** When the plantar fascia (fascial tissue on the bottom of the feet) stretches more than it should, it contracts whenever you are off your feet for any length of time. It sometimes shortens to the point that walking becomes very painful. The pain occurs as your foot first flattens during the stride, due to the weight of the body.

    This condition is often caused by TrPs in the long flexor muscles of the toes. These TrPs are found in the calf, not the foot itself. Morton's foot or any other foot deformity that causes pronation can become perpetuating factors for these TrPs. For relief, try golf ball or rolling pin foot exercisers. Unless you have a structural deformity, orthotics are usually unnecessary after the TrPs are inactivated. Buy comfortable shoes that fit and use cushioned soles when standing or walking on hard surfaces.

17. **Do you have burning feet?** This can have many possible causes, including TrPs. Tight shoes, circulatory dysfunction, and neuropathy can all contribute. Blood sugar problems, medications, pollutant exposure, and liver problems may add to this symptom. Burning feet at night that cause you to kick off the covers, followed by relief, has been considered a sign of neurotransmitter imbalance.[43] In this instance, the feet are not the origin of the pain, only the area to which the pain is referred. Choose comfortable shoes that can "breathe." Make sure they fit well and are in good repair. Exercise your feet, and soak and massage them periodically.

Endnotes

1. Travell, J., and D. Simons. 1992. *Travell and Simons' Myofascial Pain and Dysfunction: The Trigger Point Manual, Vol. II*, First edition. Baltimore: Williams and Wilkins, p. 440.

2. Burgunder, J. M. 1998. Pathophysiology of akinetic movement disorders: a paradigm for studies in fibromyalgia? *Z Rheumatol* Suppl 57(2):27-30.

3. Personal communication 1999. Simons, David. April 16.

4. Cantu, R. L., and A. J. Grodin. 1992. *Myofascial Manipulation: Theory and Clinical Application*. Gaithersburg, MD: Aspen Publishers Inc.

5. Simons, D. G., J. G. Travell, and L. S. Simons. 1999. *Travell and Simons' Myofascial Pain and Dysfunction: The Trigger Point Manual, Vol. I*, Second edition. Baltimore: Williams and Wilkins, p. 399.

6. Enestrom, S., A. Bengtsson, and T. Frodin. 1997. Dermal IgG deposits and increase of mast cells in patients with fibromyalgia-relevant findings or epiphenomena? *Scand J Rheumatol* 26(4):308-313.

7. Bassoe, C. F. 1995. The skinache syndrome. *J R Soc Med* 88:565-569.

8. Deodhar, A. A., R. A. Fisher, C. V. Blacker, and A. D. Woolf. 1994. Fluid retention syndrome and fibromyalgia. *Br J Rheumatol* 33(6):576-582.

9. Mense, S. 1998. Descending antinociception and fibromyalgia. *Z Rheumatol* 57(Suppl 2):23-26.

10. Kabongo, M. L., and A. W. Bedell. 1987. Nail signs of systemic conditions. *Amer Fam Physician* 36(4):109-116.

11. Starlanyl, D. J. 1998. *The Fibromyalgia Advocate*. Oakland, CA: New Harbinger Publications.

12. Helme, R. D., G. O. Littlejohn, and C. Weinstein. 1987. Neurogenic flare responses in chronic rheumatic pain syndromes. *Clin Exp Neurol* 23(1):91-94.

13. Kasteleijn-Nolst Trenite, D. G., A. M. da Silva, S. Ricci, C. D. Binnie, G. Rubboli, C. A. Tassinari, et al. 1999. Video-game epilepsy: a European study. *Epilepsia* 40(Suppl 4):70-74.

14. Donaldson, I. M. 2000. The functions of the proprioceptors of the eye muscles. *Philos Trans R Soc Lond B Biol Sci* 29:355(1404):1685–1754.

15. Russell, I. J. 1999. Personal communication. April 15.

16. Simons, Travell, and Simons. 1999. *Travell and Simons' Myofascial Pain and Dysfunction: The Trigger Point Manual, Vol. I,* Second edition. Baltimore: Williams and Wilkins, p. 117.

17. Grahame, R. 2000. Pain, distress and joint hyperlaxity. *Joint Bone Spine* 67(3):157-163.

18. Simons, Travell, and Simons. 1999. *Op. cit.,* p. 369.

19. Lockwood, A. H., R. J. Salvi, M. L. Coad, M. L. Towsley, D. S. Wack, and B. W. Murphy. 1998. The functional neuroanatomy of tinnitus: evidence for limbic system links and neural plasticity. *Neurology* 50(1):114-120.

20. Simpson, J. J., and W. E. Davies. 1999. Recent advances in the pharmacological treatment of tinnitus. *Trends Pharmacol Sci* 20(1):12-18.

21. Starlanyl. 1998. *Op. cit.*

22. Goldstein, L. B., F. C. Last, and V. M. Salerno. 1997. Prevalence of hyperactive digastric muscles during swallowing as measured by electromyography in patients with myofascial pain dysfunction syndrome. *Funct Orthod* 14(3):18-22.

23. Simons, Travell, and Simons. 1999. *Op. cit.,* p. 241.

24. Travell, J. G. 1960. Temporomandibular joint pain referred from muscles of the head and neck. *J Prosthet Dent* 10(4):745-763.

25. Aurora, S. K., and K. M. Welch. 2000. Migraine: imaging the aura. *Curr Opin Neurol* 13(3):273-276.

26. Pappagallo, M., Z. Szabo, G. Esposito, A. Lokesh, and L. Velez. 1999. Imaging neurogenic inflammation in patients with migraine headaches. *Neurol* 52(Suppl 2):A274-275 (abstract).

27. Simons, Travell, and Simons. 1999. *Op. cit.,* p. 242.

28. *Ibid.,* p. 792.

29. *Ibid.,* p. 792.

30. *Ibid.,* p. 875.

31. Lurie, M., K. Caidahl, G. Johansson, and B. Bake. 1990. Respiratory function in chronic primary fibromyalgia. *Scand J Rehabil* Med 22(3):151-155.

32. Simons, Travell, and Simons. 1999. *Op. cit.,* p. 851.

33. Ling, F. W., and J. C. Slocomb. 1993. Use of trigger point injections in chronic pelvic pain. *Obstet Gynecol Clin North Am* 20(4):809-815.

34. Slocomb, J. C. 1984. Neurological factors in chronic pelvic pain: trigger points and the abdominal pelvic pain syndrome. *Am J Obstet Gynecol* 149(5):536-543.

35. Travell, J., and D. Simons. 1992. *Myofascial Pain and Dysfunction: The Trigger Point Manual, The Lower Extremities. Vol. II.* Baltimore: Williams and Wilkins, p. 127.

36. Starlanyl, D. J. 1998. *The Fibromyalgia Advocate.* Oakland, CA: New Harbinger Publications.

37. Rosomoff, H. L., and R. S. Rosomoff. 1999. Low back pain. Evaluation and management in the primary care setting. *Med Clin North Am* 83(3):643-662.

38. Travell and Simons. 1992. *Op. cit.,* p. 38.

39. Simons, D. G., and S. Mense. 1998. Understanding and measurement of muscle tone as related to clinical muscle pain. *Pain* 75(1):1-17.

40. Prateepavanich, P., V. Kupniratsaikul, and T. Charoensak. 1999. The relationship between myofascial trigger points of gastrocnemius muscle and nocturnal calf cramps. *J Med Assoc Thai* 82(5):451-459.

41. Shankland, W. E., II, J. A. Negulesco, and B. O'Brian. 1996. The pre-anterior belly of the temporalis muscle; a preliminary study of a newly described muscle. *Cranio* 14(2):106-112.

42. Simons, and Mense. 1998. *Op. cit.*

43. Birkmayer, W., and P. Riederer. 1989. *Understanding the Neurotransmitters: Key to the Workings of the Brain.* Translated from German by Karl Blau. New York: Springerer-Verlag.

CHAPTER 9

Chronic Pain

I know as much as I do about fibromyalgia (FMS) and chronic myofascial pain (CMP) because I have them in such a severe form. They have been great teachers, but I don't remember enrolling in this particular course. Pain is a personal and an emotional issue. No one else can know just how much *you* hurt, nor understand how overwhelming it can be when pain seeps through the tiniest cracks in your support structure, threatening your stability, your health, and sometimes your life itself. By itself, pain can suppress the immune system and can encourage the growth of some forms of cancer. It can affect blood pressure and many other body functions. In this chapter we will be looking at why chronic pain is so different from acute pain.

Pain 101

Acute pain can be a blessing when it serves as a warning of possible tissue damage because it can help prevent further injury. Special nerve endings in your skin and muscles, those nociceptors you met earlier in this book, respond to biochemicals that are released by damaged cells, such as histamine. The nociceptors send signals racing to your brain, letting it know that immediate action is required. Danger is threatening and damage is occurring. This biochemical pain response takes place even in surgical patients under general anesthesia. These signals travel from nerve to nerve. Nerves are not physically connected to one another, so each nerve cell must release a neurotransmitter, which travels to the next nerve. These physical processes are fluid, multidimensional, and change constantly, affecting other physiological events.

Endorphins and Pain

Physical and emotional trauma releases the body's own painkillers, the endorphins, which are produced in response to orders from the hypothalamus and the pituitary glands (plus a type of gray matter in the nervous system). These glands, with the adrenals, form the HPA axis, the functioning of which is disrupted in FMS. When the stress response is triggered by acute pain, endorphins flood the body, dampening the pain to allow response to the threat. This does not happen with chronic pain. You don't get "used to the pain." Chronic pain becomes harder to endure.[1] After a time, fewer endorphins are produced to counter the same amount of pain. The body cannot remain in a fight or flight mode for long without succumbing to exhaustion. The mechanism for dealing with physical pain is subject to malfunction just like any organ system.

Chronic Pain States: A Different Animal

When you know your pain is eventually going to end and that you will recover, it is easier to tolerate. Hope helps you to carry the burdens. If you have chronic pain, you may feel hopeless and helpless, and your medical team may feel the same, until you get a diagnosis and some specific help. Chronic pain institutes an extended and destructive cascade of neuroendocrine dysregulation, fatigue, general discomfort, muscle aches, and decreased mental and physical function. When you feel the pain is uncontrollable, a sense of hopelessness adds to your stress. If your job, family, and social life changes, your identity is damaged. Your doctor can help prevent this from happening by controlling your pain.[2]

> In chronic pain, your doctor can't put a finger on an obvious reason for your pain. That does not mean it does not exist. Your doctor must understand that chronic pain is not the same as acute pain, and cannot be managed in the same fashion. Lack of understanding on the part of the physician has too often caused chronic pain patients to be branded with the labels "neurotic" or "malingerer.[3]

Chronic Pain and Your State of Mind

Depression is a *normal* response to chronic pain. If you are already depressed, chronic pain will intensify normal depressed reactions and must be dealt with, and not just in the obvious, psychological way. The same biochemicals that intensify pain can also cause or intensify depression. Research shows that it is the stress of living with chronic pain, not personal or family predisposition, that causes depression.[4] Depressed mood is more closely tied to ability to function than to the experience of pain.[5] If you feel that you can't cope with your chronic pain and still maintain function, you're more likely to become disabled and/or depressed.[6]

If the members of your medical team say things like, "It's not going to kill you," "It couldn't hurt that much," "Forget the pain. You are too preoccupied with your illness. Get a life," these are signs that your medical team is in denial. What they don't know can hurt you. Chronic pain itself can also cause fatigue, difficulties concentrating, changes in appetite, and withdrawal from life. Chronic pain is an aggressive condition that must be vigorously treated as soon as possible, before it leads to central nervous system hypersensitivity and muscle tightness, and thus to even more pain.

Leveling with the Pain

Like most people, you were probably unprepared for the totality of chronic pain or for the way in which pain takes over your whole life. Chronic pain means that your old life died and the new life that was born is prickly, with sharp edges that can wear away the spirit and endurance of the unprepared.

Jan Dommerholt, a specialist in pain management, made an important point about pain in his presentation at the Focus on Pain 2000 Seminar. He asked, From whose perspective is pain assessed? Can your health care provider decide how much pain you have, or an insurance company, or a lawyer? Only you can judge how bad your pain is, and if others disagree, *you should not suffer because of that*. Jan Dommerholt explained that medical professionals must provide relief and hope. Hope activates the body's own opioid system. In FMS patients, hope is the light at the end of the tunnel that has all too often been turned off. It is the clinician's job to turn that light back on.

People who are frequent visitors to the emergency room and who are regularly in a crisis state due to pain may have poor coping behavior and/or an ineffective support strategy, or they may have been provided with inadequate pain control. When people are in pain, there is no excuse for blaming them. Patients may need extensive counseling and/or other intervention, but they are doing the best they can. That's all that can be asked of anyone.

Treating Chronic Pain

There are many nonmedicinal treatments for pain and these should be explored first. You may be able to cut your pain burden indirectly by dealing with contributing factors, such as lack of sleep, or stress. This may diminish your need for pain medication. Many different neurotransmitters may be involved in your chronic pain state, so you may have to try a number of different medications before finding the combination that works for you. Many physicians give up to soon and their patients suffer. Of course, you must do what you can to minimize your pain by being good to your body, avoiding overwork, and refusing to perform activities when you are exhausted or in pain. Often, however, such preventive measures aren't enough.

> One woman with FMS I spoke with could not get any pain relief from Darvocet or other more standard medications. Her doctors didn't want to prescribe anything stronger, but she couldn't sleep because of the pain she was experiencing. When her doctors found cancer, suddenly she was prescribed all the pain medications she needed. The pain hadn't changed at all—only her *doctors'* perception of it.

The Dependency Factor

With FMS and CMP, you need a primary care doctor who understands how to treat chronic pain and a pharmacist to match. They must understand and agree that physical dependency is the body's natural adaptation to some types of medication. If you stop taking a medication that has been taken regularly for some length of time, a withdrawal effect will occur; but this is not an addiction. It was once thought that addiction was both psychological and physiological dependence. Now physiological changes from repeated use of narcotics are recognized and treated as separate processes.[7]

If you suffer from chronic pain, you should not be denied adequate pain control because of fear that you will become addicted. Adding the burden of guilt to your life does nothing to ease your pain. It is not unusual for a well-educated patient to be aware of the times they require medication and what medication they may require. If you are continuously going to the emergency room for relief of pain, this is a signal that your pain is inadequately treated. Being relieved that you are no longer in pain is not the same as being high on a drug.

As a rule, FMS and CMP patients save the strong pain medications they receive after a surgery or an injury for the times when they will really need them, those times when they have a flare (see chapter 13). If you are doing this, it is another sign that your doctor is not managing your pain adequately. To ask your doctor for a small amount of stronger medication to have on hand for short-term use when you really need it is responsible behavior, not a sign of a drug addiction.

> I would not have been able to write this book without the help of adequate pain medications, other medications, and tons of physical therapy. I am looking forward to the time when I can cut back on the medications and still improve my quality of life.

Chronic pain is exactly that, *chronic*. For some reason (could it be financial?), insurance companies and other third-party payers set arbitrary limits on when we "should" no longer need physical therapy, medications, etc. Doctors put chronic pain patients through drug counseling and treatment programs, to try and "taper them off" the very medications they need to allow them to continue to function! We need to improve education about painkillers at the medical school and continuing education level, so that doctors will have the knowledge and desire to change prevailing opinions about drugs that relieve pain. Doctors are supposed to "do no harm," and one of their primary functions is to alleviate unnecessary pain. Changing attitudes will take time, education, and concern. It is unethical, even criminal, that conflicting interests can have an impact on peoples' lives to such an extent that they are denied the very medication that would permit them to get out of bed and function.

Using Opioids to Treat Chronic Noncancerous Pain

Nonsteroidal anti-inflammatory drugs (NSAIDs) can cause gastric ulcers, increased bleeding time, and kidney problems. Regardless of dosage form, NSAIDs inhibit the prostaglandins that are necessary to maintain the protective barrier in the gastrointestinal (GI) tract. The use of antacids with NSAIDs can lessen this GI damage, but it also reduces the absorption and effectiveness of the NSAIDs. Most patients with gastric lesions from NSAIDS have no symptoms until bleeding or perforation occurs.

The most common side effect from long-term use of opioids is constipation. But, contrary to current medical research, many doctors still refuse to prescribe opioids for noncancerous pain. Patients in chronic pain from a noncancerous source deserve as effective pain control as those whose pain derives from cancer. Medical providers in the United States and around the world have not been as effective as they should and could be because they are reluctant to use opioid analgesics for moderate to severe pain.[8]

Reluctance to use narcotics for selected patients with nonmalignant painful medical conditions stems from the mistaken belief that they will become addicted. Data from the medical literature refutes this misconception.[9] "Currently opiates are the most effective medications for managing most chronic pain states. Their use in fibromyalgia and other non-malignant chronic pain conditions is often condemned out of ignorance regarding their propensity to cause addiction, physical dependence and tolerance. Opiates are seldom the first choice of analgesia in chronic pain states, but they should not be withheld if less powerful analgesics have failed."[10]

In order to provide satisfactory pain relief and prevent the possible results of untreated pain, physicians must possess both knowledge and expertise in the use of opioid and nonopioid analgesics. Opioid analgesics have been underused in the management of pain. They have a higher analgesic potency and wider range of indications than any of the other currently available medications for pain control.[11]

Opioids are a necessary and effective component of the management of chronic noncancer-related pain in some patients.[12] As more doctors become educated in the use of chronic pain management, more doctors are using opioids for noncancer chronic pain.[13] Used appropriately, opioids may represent the only source of relief for many patients.[14]

Inadequate treatment of pain continues to be a problem despite greater knowledge about its causes and control. Scientific data show that almost all patients with painful medical conditions requiring opioids for treatment have discontinued their use after the medical condition for which the opioids were needed no longer exists. In all situations, relief of pain, either acute or chronic, must be the standard for success.[15]

If a patient receiving chronic opioid therapy experiences an intolerable side effect or if the drug is ineffective, changing to a different opioid may result in a lessening or elimination of that side effect and/or improved analgesia.[16] In addition to preventing central nervous system sensitization, coadministration of NMDA-receptor antagonists with an opioid may prevent tolerance to opioid analgesia.[17]

The interpretation of the regulations that establish standards for prescribing opioids by government regulatory boards and drug-enforcement agencies is more restrictive for treatment of nonmalignant pain than it is for malignant pain. The boards and agencies determine standards of practice for opioid use are based on myths, prejudices, and misinformation about opioids and the unexamined belief that mere exposure to these drugs causes psychological dependence.[18]

Describing Chronic Pain to Your Doctor

Pain is a way your body has of warning you that there is a threat. Perceived threat leads to negative emotions. The negative emotions may not have caused the pain, but they can add to the pain. Dealing with the negative emotions may help you gain some control over the pain. You must communicate to your health care team what the pain means to you in the context of your life.

How is it changing your life? How is it interfering with your functioning? What do you want to do that you can't do because of the pain? Bring your medical team into *your* frame of reference. Pain has no external reference. Your motions are also important. A man describing a crushing pain may clench his arms tight to his body. A woman describing a radiating pain may spread her fingers in the direction of the radiation.

You need to learn how to communicate to others, especially to your doctors, what you are feeling. You need to understand the language of pain. The words you choose are important because they provide your doctor with clues as to what your pain is like.

It may be very hard for you to tolerate being hugged or even touched on some days. It you ache for days (or longer) after a "range of motion" test or other office procedure, let your doctor and bodyworker know. They may not understand how much pain the visit caused. In the future, you may need extra medication before such exams to help avoid this added stressor. You need to communicate this fact.

The Language of Pain

There are many words to describe pain. Words such as pulsing, throbbing, pounding, shooting, prickling, stabbing, lancing, electrical, sharp, pinching, pressing, gnawing, cramping, crushing, tugging, wrenching, hot, cruel, vicious, killing, blinding, intense, unbearable, spreading, radiating, piercing, tearing, agonizing, and torturing all describe different types of intense pain.

Tingling, itchy, smarting, stinging, dull, sore, aching, heavy, tender, taut, tiring, exhausting, sickening, suffocating, frightful, annoying, troublesome, miserable, tight, rigid, numb, drawing, squeezing, cool, cold, icy, and nagging are other words to describe different kinds of pain more precisely.

There is also the kind of pain that brings on other symptoms such as vomiting, shaking, distractibility, and/or an inability to concentrate. Important questions to ask your doctor may be: "Do you believe that I have this pain?" "Do you understand its severity and the disrupting influence it has on my life?" "Do you understand that it is important to me to regain as much function as possible?" "What are my options?"

Narcotics, or opioids, work because their chemical structures are similar to the shapes of some neurotransmitters. They block the pain receptors and stop the pain messages from getting through. New research indicates that aggressive pain management may eventually reverse the physiological effects of heightened pain sensitivity, such as central nervous system sensitization. In the future, we may have better medications. Right now we must use what we have wisely and effectively.

Posttraumatic Hyperirritability Syndrome (PTHS)

Posttraumatic hyperirritability syndrome (PTHS) is the result of extreme sensitization. It can occur after the severe sudden onset FMS and CMP associated with physical trauma.[19] It can also occur when a patient with FMS and/or CMP or another coexisting condition experiences major trauma that may be sufficient to damage the sensory modulation mechanisms of the spinal cord or brain stem.

Posttraumatic hyperirritability syndrome is an altered state of constant pain, which may be worsened by the vibration of a passing car, the slamming of a door, a ringing phone or other loud noise, by jarring, mild thumps, pain, prolonged physical activity, and by emotional stress. Recovery from such stimulation is slow. It may take hours, days, or weeks to return to your baseline pre-stimulation pain level.

Most people with PTHS were coping well before their initiating traumas. The changes they experienced after the initiating trauma were extreme. They experience extreme sensory overload. They suddenly find themselves walking a tightrope, trying to live while avoiding much of the stimuli that life brings. Their activity may be severely limited. The fragility and hypersensitivity of their autonomic nervous systems can cause rapid skin temperature changes and swellings that may be resolved by inactivating specific trigger points (TrPs). Some of these patients move into survival mode and respond to any stimuli with anger, violence, or other strong emotions.

Patients with PTHS are often considered "crocks" and are dismissed.[20] This may be the ultimate abuse. Any additional fall or other stressor that would ordinarily be considered minor can severely worsen this condition for years. If you have *PTHS*, you need your space and you need expert care. It is vital that you learn protective mindwork controls (see chapter 20) and that you regulate the amount of stimuli you experience.

Posttraumatic hyperirritability syndrome is also called cumulative trauma disorder, stress neuromyelopathic pain syndrome, and jolt syndrome. Some researchers say that FMS is the end stage of a number of chronic pain conditions. I believe that PTHS is such an end state. We need greater recognition of this condition and we need a great deal of research. It can be incapacitating. We need to know how to halt the progression, how to reset the nervous system, and how to reverse the symptoms.

The Suicide Factor

A suicide attempt must be taken seriously. The serious suicide attempt is an overwhelming desire for death. Fate, in the form of others who intervene, prevents this desire from being consummated. The desire is still there, but the desperate need is not met. Yet some doctors will use even a suicide attempt as an excuse to withhold adequate medications from their patients. How long this state of affairs will continue to be tolerated will, in some way, be a measure of the quality of our medical care system.

In one study of 204 people with chronic nonmalignant pain, only 50 percent reported receiving adequate pain relief. They identified depression as one of their worst problems caused by their chronic pain: Fifty percent reported that they had considered suicide due to feelings of *hopelessness* associated with their pain.[21]

All chronic pain patient suicide rates are significantly greater than that of the general population.[22] This, to me, is the greatest indicator that the needs of chronic pain patients are not being met.

I had the sad honor of facilitating a memorial service over the Internet for one woman who could no longer bear her suffering. She was not getting the symptom relief she needed, and she took her own life. Her own minister refused to do that service. He insisted that because of the manner of her death, she went to hell. It is my own belief that this minister may be very surprised when *he* arrives at that destination and *she* isn't there. She had already served her time in hell. I believe that religion is about healing and compassion, not about judgment.

At about the same time, I heard about a woman living near Chicago who was suffering from unbearable pain. Her doctor had examined her and had diagnosed myofascial pain. Then he told her she'd have to "learn to live with it," because there was *nothing* she could do. Her husband could not stand to see her in so much pain, so he shot her and then he killed himself. Does her doctor understand what he has done?

Some researchers have written that patients with FMS have a lowered pain *threshold*. This statement has been used to belittle and even to victimize FMS patients. It is important to make something very clear here. People with FMS experience a lot more pain from any given stimulus than a healthy person would. But, based upon my observations, many patients with FMS and CMP have a high pain *tolerance*, even though they feel pain more readily. The amount of pain some of us endure is amazing. The only way we will get to that light at the end of the tunnel is for our care providers to become enlightened and educated in the options available for the treatment of chronic pain. We deserve no less.

Endnotes

1. McCaffery, M., and C. Pasero. 1999. *Pain: Clinical Manual.* St. Louis: Mosby.

2. Chapman, C. R., and J. Gavrin. 1999. Suffering: the contributions of persistent pain. *Lancet* 353(9171):2233-2237.

3. Bennett, R. M. 1999. Emerging concepts in the neural biology of chronic pain: evidence of abnormal sensory processing in fibromyalgia. *Mayo Clin Proc* 74(4):385-398.

4. Gallagher, R. M., and S. Verma. 1999. Managing pain and comorbid depression: A public health challenge. *Semin Clin Neuropsychiatry* 4(3):203-220.

5. Kuch, K., B. Cox, R. J. Evans, P. C. Watson, and C. Bubela. 1993. To what extent do anxiety and depression interact with chronic pain? *Can J Psychiatry* 38(1):36-38.

6. Arnstein, P., M. Caudill, C. L. Mandle, A. Norris, and R. Beasley. 1999. Self-efficacy as a mediator of the relationship between pain intensity, disability and depression in chronic pain patients. *Pain* 80(3):483-491.

7. McCaffery, M., and C. Pasero. 1999. *Op. cit.*

8. Parrott, T. 1999. Using opioid analgesics to manage chronic noncancer pain in primary care. *J Am Board Fam Pract* 12:293-306.

9. Fishbain, D. A., H. L. Rosomoff, and R. S. Rosomoff. 1992. Drug abuse, dependence, and addiction in chronic pain patients. *Clin J Pain* 8(2):77-85.

10. Bennett, R. 2000. Understanding chronic pain and fibromyalgia. *Inland Northwest Fibromyalgia Association News.* Winter edition, p. 11.

11. Pappagallo, M. 1998. Aggressive pharmacologic treatment of pain. *Rheum Dis Clin North Am* 25(1):193-213, vii.

12. Savage, S. R. 1999. Opioid use in the management of chronic pain. *Med Clin North Am* 83(3):761-786.

13. Portenoy, R. K. 2000. Current pharmacotherapy of chronic pain. *J Pain Symptom Mange* 19(1 Suppl):S16-20.

14. Passik, S. D., and H. J. Weinreb. 2000. Managing chronic nonmalignant pain: overcoming obstacles to the use of opioids. *Adv Ther* 17(2):70-83.

15. Hill, Jr., C. S. 1995. When will adequate pain treatment be the norm? *JAMA* 274(23):1881-1882.

16. Quang-Cantagrel, N. D., M. S. Wallace, and S. K. Magnuson. 2000. Opioid substitution to improve the effectiveness of chronic noncancer pain control: a chart review. *Anesth Analg* 90(4):933-937.

17. Bennett, G. J. 2000. Update on the neurophysiology of pain transmission and modulation: focus on the NMDA-receptor. *J Pain Symptom Manage* 19(1 Suppl):S2-6.

18. Hill, Jr., C. S. 1996. Government regulatory influences on opioid prescribing and their impact on the treatment of pain of nonmalignant origin. *J Pain Symptom Manage* 11(5):287.

19. Simons, D. G., J. G. Travell, and L. S. Simons. 1999. *Travell and Simons' Myofascial Pain and Dysfunction: The Trigger Point Manual.* Second edition. Baltimore: Williams and Wilkins, p. 44.

20. *Ibid.*, p. 545.

21. Hitchcock, L. S., B. R. Ferrell, and M. McCaffery. 1994 The experience of chronic non-malignant pain *J Pain Symptom Manage* 9(5):312-318.

22. Fishbain, D. A., M. Goldberg, R. S. Rosomoff, and H. Rosomoff. 1991. Completed suicide in chronic pain. *Clin J Pain* 7(1):29-36.

CHAPTER 10

Sleep and Fatigue

Sleep plays a vital role in memory. Many people seem able to solve some of their problems in their dreams, and new skills can be consolidated while asleep. Sleep dysfunction is an integral part of many illnesses. Disorganization, fragmentation or loss of the healthy sleep-wake cycle is accompanied by changes in immunological, neuroendocrine, and thermal functions. Even a partial night's sleep deprivation reduces natural killer cell and other cellular immune responses![1]

Even during sleep, the body and mind are continually communicating at a rate that can be difficult to grasp. Picture the thin, convoluted surface of the brain, the outer part that resembles the surface of a walnut kernel. This area is called the cerebral cortex. In this part of the brain alone, there are about 10 billion nerve cells. Each of these nerve cells is communicating by neurotransmitter with at least 10,000 other nerve cells next to it, and sending between 100 and 300 communications a second. Each of them, no matter whether we are awake or asleep, is active to that degree.[2]

Fibromyalgia (FMS) and perhaps chronic myofascial pain (CMP) can create a great deal of extraneous noise along these transmission lines. This can contribute to chronic sleep deprivation, a dangerous condition.

Sleep and Fibromyalgia

The quality of our sleep has an impact on every facet of our lives. Sleep deprivation affects the activity of the hypothalamus-pituitary-adrenal (HPA) axis and growth axis. Sleep deprivation for one night results in significant changes in adrenal secretion the next day. Healthy deep sleep inhibits the HPA axis and enhances the growth hormone axis.[3] FMS patients have low levels of somatomedin C, a growth hormone that is stimulated in sleep.[4]

There seems to be a problem with the microstructure of sleep in FMS.[5] This means that in healthy people the sequence of sleep stages progresses in an orderly pattern. In FMS, there is no orderly pattern. The stages are fragmented. Our nighttime biological circadian rhythms may be out of sync and this contributes to our daytime symptoms. If sleep is fragmented and unorganized, this can cause a burst of alertness when you should be getting sleepy.[6] Deliberately keeping yourself awake when your body and mind want to sleep can be dangerous.

If you start yawning and need to rub your eyes, these are the early warning signs of approaching sleepiness. Go to bed and settle in your preferred going-to-sleep position. If you don't get right to bed, the reflex arousal will put you into an alert state again. (The reflex arousal occurs when you are sleepy, but your actions signal that you aren't going to sleep. Then, you start manufacturing biochemicals to overcome the sleepy feeling.) It is a temporary feeling and it can be dangerous. The moment you relax the hypervigilant state that put you into arousal, you can fall asleep *instantly*. If you are doing something that requires you to be awake at this time, like driving, you are in trouble. Avoid arousing situations before you go to bed. You may need to avoid sexual intercourse immediately before sleep time. Discuss options with your partner. Avoid doing homework, paying bills, eating late, or checking your email before retiring for bed. Also avoid TV programs that leave your heart racing (this is especially important for children).

Forget about tomorrow. You will cope with tomorrow even better if you don't try to deal with it the night before. Don't fight sleep if it comes early. If you start to yawn, get to bed. This is a good time to try meditation, self-hypnosis, or some other form of mindwork. Too often we push the envelope in the hours that we work. Sleep is often viewed as an enemy. Treat it as a friend, and it will come to visit you more often. According to a Cornell University Medical Center study, by Daniel Wagner, M.D., it takes four to six weeks of getting enough sleep to fully recover from prolonged sleep deprivation.[7] If, like many people with FMS and CMP, you have had years of sleep deprivation, you have a lot of catching up to do.

Sleep and Myofascial Pain

As your muscles work during the day, they gain a momentum, an electrical loading, that doesn't stop even when you're asleep. Even slightly tensed muscles send nerve impulses through the spinal cord to your brain. There, these impulses activate thoughts that can be persistent and annoying when you are trying to sleep.

During the night, parts of your body may become numb if they have the slightest weight on them. Nerve entrapments may also occur because of pressure on the nerves by the palpable bands of taut muscle fibers that are associated with trigger points (TrPs). When a nerve passes through the muscle between taut bands of myofascia, or when it is compressed between such a band and bone, the result may be loss of nerve conduction. People who have had TrPs for months or years are likely to have sleep problems. Your doctor and bodyworker should give top priority to inactivating those TrPs that contribute to your sleep problems.

The Stages of Sleep

Sleep is different for each individual, but to a greater or lesser extent, most people experience specific stages while they are sleeping. Just before you fall sleep, you pass through a period known as the hypnogogic stage. It is matched by an after-sleep awakening period known as the hypnopompic stage. Unusual things can happen to you at these times. You are more suggestible and, if you can focus on them, affirmations work particularly well at this time. Some people even hallucinate during this stage. The onset of sleep is often heralded by a feeling of floating or falling and sometimes this stage ends abruptly with a startled wakefulness. Your whole body can twitch or jump. These actions are called sleep starts. Myoclonus (the plural is myoclonia) is a term that includes sleep starts, periodic leg movements, and hiccups. Sleep starts include explosions of noise and light, seeing lights, vocalizations, and falling sensations. These happen occasionally to everyone but they occur more often when you are exhausted or under stress. There is another condition called "the exploding head syndrome." This is characterized by unpleasant and even terrifying sensations of flashing lights and/or sounds during your sleep. You might even make animal noises. The patients in this study were relieved by clomipramine.[8]

Rapid Eye Movement (REM) Sleep

Dreaming takes place during rapid eye movement, or REM, sleep. Stage One sleep is a drowsy non-REM sleep. (It is called NREM sleep.) Stage Two is a light NREM sleep. There are also deeper stages of NREM sleep, times of delta-brain wave rhythm, when much of the body's regulatory work and biochemical balancing take place, and when antibodies are produced in greater numbers. These stages are punctuated by periods of REM sleep.

During REM sleep, there is a complete loss of muscle tone, called flaccid paralysis. You cannot move. This prevents you from physically acting out your dreams. If you wake suddenly from this stage of sleep, you can have a residual paralysis that can be very frightening. This happens more often with disorders of sleep fragmentation, which seem to be common in FMS. Body movement takes place in the lighter stages of sleep, but not in the deep ones. In healthy people, NREM sleep is always the first stage in each sleep cycle. At the onset of REM sleep, you may have small convulsive twitches of your face and fingers similar to the movements you can see in a sleeping cat or dog. Snoring occurs during NREM sleep.

Chronic Pain, Stress, and Insomnia

Insomnia is not a disease. It is a symptom. A *symptom* is something you experience and communicate to your doctor. *Signs* are what the doctor can observe. It is the doctor's responsibility to search for the cause of the symptoms like insomnia, but too often the symptom—and you—are dismissed with a pill.

Insomnia is a frightening and life-altering symptom. You feel trapped, knowing that you must get some sleep if you are to function at all the next day. But with FMS and CMP, sleep often remains elusive. Chronic pain worsens sleep difficulties. In chronic pain conditions, alpha rhythms often intrude, especially into delta sleep, disrupting slumber. (Alpha waves are normally generated during waking hours. Delta brain waves are associated with deeper levels of sleep.) A high proportion of alpha waves during sleep means that there will be a more sensitive perception of pain. More delta waves during sleep lessen pain sensations and improve energy levels.

Stress and Sleep

Stress is a leading cause of insomnia. Stress causes sleep loss that then causes further stress, which causes further sleep loss, and so on. Stress itself is a symptom with many causes, such as illness, psychological problems, medications, the environment (noise, interruptions, etc.), sleep disorders, jet lag, shift work, and more. Drinking alcohol may cause temporary drowsiness. It depresses the central nervous system. You don't get a healthy sleep, and then your body rebounds from the carbohydrate infusion you got from the alcohol—it hits the bloodstream fast and interferes with the workings of your gastrointestinal tract on the way.

Forms of Insomnia

There are three main forms of insomnia. Difficulty in falling asleep is called *sleep onset insomnia*. Waking up many times during the night is called *maintenance insomnia*. Waking very early and being unable to go back to sleep is called *early A.M. insomnia*. There is also *mixed insomnia*, which is some combination these forms. *Conditioned insomnia* can occur after a period of interrupted or poor sleep, such as might happen with a new baby. *Compulsive urination insomnia* appears to be very common in FMS and CMP. Most people urinate before they go to bed, and a small amount of urine is usually left in the bladder. Because people with FMS have hypersensitive nerve endings, they feel the bladder pressure, so they soon get up to urinate again. Whenever they wake, which can be often, they visit the bathroom. This can happen more than thirty times a night! This can be aggravated by yeast or low-grade bacterial infection, so see your doctor. Ask about a topical anesthetic to use on the urinary opening to decrease some sensitivity. Another type of insomnia called *dream-interruption insomnia* is caused by deep anxiety. You awaken during REM sleep and experience residual paralysis. In some cases, a person may wake up with laryngeal muscle spasms and be unable to speak. This can be terrifying.

In *delayed sleep phase syndrome (DSPS)*, which can be mistaken for insomnia, the circadian rhythm is out of phase. You feel as if you aren't ready for sleep when the clock tells you that you should be. At times you may not get to sleep until early in the morning. When you sleep, you do sleep well and you wake refreshed, unless you have a coexisting sleep disorder. Most DSPS people are night owls. They are sleepy during the day and have very bad mornings. On days off, they may stay in bed until noon to clear up their sleep debt. Delayed sleep phase syndrome may start in infancy.

Factors Affecting Sleep

Nicotine can play a role in insomnia. Nicotine is a stimulant that causes the release of epinephrine, a neurotransmitter, which interferes with sleep. Withdrawal from nicotine begins two or three hours after smoking and can also promote insomnia. Your diet and the time you eat may be factors in the quality of your sleep. Give your body time to digest your evening meal before going to bed. Ensure that your room is at a comfortable temperature for sleeping and that you will have no interruptions.

Climatic conditions can prevent sleep or promote it.[9] Rainy weather, cool still days, and low atmospheric pressure can enhance sleepiness. Dry heat, wind and high atmospheric pressure may inhibit sleep and lead to restlessness.

Noise can be another factor that keeps you awake. I use industrial-strength ear plugs recommended to me by Hal Blatman, M.D. I keep some handy by my bed, in case my spouse or cats snore. Electric lights can confuse your internal clock. Try moderating the lights in your house an hour before going to sleep. Keep regular times for going to sleep. Go to bed only when you are sleepy, but get up at a regular time. Don't vary your routine by more than an hour. You may need medication to help you sleep. Don't give up until you find the right combination that works for you.

Some people don't *want* to go to bed. Some of these are high-energy achievers or high-anxiety worriers who don't want to "waste time" sleeping. Some are having marriage problems. Some were abused in bed. It is important that you get to the root of your problem and deal with it. Find out what it is about going to bed that you don't like. Meditation and mindfulness, relaxation techniques, breathing exercises, and affirmations may help.

Rotating shift work is a severe sleep disruptor. Rotating shift workers experience more sleep-wake cycle disruption and nod off more at work. They have twice the odds of falling asleep while driving to or from work, and twice the odds of a reported accident or error related to sleepiness.[10] Daytime sleep and nighttime work are associated with endocrine dysfunctions.[11] This could mean that people with the genetic tendency to develop FMS could do so if they have to work shift work. One study of healthy young men found that they awoke feeling less rested if they slept in a 60 Hz magnetic field.[12] We need more research on this.

Anything that upsets the circadian rhythm, such as a change in time zones or the switch to daylight savings time, can significantly alter immune function.

One sleep expert, David Nye, M.D., has kindly given us permission to describe his plan to minimize sleep disruption during the time changes in the spring and fall. He suggests that you should begin to prepare a week or so before the time change goes into effect. In the fall when the clock moves back, start your night medications and bedtime preparations fifteen minutes or so earlier than usual, and increase the time by fifteen-minute increments until you are on a winter-time schedule. In the spring, a week before the clock moves forward, start your bedtime preparations and medications fifteen minutes later than you do in winter and increase the time by fifteen-minute increments until you are on daylight savings time. This will ease you into the change.

One study showed that the pillow you use may be as important as the bed. Proper selection of a pillow can significantly reduce pain and improve the quality of sleep.[13] You may need a number of pillows in assorted shapes and sizes to help you through the night.

Sleep Phenomena

There is no magic pill that will provide normal restorative sleep for us all. There are many coexisting conditions that can add to FMS and CMP sleep difficulty. Dealing effectively with any of these may improve your sleep considerably.

Sleep Apnea

Sleep apnea is not a significant cause of FMS symptoms in women. In men with FMS, sleep apnea is very common.[14] If you have sleep apnea of any type, you usually snore when you breathe in. Snoring is a sign of an incomplete obstruction. If breathing is blocked for more than ten seconds, snoring is followed by gasps and snorts as you try to get your breath back. This sign tells your sleeping partner that you either have sleep apnea or you are developing it. If you sleep alone, you may be totally unaware that this is happening. Sleep apnea must be taken seriously. It is a life-threatening condition. There is a continuous positive air pressure (CPAP) machine that ensures you continue to breathe if you have sleep apnea, even while you sleep. For those of us with FMS as well, having to hook up to CPAP can be a daunting prospect. The machine isn't quiet, and you are attached to it either with a mask over your face or with a tube that has little insertions that fit into your nasal passages.

Obstructive sleep apnea can sometimes be eased by removing some of the soft tissue in the area. This can now be done in the doctor's office. Somnoplasty shrinks the swollen tissue at the back of the throat and nasal cavity using radio frequency vibration. The treated tissue sloughs off naturally. Some coexisting conditions, such as obesity, can cause or worsen sleep apnea. Insulin resistance can also have an impact on sleep apnea.[15]

Restless leg syndrome (RLS) is a condition that occurs as you are trying to fall asleep. It is not the same as periodic leg movements. If you have RLS, you can't hold your legs still (see chapter 6). Restless leg syndrome can also begin with fasciculations; these are rapid-firing motor neurons that feel like mini-twitches. These may lead to bigger twitches. Restless Leg Syndrome becomes worse after you sit for long periods or if you become cold. You can relieve RLS by shaking or moving your legs, or by walking. Lying on a surface with many hairlike extensions, such as wool, also seems to help, although we don't know why. Ropinirole,[16] used in Parkinson's disease, has been of help to some people with RLS.

One person developed tremors when she woke up in the morning. She experienced head-to-toe shakes and muscle spasms all over throughout the day, even in her toes. Some people are okay until they stretch in the morning, and then the tremors take over. Sometimes, one limb will keep jerking for a while. RLS can involve the genital area.

A *hypnic jerk* is a sudden twitch of your whole body, which can occur in healthy people but may be more common in FMS because it indicates a high arousal state. Hypnic jerks also accompany anxiety states and indicate a need for relaxation. Some studies have found that if serotonin is inhibited (as it is in FMS), animals are able to learn to sleep without it, but they develop twitching muscles.[17]

Nocturnal cramps are often strong contractions of leg and foot muscles. You can sometimes relieve them by flexing your foot upward or by leaning forward against a wall with your feet flat. With CMP, any muscle can cramp. Electrical muscle stimulation and other bodywork may relieve this.

Perchance to Dream

Chronic pain states often cause more dreaming than normal. Some medications, and withdrawal from some medications, can cause nightmares. Nightmares and bizarre dreams usually take place in the second half of sleep during long REM periods. From what I have heard, people with FMS seem to have especially vivid dreams. They aren't necessarily bad dreams, just vivid. It may be hard to distinguish what occurred in dreams from what actually happened in your life. You may go to pick up a library book that you believe is on reserve, only to find that the library called you "in your dreams." Several people have told me that Flexeril seems to cut down on these dreams.

The changing balance of informational substances and the related shift of blood flow in the brain may help to shape your dreams.[18] One reader told me that her dreams would stick with her all day, along with their emotional components. When she had a sleep study done, she discovered she was in REM sleep most of the night.

If you are afflicted by recurring nightmares, try rewriting your script. Write down the details of the nightmare and then change them to program a positive outcome. Go over the new dream script a few times a day. Your dreams may change. Sleep terrors are different from nightmares. They are actually partial arousals from NREM sleep, similar to sleepwalking and to talking in your sleep. If you are able to program your dreams to some extent, you are part of the lucky 5 percent of the population with lucid dreams.[19] Lucid dreaming has great potential to correct bad habits and program your subconscious during sleep.

Sleep-Inducing Techniques

When you can't sleep, that's a good time to make a journal entry. Write down what you are feeling; you don't have to analyze it. The wee hours are a good time for meditation, breathing exercises, body scans, affirmations, and subliminal tapes. (See chapter 20.) Create a routine that prepares your body/mind for sleep. One hour before bedtime, unwind. Before this hour, make a list of your tasks for the next day. This will give you a head start. Then put the list where you have breakfast and forget it until tomorrow morning. Make sure you have the type of bed you need. Many people with FMS or CMP need a waterbed. There is no bed too soft for them. Some use a Select Comfort or other airbed. Some use futons. Some people need an especially hard mattress. Find out what works for you.

Fatigue

Over 75 percent of FMS patients in one study reported experiencing substantial fatigue.[20] It is hard for healthy people to understand what "substantial fatigue" means. They have never gone food shopping and had to leave their cart in the checkout lane to get to their car before they collapsed. Fatigue is common in CMP as well. There are many possible causes for fatigue. One cause is the lack of adequate, restorative sleep. Once the factors are changed to allow you to wake up feeling refreshed, fatigue often diminishes greatly. Paradoxical breathing is another common cause of fatigue: People with FMS and CMP are often oxygen starved. Proper, deep "belly" breathing must be restored, with the belly expanding with the inhale and contracting on the exhale. Trigger points in the respiratory muscles and accessory muscles may need attention. Lack of oxygen may also be caused by allergy, fluid retention, or microcirculation difficulties. You may also have chemical toxins and wastes that exhaust your body's ability to process them, and your body uses up a lot of energy in this process.

Fatigue can also stem from the constant effort to function in spite of your pain. The pain caused by the trigger points of chronic myofascial pain takes a lot of energy. Fatigue can also be a result of insulin resistance and reactive hypoglycemia, especially if you haven't been careful about your diet. Following the Barry Sears' "Zone" type diet with 30 percent of your calories coming from protein, 30 percent from fat, and 40 percent from carbohydrates often relieves this fatigue (see Appendix B). Avoiding excess carbohydrates is important to combat fatigue.

At least some of the fatigue in FMS may be due to your body's lack of usable fuel in the form of adenosine triphosphate (ATP). Some of this lack may be due to problems in your bowel function, including difficulties with absorption (see chapter 23). There are many steps in the process of creating energy, and if any of them lack a necessary biochemical, energy is not produced.

Now, take a moment to list your fatigue perpetuating factors. Some of them may include:

- Lack of restorative sleep • Stress • Pain • Overwork and lack of pacing • Lack of exercise • Emotional depression or suppression • Clutter in your life and surroundings • Frustrations • Sensory overload.

Fatigue is a challenge. Find out why you are fatigued and create a new world for yourself where those "whys" don't exist, or are modified. Pace yourself. Huge tasks that seem daunting can be divided into manageable pieces. Delegate, delete, or modify your tasks so that your life is more rewarding and fun. Don't be shy about asking for help.

Consult various members of your medical team. Check with your doctor, social worker, occupational or physical therapist, myotherapist, psychologist, or counselor. They may be able to supply other resources. Talk to your librarian. There is a world of books at your fingertips, waiting to help you. Solving at least some of your sleep and fatigue problems may ease your symptom load of pain and depression. If you cannot solve all of your problems, you can probably diminish the intensity of some of them.

Exciting new research has confirmed that "arousal biochemicals" have been identified as hypocretins (also called orexins). These biochemicals activate the HPA axis in rats.[21] Two independent groups of researchers have found that these peptides, which are secreted in the lateral hypothalamus, stimulate appetite and autonomic function, and are the physiological regulators of the arousal state.[22] This research holds great promise for future relief of insomnia, as well as for insights into FMS itself.

Endnotes

1. Irwin, M., J. McClintick, C. Costlow, M. Fortner, J. White, and J. C. Gillin. 1996. Partial night sleep deprivation reduces natural killer and cellular immune responses in humans. *FASEB J* (Federation of American Societies for Experimental Biology) 10(5):643-653.

2. Alvarez, A. 1995. *Night: Night Life, Night Language, Sleep and Dreams*. New York: W. W. Norton.

3. Vgontzas, A. N., G. Mastorakos, E. O. Bixter, A. Kales, P. W. Gold, and G. P. Chrousos. 1999. Sleep deprivation effects on the activity of the hypothalamus-pituitary-adrenal and growth axes: potential clinical implications. *Clin Endocrinol* (Oxford) 51(2):205-215.

4. Bennett, R. M., S. R. Clark, S. M. Campbell, and C. S. Burckhardt. 1992. Low levels of somatomedin C in patients with the fibromyalgia syndrome: a possible link between sleep and muscle pain. *Arthritis Rheum* 35(10):1113-1116.

5. Drewes, A. M., K. D. Nielson, S. J. Taagholt, K. Bjerregard, L. Svendsen, and J. Gade. 1995. Sleep intensity in fibromyalgia: focus on the micro-structure of the sleep process. *Br J Rheumatol* 34(7):629-635.

6. Dement, W. C., and C. Vaughan. 1999. *The Promise of Sleep*. New York: Delacorte Press, p. 85.

7. Wagner, D. R. 1996. Disorders of the circadian sleep-wake cycle. *Neurol Clin* 14(3):651-670.

8. Sachs, C., and E. Svanborg. 1991. The exploding head syndrome: polysomnographic recordings and therapeutic suggestions. *Sleep* 14(3):263-266.

9. Birkmayer, W., and P. Riederer. 1989. *Understanding the Neurotransmitters: Key to the Workings of the Brain*. Translated from German by Karl Blau. New York: Springerer-Verlag.

10. Gold, D. R., S. Rogacz, N. Bock, T. D. Tosteson, T. M. Baum, F. E. Speizer, et al. 1992. Rotating shift work, sleep, and accidents related to sleepiness in hospital nurses. *Am J Public Health* 82(7):1011-1014.

11. Weibel, L., M. Follenius, and G. Brandenberger. 1999. Biologic rhythms: their changes in night-shift workers. *Presse Med* 28(5):252-258. [French]

12. Graham, C., and M. R. Cook. 1999. Human sleep in 60 Hz magnetic fields. *Bioelectromagnetics* 20(5):277-283.

13. Lavin, R. A., M. Pappagallo, and K. V. Kuhlemeier. 1997. Cervical pain: a comparison of three pillows. *Arch Phys Med Rehabil* 78(2):193-198.

14. May, K. P., S. G. West, M. R. Baker, and D. W. Everett. 1993. Sleep apnea in male patients with the fibromyalgia syndrome. *Am J Med* 94(5):505-508.

15. Tiihonen, M., M. Partinen, and S. Narvanen. 1993. The severity of obstructive sleep apnea is associated with insulin resistance. *J Sleep Res* 2(1):56-61.

16. Estivill, E., and V. de la Fuente. 1999. [No title available]. *Rev Neurol* 28(10):962-963.

17. Charmes, W. 1976. *Some Must Watch While Some Must Sleep*. New York: San Francisco Book Co.

18. Hobson, J. A., R. Stickgold, and E. F. Pace-Schott. 1998. The neuropsychology of REM sleep dreaming. *NeuroReport* 9(3):R1-R14.

19. Charmes, W. 1976. *Op. cit.*

20. Hawley, D. J., and F. Wolfe. 1997. Fatigue and musculoskeletal pain. Myofascial pain–update in diagnosis and treatment. *Phys Med Rehab Clin North Am* 8(1):101-111.

21. Kura, M., Y. Ueta, R. Serino, M. Nakazato, Y. Yamamoto, I. Shibuya, et al. 2000. Centrally administered orexin/hypocretin activates HPA axis in rats. *Neuroreport* 11(9):1977-1980.

22. Samson, W. K., and Z. T. Resch. 2000. The hypocretin/orexin story. *Trends Endocrinol Metab* 11(7):257-262.

CHAPTER 11

Gender Issues

This chapter is about many of the ways your gender can affect your illnesses. This includes topics of sexuality. In this chapter, I use the medically incorrect medical term "sex" for "intercourse" at times. This is not because I want my OB/GYN friends to cringe. How many times of an evening has your partner snuggled up to you and whispered in your ear, "Wanna have coitus?"

Men and women react differently to medications. This came to light when the interactions of the antihistamine, Seldane, were found to be more dangerous to women than men. We now know that other medications, including antidepressants, are affected by gender.[1] Only recently have doctors become aware of these differences, which previously had largely been ignored. They must learn to prescribe accordingly. This is sometimes difficult because some studies on medications were done only on men.

A woman runs twice the risk of developing an irregular heartbeat than men do when they use medications that may cause this side effect. Aspirin thins a man's blood more easily than a woman's blood. Women can metabolize *some* drugs 20 percent to 50 percent faster than men.

For pain control, morphine works better in women than in men, but ibuprofen doesn't work as well for women. There appears to be both a genetic and gender-specific modulation of pain inhibition.[2] There is greater neuroendocrine response to stress in women than in men.[3] We don't yet know how much of these differences, if any, are amplified in fibromyalgia (FMS).

Women are more sensitive to pain than men. This does not mean that they complain more. They actually *experience* more pain with specific stimuli than men. This may be one of the reasons there are more women with FMS than men.[4]

Gender Issues for Men and Women

Some gender issues are of equal importance to both men and women. Some are not. This chapter begins with issues of equal importance to both sexes, moves to special issues that are of concern only to women, and ends with a discussion of special issues for men only.

Infertility in Men and Women

In FMS, the hypothalamic-pituitary-adrenal (HPA) axis is disturbed (see chapter 1). This imbalance can affect fertility profoundly in both men and women, because it affects the HPG (hypothalamus-pituitary-gonadal) axis.[5] It also affects the HPT (hypothalamic-pituitary-thyroid) axis and other axes, which, in turn, also affect the HPG axis.[6] This may seem terribly confusing. It's confusing to your doctors as well.

Any chronic pain condition can result in chronic stress. Chronic stress can cause failure to ovulate because of the interaction between the HPA and HPG axes.[7] We don't know what it might do to male fertility. There hasn't been enough research. We don't know the prevalence of infertility in people with FMS or chronic myofascial pain (CMP). It is important to remember that FMS patients are not homogenous; each of us has a unique biochemical mix. What may be true for some of us is not necessarily true for others. The affect of FMS on sexuality has implications for men as well as women, and we need more research to understand the impact of axes imbalances on both genders. There are no statistics on the prevalence of FMS among homosexuals.

One study on women with myofascial pain indicates that coexisting FMS is responsible for their lack of fertility and suggests that this may be due to the impact of dealing with chronic pain. The researchers did not understand that myofascial pain can be a widespread, chronic ailment, so that may be misleading.[8] A woman in chronic pain may decide to limit the size of her family and/or engage in sexual relations less often. In one study, myofascial pain patients with FMS did not differ from those without FMS on factors such as (a) trouble conceiving for twelve or more months, (b) previous consultation with a health care professional for trouble conceiving, or (c) irregular menses.

Some people have decided not to have children because of the fear that their children would experience the same symptoms. Often there is a great deal of guilt carried by parents with FMS and CMP who have children with the same conditions. Guilt does no one any good. Children with these conditions can do very well, especially with early diagnosis and treatment (see chapter 12).

There may be mechanical factors involved in infertility as well as biochemical ones. If you have both FMS and CMP and want to have children, be sure to deal with your perpetuating factors as well as you can. This includes a thorough check for pelvic area trigger points (TrPs). See "Special Issues for Women" and "Special Issues for Men" later in this chapter.

Melatonin may be a key factor in the regulation of seasonal variation in animal sexual activity. We don't know enough yet about its sexual impact on humans, although it is being studied. This is one reason why it is inadvisable to use melatonin in the nonadult population. Exposure to bright light, which suppresses the concentration of circulating melatonin, may be useful in treatment of both male and female infertility in couples with abnormal melatonin metabolism.[9] Guaifenesin, which some of us have found useful in FMS (see chapter 15), has been used to help women become pregnant. It thins the cervical secretions, which makes it easier for the sperm to penetrate the egg.[10]

Libido

The word "libido," as it is commonly used, means the desire to have sexual intercourse. This desire is strongly under the control of the hypothalamus. Some of us go through times when we have very strong sexual desires (especially earlier in the course of FMS), and then we drift into a time where we would "rather not bother."

You may feel undesirable at the very time you most need the reassurance and connection that intimacy can bring. Sexuality is the sum of how we see ourselves, as well as how we relate to others. When you have a runny nose, irritable bowel, irritable bladder, and water retention, sex may be the farthest thing from your mind. Teasing or offhand comments about weight, scars, or other physical "tender points" can put out the flame. Or it may be a case of, "Not tonight dear. I have a headache," and you *do* have a headache. Unexplained fatigue, lack of well-being, and diminished libido may be due to diminished testosterone in males and females. If plasma levels of *bioavailable* testosterone are low, these symptoms can be relieved by judicious administration of replacement testosterone.[11]

Chronic pain itself can decrease libido. While sexual intimacy is not confined to sexual intercourse, you may not even want to be touched. It is important to know if this feeling has a psychological basis or a medical one. Each of these categories may have a number of reasons. Tight and tender muscles may respond well to Valium or similar medication if you take them before having intercourse, but they could just as well put you to sleep. You may need specific TrP therapy to prevent pain that occurs during intercourse, and treatment of perpetuating factors for both FMS and CMP symptoms.

At times, sexual relations might cause extreme sensory overload. No, this hasn't been documented in medical studies. Yes, I have heard it hundreds of times from people with FMS and CMP. It doesn't always involve pain, but it can include a heightened sensitivity to noise and light, or at least a hyperarousal that leaves the patient with FMS wide awake all night, adrenaline racing, while their partner snores, blissfully unaware. You may have to give more attention to planning romantic interludes.

"I've Got You Under My Skin"

If you plan sexual encounters, your partner may feel that the spontaneity is gone from your relationship. But spontaneity can be elusive when you have to time your nightly medications carefully. This is especially true if you must take medications to fall sleep and they take a while to work.

You need to know ahead of time if your partner wishes some pre-sleep activity. This necessitates some form of communication an adequate time beforehand. People may need to plan ahead before they eat a dinner laced with garlic and onions, so keep a sense of humor when you deal with this issue. For successful *amore* a little sacrifice is worthwhile, yes? "Good sex" is only good sex if it is good for both of you. If one of you is taking a hypnotic and won't remember, it can still be good at the time, but it's even better if you both share the afterglow the next day. Memories are a part of good times, too, and they help to cement a relationship. Looking forward to a romantic evening can be a trip in itself: sexual intercourse can be a profound stress reliever. It can help rebalance the neurotransmitters—sort of like a reset button in a fuse box. Hans Selye used to say that it was the greatest stress reliever of all times, and he was the doctor who defined the word "stress" to mean what it does today.

Talk with your doctor. There are some medications commonly given to patients with FMS and CMP that can interfere with desire. Talk about your medicinal and nonmedicinal options. If specific TrPs or other conditions are causing painful intercourse, there may be remedies. If you lack desire, there may also be remedies. Again, it may come down to checking into your perpetuating factors. If you can get those under control as much as possible, you have a better chance of having your libido return. It is important for you and your partner to mutually support each other and work on ways to help this happen. If you have a spiritual connection as individuals and as a couple, that can be a tremendous help while you explore your options. Also, a good marriage counselor who understands the problem of chronic pain can make a world of difference to your relationship.

The inability to have an erection can happen to any man, but when you are also dealing with possible myofascial trigger points of CMP plus the vascular instabilities of FMS, the stress factor can be considerable. Some medications can contribute to impotence. Men with FMS and CMP can find intercourse painful, too. Talk to your doctor about your options. The answer isn't always a pill. Get those TrPs checked out (see chapter 8), and handle the perpetuating factors.

When Intercourse Is Painful

Painful intercourse can happen for men as well as women. Medically, it is called dyspareunia, and it can be caused by a variety of sources. Make sure any possible physical contributors are remedied as thoroughly as possible. It almost goes without saying that painful intercourse dampens desire.

If you are having internal TrP work done using topical anesthetic, remember that it will numb the area for a while, not just stop pain during treatment. I know of one couple that used a topical anesthetic as a lubricant. Perhaps it was a "fibromoment." It certainly didn't become a passionate one.

Good, clear, and compassionate communication is important in any relationship, but even more so when chronic pain is a "third partner." Can you freely tell your partner what it is you want sexually? What it is you need? If you are experiencing difficulties with intercourse, you may be hesitant to bring up yet one more symptom. Your partner may already sense that you are not enjoying sex, and s/he may be concerned about causing you pain. Talk about it. Positions or movements may have to be changed to permit orgasms to take place. This may take willingness to experiment.

Some people may be able to have intercourse without pain, but may be unable to have an orgasm. Others may find that it is pleasant to cuddle at times, but their partners don't understand that intimacy needn't always be foreplay. This can lead to frustration for both partners. Listen up! It is possible to hug, snuggle, kiss, and otherwise show affection without it being a form of foreplay. (Am I talking to the men out there?) Massaging each other can be a sharing, loving part of intimacy. Your healthy partner may even discover that s/he has an unsuspected TrP or two, or at least an area of tension that a loving massage can relieve. We all have stressors and massage is a wonderful way to relieve them, show affection, and to communicate.

Afterglow?

After sexual relations, you may be left with more than a sleepy smile and a warm sigh of contentment. Some people experience increased pain in the back and legs. This is usually caused by the activation of myofascial TrPs. Adequate treatment of the TrPs should help. A daily home stretching program is very important.

Some people with FMS feel very weak after sex. They may be unable to rise from bed to use the bathroom. They may also experience intense heat sensations. Perhaps the normal skin flushing after intercourse is amplified due to heightened FMS sensitivity. Again, there are no studies on this, just lots of comments. A few people, men and women, have mentioned that intercourse sets off abdominal TrPs. I have also heard of four cases where the woman was hypersensitive to her husband's semen. In two of these cases, FMS treatment with guaifenesin eventually resulted in the ability to have intercourse without protection. In the other two cases, the woman did not try guaifenesin therapy, and continued to use protection.

Intercourse-induced headaches are generally benign, meaning they are not caused by any specific pathology. The use of the word "benign" does not mean that the headache is any less unpleasant. This condition generally involves TrPs as part of the muscular component. Physical activity, such as sex, can activate TrPs. This means that you need to get rid of the TrPs (remember, this is not the same as letting them become latent). Latent TrPs are like time bombs waiting to go off, and the trigger can occur at the worse possible time—right before orgasm. The other component of this type of headache is vascular. Changes in the blood vessels occur when your heart is racing and your blood is pounding. Soon after orgasm, when your blood pressure lowers, the headache begins.

Headache triggered by sexual intercourse is usually localized at the back of the head, in the lower part of the skull, although sometimes your whole head can hurt. A beta-blocker like propranolol may help prevent this headache. Again, adequate timing is essential. You need to take the pill so that it can act before you do.

Special Issues for Women

Dryness of the mucosal membranes may be a cause of pain during intercourse and is often evident to both partners. Dryness may have many causes, although it is more common during and after menopause. This may be eased by water-based lubrication (ask your pharmacist for suggestions). Hormone replacement therapy may help.

Chronic pelvic congestion can cause long-term pelvic pain. This may be hormonal, but it may be circulatory, as well. This can result in pelvic varicose veins. Medical treatment is based upon hormone therapy acting upon venous receptors.[12] At least some of the circulatory congestion may be due to myofascial entrapment of nerves. This can be treated with myofascial release, myotherapy, and craniosacral release therapies. Anything that adds to the congestion of the pelvic area, such as vaginal or abdominal infections, can add to a bloated feeling. Trigger points often will cascade, with TrP activation spreading down your legs, across your abdomen and back. This may happen monthly with your menstrual period. It is important to keep fluid passages open and functional.

Breast-Related Symptoms

Galactorrhea is a discharge from your breast, usually whitish or greenish, and it can be frightening. It is important to call your doctor if you have this symptom because it may indicate malignancy, but it may be due to other causes. It may indicate too much estrogen in your bloodstream. It can be caused by a tumor on your pituitary gland. It can even be a side effect of tricyclic antidepressants, antihypertensive medication, some tranquilizers and stimulants. Hypothyroidism is a common cause as well. In half of the cases, there is no traceable cause.

Large, pendulous breasts are a perpetuating factor for myofascial TrPs. "Patients with large heavy breasts not only suffer from compression of the tissues across the shoulders by tight bra straps, but they commonly have bras that exert constricting pressure around the chest that makes deep indentations in the skin. This can aggravate and perpetuate pectoralis major TrPs."[13] I quote this because some readers have indicated that their doctors (or more likely their insurance companies) don't believe them. Heavy breasts can promote a head-forward, round-shouldered posture. In most cases, there are specific exercises (see chapter 19) such as the in-doorway stretch that can help, and special bras that may relieve pressure. In some cases, breast reduction surgery for may be a viable option, but it is not to be done lightly. It is a major surgical operation, and changes the whole balance of your body. (For those women who have large pendulous breasts in

Costrochondritis means "inflammation of the rib area," but it is often a misnomer applied to any pain in the rib areas. Two women who were diagnosed with this condition corresponded with me. When they stopped wearing underwire bras, the condition disappeared. Most likely the pain was due to TrPs. One of these women had been given several antibiotics, wiht no test to verify that there was infection present. She had developed a severe yeast infection from the antibiotics, and was in misery from the misdiagnosis and subsequent mistreatment.

need of support and who are sensitive to synthetics, see Decent Exposures in the Appendix A, Products.)

Fibrocystic breasts are often linked with FMS, but I believe that they may be due to TrPs constricting the milk ducts. There is increasingly strong evidence that, especially with FMS, the central nervous system can induce myofascial TrP activity. The smooth muscles of the breast around the ducts have motor endplates, so there is no reason for them not to have TrPs that would block the flow similar to skeletal muscle.[14]

There is a new method for breast cancer screening that is gentler and more accurate than mammography. Cancer cells are warmer than the surrounding area, because they pump out nitric oxide. This can be measured by the BioScan System photodetector.[15] It doesn't use ionizing radiation like mammograms and it is not painful or even uncomfortable. Mammograms can hurt and if the patient has FMS and CMP, they *do* hurt. The BioScan is very new, and your local hospital probably doesn't have one. There are some things you can do, however, to ensure minimum aggravation during a mammogram. Make sure you have any pectoral TrPs treated before mammography. You may need some extra medication beforehand as well. Concern about pain should not prevent you from having this important diagnostic test. Be sure to tell the mammography technician that you have FMS and CMP and explain that might mean a little extra gentleness is required.

Trigger points can cause phantom limb pain in remaining myofascia. This is true after mastectomy as well. I know of several patients who have experienced this who were relieved by proper TrP therapy and, in one case, by TrP injection of scar areas. Much of the range of motion for arms and neck may also be regained if the TrPs are properly treated. Vodder manual lymph drainage (see chapter 5) may greatly help *lymphedema*, which may occur if lymph nodes have been removed.

Genital Symptoms

Pain in the external female genitalia is called vulvodynia. There are many possible contributory causes of this, including myofascial TrPs. The Vulvar Pain Foundation (see Resources) has a newsletter for women who experience pain in this area. They have found that a low oxalate diet may help ease this pain. A diet low in oxalates would avoid spinach, sorrel, tofu, peanut butter, cocoa, baked beans, green beans, beets, chives, celery, sweet potatoes, parsley, summer squash, grits, soybeans, and citrus peel.

A precancerous condition called *lichen sclerosis* may cause pain, soreness, and even bleeding in the vaginal area for days after intercourse. This condition may occur at any age, and may go unrecognized unless a doctor knows what it looks like. It may also cause itching. It has a typical ivory or other light discoloration accompanied by edema, inflammation, and fibrosis, and may be also accompanied by atrophy and erosion.[16] If bodywork, guaifenesin therapy, and other treatments create acid urine (see chapter 15), it would be wise to prevent irritation of the contact areas of the back of the vulva by using a protective lotion. I may be taken to task for this recommendation, because this is connection has not been proven (yet), but if I can save one person from cancer, or even from painful intercourse, I willingly accept the slings and arrows from a few critics. I don't write books for them.

Premenstrual Syndrome

Remembering that FMS can amplify all sensations, it makes sense that life can seem intolerable for some FMS women who suffer from premenstrual syndrome (PMS). Like FMS, PMS seems to be a neuroendocrine imbalance.[17] The hormonal shifts disrupt multiple brain centers, and your life. The physical symptoms, which include bloating, nausea, and water retention, can be coupled with an emotional roller-coaster ride that can include mood swings which have you crying one minute and screaming the next. You can experience free-floating anxiety that feels like impending doom, or suicidal desires, even though everything in your life is rosy, except your neurotransmitters. You may even react differently to medications at this time.

It has been shown that ovarian steroids have direct effects on neurotransmission.[18] This research was a pilot study, which means it was small, but it showed that PMS patients had reduced sensitivity to benzodiazepine medications. Immediately before the menstrual period estrogen and progesterone levels fall rapidly. It may be that the fall causes at least some of the symptoms of PMS, rather than the levels of the hormones themselves.

If you have PMS, I strongly recommend the book *Screaming to Be Heard*, by Elizabeth Lee Vliet, M.D. Barry Sears, in *The Anti-Aging Zone*, mentions that about 5 to 10 percent of childbearing-age women have severe PMS, and that the Zone diet helps them. Hormone replacement therapy (HRT) is one option that is, itself, many options.

Hormone Replacement Therapy (HRT)

There are many kinds of HRT and there have been many books written about it. It is hard to believe that so many women are still automatically given a "standard" preparation of horse hormones. Often there is no testing to see what hormones were lacking in what proportion. Estriol is routinely used in Europe for menopausal symptoms. Progestins, often prescribed in the United States, are not the same as natural progesterone. The human body does not know how to use progestins.[19]

Estrogen therapy is a double-edged sword. Estrogens raise glucose levels, which might add to the risk of insulin resistance. They boost sodium levels and may increase fluid retention. Progesterone regulates temporary water retention. There appears to be a significant subgroup of women whose sexual difficulties respond initially to estrogen replacement therapy but who subsequently revert to their initial problems, especially when the problem has been a loss of libido. For these women, the addition of androgen has proved helpful.[20] Some of these women do well with DHEA, which converts to testosterone. Lack of estrogen has a significant effect on carbohydrate and lipid metabolism.[21]

Sex steroids have potent effects on mood, memory, and mental state in humans.[22] In some studies, menopausal women experienced enhanced short- and long-term memory and learning capacity with estrogen replacement therapy.[23] Some women may be unable to absorb oral estrogen, which may mean that some research is skewed. Human estrogen is a complex biochemical that is made up of the following three components:

- Estriol   1.0 mg

- Estrone   0.25 mg

- Estradiol   0.25 mg

A compounding pharmacist can formulate this in a transdermal (topical) preparation. This mixture at 0.1 cc per day, days 1 through 25 of your cycle, is roughly equivalent to human estrogen. Progesterone transdermal cream can be added on days 12 through 25, if you need it. Progesterone may cause greater insulin resistance. I've observed that there is a subset of women with FMS who can't tolerate progesterone.

Menstruation

Some women report that FMS symptoms worsen dramatically during their period. They are more sensitive to heat, cold, light, noise, and other stimuli at those times. There are frequent reports of irregular blood flow, cramping, membranous discharge, often with blood clots, and occasional extreme blood flow. This is not surprising, due to the HPG axis imbalances in FMS. It *is* surprising to me that there aren't more studies on this. But it happens, with regularity, because I'm told about it. When I mention it in talks, women recognize it. Their doctors need to know about it.

Painful menstrual periods should *never* be accepted as something you have to live with! There may be perpetuating factors, such as endocrine imbalance (get that thyroid checked!), or contributing myofascial TrPs that can be remedied. No woman should have her whole life shaped by the tyranny of painful menses. The pain can be pervasive, and can last long enough that the effects of one period are not over before the premenstrual symptoms of the next period start.

I am not writing from medical references. I am writing from memory. That memory resonates with every letter I have received on this. It is virtually impossible to concentrate in school or at work while you are being skinned alive from the inside. The combination of activated TrPs and FMS amplification of menstrual pain can be overwhelming. The pain and accompanying nausea can be so severe you vomit. This happened to me during a chemistry final exam. I had to leave the examination room and was not allowed to return to finish the test. I couldn't explain the intensity of the symptoms then, and no one would have believe me if I had tried. Teachers must learn to understand. This type of abuse is not acceptable.

You may have hormonally activated migraines. Your weight may swing wildly (even from hour to hour), and you may need to have several sizes of clothing in your closet. The bra that fits in the morning may cut into you cruelly in the afternoon. Of course, during all this, you look just fine, and people expect you to behave accordingly. You may also experience "mittelschmirtz," which is pain during the time of ovulation. It isn't unusual to be able to tell which ovary is ovulating, due to the activation of TrPs. You may experience TrP-related pain shooting down your legs, as well as other myofascial activation. Diet can figure prominently in these symptoms, as can sleep and other perpetuating factors. If your daughter is going through this ordeal, speak up in a parent-teacher conference. Make sure the teacher understands. Get those perpetuating factors addressed and get an experienced myotherapist or myofascial release therapist to work on the TrPs. Ensure that there is adequate medication on hand to allow function. This pain can be enough to drive someone to suicide. It must be taken seriously.

The menstrual cycle affects the number of FMS tender points. One study showed that the number of tender points by palpitation was greater *after* the menstrual cycle as compared to during menstruation, but not in users of oral contraceptives.[24] There is also a change in the pattern of pain and other symptoms related to FMS.[25]

Body temperature, bile pigments, neurotransmitter production, thyroid and adrenal hormone production, red and white blood cell counts, fluid balance, respiration, acid/alkaline blood values, brain wave patterns, heart rate and rhythm, balance, fine motor coordination, pupil size and reactivity, platelet counts, blood protein levels, blood levels of adrenaline, body weight, basal metabolism rate, galvanic skin resistance, memory and concentration, pain threshold, energy levels and sleep patterns, pulmonary vital capacity, visual/auditory/olfactory acuity, and many other values are influenced by the changing menstrual cycle.[26] This can make research exciting. It also casts a shadow on research done in the past, which rarely took these effects into consideration.

There are times when the pains of a period can be relieved by heat or ice on your back or legs or groin. If this is the case for you, TrPs may be at work, and you need to do more tennis ball work and stretching daily, especially between your periods. You may need to carefully review your perpetuating factors. I have heard from several doctors and patients that the low-dose Climera patch can help hormonally induced migraines. If you are irritated by regular commercial menstrual pads and cannot tolerate tampons, Glad Rags offers a natural cotton alternative (see Appendix A, under Products).

Infertility Issues for Women

Pregnancy and infertility may be affected by torsion of the pelvis, according to my observations and those of others in the field. This is often caused by myofascial TrPs. Often, when the pelvis is stabilized, the patient will be able to get pregnant. I have not seen anything in the medical literature on this, but those women who wish to become pregnant need to know about this treatment option. Also, insulin resistance may cause decreased fertility.[27]

Pregnancy

Some women already stressed by FMS or CMP also struggle with the formidable demands of pregnancy. This is a time in their lives when women most need support, yet most of the medications that can help them deal with difficult FMS and CMP symptoms are not safe for pregnant or lactating women. Even NSAIDs (non-steroidal anti-inflammatory drugs) such as ibuprofen are not recommended for use during pregnancy. During the third trimester, salicylates and NSAIDs should be avoided because they can delay the onset of labor, as well as increasing the danger of bleeding. Some pregnant patients have reported that Inderal helped their pain.

If you are thinking of becoming pregnant, consult your doctor. It may be necessary to go off medication three months before conception, to ensure that your developing child is not harmed. If you plan on nursing your baby, you also may be required to stay off medications until your child is weaned. Explore your nonmedicinal options. Make sure your doctor is familiar with both FMS and CMP. Have a good bodyworker nearby, watch your diet, and pay attention to your sleep habits, mindwork, exercise, and stretching routines. Make sure that your support structure is online and functioning at peak efficiency.

Studies[28] indicate that stress response biochemicals from the pregnant woman can lead to later HPA axis imbalance and coping problems in the child (see chapter 12). This is a time when all your coping skills should be working at full force. Focus on mindwork, gentle exercise like t'ai chi, and gather as much support and happiness as you can at this time.

The HPA axis response changes during pregnancy and lactation. These are times of prolonged physiological changes affecting neuroendocrine and immunological systems, yet stress doesn't affect you as strongly during these times.[29] This may be part of the reason many women feel that their FMS gets so much better during pregnancy.

If you are on thyroid supplementation, it may need to be increased during pregnancy. Late pregnancy may be a time of rising concentrations of several diabetogenic hormones, and increased insulin resistance,[30] so if you have reactive hypoglycemia, be extra strict about following a balanced, healthy diet.

One woman said her FMS went into remission for most of her pregnancy but that in the last few months, it returned with a vengeance. When it came back, the headaches, depression, and pain were particularly severe. This is not unusual. Many readers have reported partial remission of FMS symptoms during pregnancy, but they also reported they went into flare after the birth of their child. Trigger points can worsen during pregnancy, as your body changes to accommodate the added burden. One study[31] indicated that the gluteus medius TrPs may cause hip pain in the later stages of pregnancy and also may simulate the pain of sciatica (see chapter 8). Several women noted that they experienced more joint pains during the night. These pains were mostly in their shoulders, hips, and knees. They had to use extra pillows to prop themselves up and to maintain comfortable positions.

Some of these women complained of sacroiliac joint dysfunction. These "joint" pains may often be TrP-referred pain and can be treated with gentle physical therapy. The unusual muscle tensions due to differently distributed weight during pregnancy can force your muscles and joints into displaced positions. The sacroiliac joint, especially, can then become locked in place. For proper functioning and for an easier delivery, it must be mobilized again. This can be accomplished with specific bodywork and maintained with stretching. One woman found that if she got on her hands and knees, the developing babies (twins) hung away from her vertebrae and she got relief from the pains that had been troubling her.

Great care must be taken to avoid sternocleidomastoid and gluteus minimus TrPs. (See Figs. 8-2 and 8-31 in chapter 8.) There is the added danger of falling because of the dizziness and imbalance that these TrPs cause. Pregnancy and resultant changes in weight distribution can magnify these problems. Be aware of foot slap, foot drop, buckling knee, and buckling ankle TrPs. If you start to feel as if you are falling over your own feet, take action and get some bodywork.

During pregnancy, your quality of sleep changes. So does your dreaming. Often there is an increase in dreaming, including the appearance of many dreams that deal with body changes. You also may need to take more naps as you may feel sleepier during the first two trimesters. Starting in the fifth month, fetal movements can disturb your sleep, so sleep when you can. Body changes in late pregnancy, such as bladder pressure and an inability to assume your preferred sleep position, may further impact the depth and quality of your slumber. Insomnia may worsen, especially in the last trimester. You may need to use body pillows to get comfortable. Sleeping in the fetal position, with your legs drawn up, can perpetuate the psoas TrPs, and back pain with psoas involvement is common in pregnancy. You may need to place a small pillow under your knees when sleeping on your back, or between your knees when lying on your side. Special bands, such as Mother-to-Be (see Mother Wear in Appendix A, under Products), can help support the weight of your developing baby when you are standing or sitting. During normal pregnancy your total body water increases by six to eight liters, four to six liters of which are extracellular, and at least two to three liters are interstitial (see chapter 5). This is due to changes in hydration of your connective tissue ground substance.[32] If you are beginning a pregnancy with pre-existing edema, insulin resistance, or diabetes, these conditions must be monitored very closely.

Nighttime leg cramps can increase during pregnancy. One woman found that she had less of a problem with leg cramps if she consumed a small amount of milk and cheese before going to bed, but not enough to cause reflux. Other women have reported that extra calcium and magnesium decreased or eliminated the leg cramps. Restless leg syndrome often becomes worse with pregnancy, especially at night. Reflux also may get worse and may start early in pregnancy. Avoid eating two to four hours before going to bed. Use gentle finger acupressure on contributing TrPs in the area under your breastbone. Some women have reported that fresh lemon juice diluted with water and taken as soon as they get out of bed helps to curb morning sickness. Ginger or mint tea may also help diminish nausea. Trigger points may be involved in perpetuating or increasing nausea (see chapter 8), and should be treated promptly.

Pregnancy-induced hypertension is the most common complication of pregnancy. Insulin resistance can cause this.[33] Heat-intolerance may be a problem during pregnancy. This has not been documented, but it is logical. People generate heat, and the tiny being growing inside generates heat, too. Since heat intolerance is not uncommon in FMS, it may be magnified during pregnancy.

I have had many letters and emails (more than twenty in the last five years) concerning pregnancies lasting ten months in women with FMS. All delivered healthy children. I know of at least two women of Asian-American ancestry who have arranged their current pregnancy to allow for another possible ten-month gestation. They wanted to be sure that their baby was born in the Year of the Dragon. They have each had one baby with a ten-month gestation, have FMS, read my book, and wanted to ensure their present child was born under this sign of good fortune. Yes, I know. There is no medical literature on FMS and ten-month pregnancies. Do you want to argue with a dragon?

Ripening of the cervix, which occurs before labor begins, requires the cervical collagen to change from highly organized and tightly bound to a much looser arrangement. This allows the tissue to become more compliant and is associated with profound changes in the composition of the ground substance.[34] When FMS and CMP are present and the ground substance is involved, as we have discussed in previous chapters, don't expect changes to proceed normally.

A ten-month gestation period may also be related to altered hormone levels, other FMS biochemical irregularities, or even to myofascial tightening. Serotonin is one of the hormones that start the delivery process. Relaxin, another pregnancy hormone (see chapter 15), also may be involved. This hormone eases the tension in the pelvic floor muscles, allowing the opening to widen enough for the baby's head to pass through. Your hips must angle forward and go into extra extension for delivery. A woman whose hips are locked in flexion (which is a condition all too common to both sexes) is likely to have trouble during delivery.[35]

Labor of Love

If FMS and CMP are part of your life, common sense would indicate that you may need pain medication earlier in labor than a healthy woman and you may also need something to start the labor. Some healthy patients develop *tachycardia* (usually defined as a heartbeat rate of over 100 beats per minute) during pregnancy and this symptom may also occur in FMS. A little extra monitoring in the labor room may be warranted. Myofascial pain can exist during pregnancy and exceed the analgesia provided by an epidural for labor. Trigger point injections, even when used with a functioning epidural infusion, can be a valuable aid for providing complete analgesia during labor,[36] and can prevent TrPs from lingering to complicate the postpartum period.

After Birth

Many patients initially thought to have postdural puncture headache may actually have postpartum cervical myofascial pain.[37] In addition, 10 to 28 percent of women are affected by an intense emotional response commonly called *postpartum depression*. There are as yet no studies that show the percentage of women with FMS who develop this condition. Postpartum depression can include crying, confusion, fatigue, depression, insomnia, difficulty caring for the baby and yourself, and even suicidal thoughts.[38] Right after giving birth, women are at increased risk for HPA and hypothalamic pituitary thyroidal axes dysfunction.[39] This last study indicates to me the need for more research on FMS mothers.

A critical period may occur right after you return home with your baby, especially if you and your child leave hospital care quickly. Around-the-clock new baby care disrupts anyone's sleep. You must recover from labor and delivery with all the stresses and new TrPs that may have resulted. Your hormones are fluctuating and your usual routines are disrupted. It is no surprise that many deliveries are followed by an FMS flare response. Many new mothers who have both FMS and CMP need much greater life support. Talk to your bodyworker in advance to learn how to lift an infant without hurting your body. Good habits will save you when your little one is no longer so little.

Because having a new baby at home is usually an exercise in sleep deprivation, it may be difficult for a mother with FMS and CMP to breast-feed. The usual FMS and CMP medications get into breast milk. If you are breast-feeding your infant, before resuming any medications after delivery, first check with your doctor.

Some women reported a problem I have not seen in the literature. These women nursed their babies and at first everything went fine. Then, after three or four weeks, the milk flow seemed to slow or stop. One mother reported that if she closed her eyes and concentrated on the process, the milk flow improved. Some women increased their fluid intake and others tried massage. Most were able to resume nursing.

One study showed that mice lacking norepinephrine and epinephrine exhibited impaired mothering instincts. Norepinephrine, a neurotransmitter, is responsible for long-lasting changes that promote maternal behavior during both development and parturition in mice.[40] Mothers, if you don't develop the normal healthy bonding and maternal instinct for your child, tell your doctor. If you feel anger or resentment that is out of control when your baby cries or needs attention, *you* get attention—immediately. The demands of a new baby can stress anyone. Fibromyalgia amplifies stress. Please don't take your frustration out on your child. Talk to your doctor right away. You may only need a friend to come over and give you a break once in a while. You may need medication. If you are nursing, you may have to stop, but your neurotransmitters—and your emotions—*must* be brought under control. I have no medical studies to back up my feeling that some FMS mothers may harm their children. I *have* talked to FMS mothers who have lost their children due to neglect or abuse. It isn't common, but even one is one too many. Lack of control may be neurotransmitter-related and must be treated. This is not the time for a blame-game, or for feelings of guilt. Recognize your feelings and get help.

Menopause and Perimenopause

Technically, menopause begins after your period has ended for a year. This doesn't occur overnight. Menopause is preceded by perimenopause, when you aren't in full menopause yet, but your periods are sporadic, and your hormones fluctuate like a spinning top running down, wobbling this way and that, and causing no end of symptoms. The perimenopausal phase can last as long as ten years and can begin very early. Some women enter perimenopause in their middle thirties.

The wild hormonal swings of perimenopause produce hot flashes, night sweats, irritability, dryness of the vagina, loss of libido, and osteoporosis. Some women with FMS start menopause very early. Menopause resulting from the removal of your ovaries may start abruptly, even though other parts of your body still produce estrogen.

It is important to find out exactly what your hormone levels are before you consider hormone replacement therapy (HRT), and then the hormones should be replaced to your normal level. Effects of estrogen decline include vaginal burning, pain with intercourse, recurrent bladder infections, urethral infection, recurrent vaginal infections, incontinence, painful urination, urinary frequency, or urinary urgency. If you have adequate replacement therapy and these symptoms still occur, check into the possibilities of TrPs and get treatment. It isn't unusual for my myotherapist to restore function to people who are incontinent.

Although hot flashes can last up to five years for most postmenopausal women, some have hot flashes for fifteen years. Hot flashes tend to last longer and be more severe in surgically menopausal women.[41] Insomnia can be intensified by hot flashes, because they certainly can wake you up. Hormone replacement therapy, properly balanced, may provide relief. Another promise of relief for those with hot flashes is gabapentin.[42] Patients experienced an average 87-percent reduction in the frequency of hot flashes.

Hot flashes result from a temporary lowering of the body's hypothalamic temperature regulatory set point. This results in a sudden perception of heat and the activation of cooling processes, such as sweating and dilation of blood vessels. This may be caused by overactivity of brain cells in this area. Gabapentin may decrease the cellular activity in the hypothalamus. It is sometimes given to patients with FMS to reduce central nervous system sensitization. Another possible remedy is Paxil. A pilot trial indicated that it helped with hot flashes in breast cancer survivors.[43]

Many postmenopausal women find their symptoms are eased by androgen therapy. If tests indicate a low bioavailable circulating testosterone level, replacement therapy may ease fatigue, restore libido, and improve the sense of well-being.[44]

Special Issues for Men

I apologize that this "special issue" section for men is so small compared to the women's section, but one reason is that women have to deal with a lot of special issues. The other reason is that there hasn't been a lot of research done on men in this area.

We don't know what effects some medications have on patients who wish to father a child. Studies on fertility in males have mostly been done on animals. Not enough physicians recognize that FMS is a problem for men, too. Men often get short shrift when it comes to FMS and research, although there are now fewer doctors insisting that FMS is the hysterical complaint of middle-aged women and men don't get it. Men also have specific myofascial pain issues that can be terribly destructive to their quality of life. Some researchers who have studied FMS in men have found that male FMS patients have fewer symptoms and fewer tender points, and less common "hurt all over" fatigue, morning fatigue, and IBS, compared with female patients.[45] They found significant differences between men and women in the number of tender points.

Sleep apnea is very common in men with FMS, and no more so in women with FMS than in healthy women (see chapter 10). We don't know why this is so. One doctor found that 34 percent of his total FMS patients were men. He found that his male patients responded more to behavior modification or to a change in their work conditions than to medications, unlike his women patients.[46]

The over-the-counter supplement yohimbine is sometimes taken to increase libido. It can have profound effects on the heart. It can also severely worsen cases of anxiety and panic, and should not be used by men with posttraumatic stress disorder.[47]

Myofascial pain can often mimic or contribute to prostate pain. Any surgical intervention in the thigh or groin area can result in myofascial entrapment pain that mimics prostate pain. In one study, continuous pain in the testes, groin, and inside the thigh and knee after surgical intervention was attributed to myofascial pain.[48]

Impotence

Sexual dysfunction in men with FMS may be due in part to the need to improve communication between hormones. Men, your sex urge starts in the hypothalamus. Surprised? You need this gland to do its thing before an erection can take place. Many medications, such as serotonin reuptake inhibitors (SSRIs), antihistamines, and reflux medications such as Tagamet, Pepcid, Axid, and Zantac can interfere with the action of these nerve impulses and block the action.[49] Another major cause of impotence is lack of blood flow to the genital area, because the penis works by hydraulics. Impotence may occur in men with type II diabetes and in men with hypertension who are taking diuretics or beta-blockers that increase insulin. Reactive hypoglycemia and insulin resistance are steps on the way to type II diabetes. Watch your diet. Those extra car-bohydrates could block your way to sexual fulfillment. Then there are (you guessed it) myofascial TrPs.

Impotence Occurring Secondary to Myofascial Trigger Points

The following information is taken from *Myofascial Pain and Dysfunction: The Trigger Point Manual, Volume II*, by Janet G. Travell and David G. Simons.[50] I include page references because so many patients have told me that their doctors "don't believe" that this is in the *Trigger Point Manual*s. It is. Read it again, docs!

This information is, by necessity, technical. You can take it to your urologist, say, "See!" and then get a prescription for some specific trigger point myotherapy. Impotence is *not* just part of getting older.

To understand how impotence can occur secondary to myofascial TrPs, it is necessary to understand the basic anatomy of the region. Both the bulbospongiosus and ischiocavernosus muscles enhance erection of the penis. These muscles can develop TrPs. The bulbospongiosus essentially wraps around the corpus spongiosum of the penis, which is the central erectile structure through which the urethra passes. The anterior and middle fibers of the bulbospongiosus and ischiocavernosus muscles contribute to erection by reflex and voluntary contraction that compresses the erectile tissue of the bulb of the penis and also its dorsal vein. Contraction of the ischiocavernosus muscle maintains and enhances penile erection by retarding the return of blood through the penis. Trigger points in the bulbospongiosus muscle can cause impotence.[51] Trigger points in scar tissue produced by surgical incision are well-known.[52] Trigger points in the pelvic floor muscles are sometimes activated by surgery in the pelvic region.[53]

The piriformis is a major intrapelvic muscle, which is a frequent site of TrPs. The nerves and blood vessels that pass through the greater sciatic foramen along with the piriformis are subject to myofascial entrapment.[54] Exiting the pelvis along the lower border of the piriformis are the pudendal nerve and blood vessels. The pudendal nerve innervates the bulbocavernosus, ischiocavernosus, and sphincter urethrae membranacea muscles and the skin and corpus cavernosus of the penis. Innervation of these structures is essential to normal sexual function.[55] "Patients may complain of . . . sexual dysfunction."[56] "Pudendal nerve entrapment may cause impotence in men."[57] The piriformis TrP is most commonly found with a complex of other TrPs.[58] This is a complex area with multiple layered muscles and opportunities for entrapment. After a surgical procedure, such as a hernia repair, a regimen of stretches can often help prevent adhesions and TrPs.

Endnotes

1. Kornstein S. G., A. F. Schatzberg, M. E. Thase, K. A. Yonkers, J. P. McCullough, G. I. Keitner, et al. 2000. Gender differences in treatment response to sertraline versus imipramine in chronic depression. *Am J Psychiatry* 157(9):1445-1452.

2. Mogil, J. S., S. P. Richards, L. A. O'Toole, M. L. Helms, S. R. Mitchell, B. Kest, et al. 1997. Identification of a sex-specific quantitative trait locus mediating nonopioid stress-induced analgesia in female mice. *J Neurosci* 17(20):7995-8002.

3. Jezova, D., E. Jurankova, A. Mosnarova, M. Kriska, and I. Skultetyova. 1996. Neuroendocrine response during stress with relation to gender differences. *Acta Neurobiol Exp (Warsz)* 56(3):779-985.

4. Mense, S., and D. G. Simons. 2000. *Muscle Pain: Understanding Its Nature, Diagnosis and Treatment*. Baltimore: Lippincott, Williams and Wilkins p. 3.

5. Hendrick, V., M. Gitlin, L. Altshuler, and S. Korenman. 2000. Antidepressant medications, mood and male fertility. *Psychoneuroimmunology* 25(1):37-51.

6. Achermann, J. C., and J. L. Jameson. 1999. Fertility and infertility: genetic contributions from the hypothalamic-pituitary-gonadal axis. *Mol Endocrinology* 13(6):812-818.

7. Berga, S. L. 1998. Hypothalamus pituitary gonadal axis: stress-induced gonadal compromise. *J Musculoskel Pain* 6(3):61-70.

8. Raphael, K. G., and J. J. Marbach. 2000. Comorbid fibromyalgia accounts for reduced fecundity in women with myofascial face pain. *Clin J Pain* 16:29-36.

9. Partonen, T. 1999. Melatonin-dependent infertility. *Med Hypotheses* 52(3):269-270.

10. Check, J. H., H. G. Adelson, and C. H. Wu. 1982. Improvement of cervical factor with guaifenesin. *Fertil Steril* 37(5):707-708.

11. Davis, S. R. 1999. Androgen treatment in women. *Med J Aust* 170(11):545-549.

12. Charles, G. 1995. [Congestive pelvic syndromes]. *Rev Fr Gynecol Obstet* 90(2):84-90. [French]

13. Simons, D. G., J. G. Travell, and L. S. Simons. 1999. *Travell and Simons' Myofascial Pain and Dysfunction: The Trigger Point Manual, Volume I*, Second edition. Baltimore: Williams and Wilkins p. 839.

14. Simons, D. G. 2000. Personal communication. February 17.

15. Lovato, N. 2000. Breast cancer screening aid cleared for diagnostic use. JPL, Pasadena, CA: NASA News Release #00-17. (818-354-0474)

16. Cattaneo, A., A. De Marco, L. Sonni, G. L. Bracco, P. Carli, and G. L. Taddei. 1992. [Clobetasol vs. testosterone in the treatment of lichen sclerosus of the vulvar region.] *Minerva Ginecol* 44(11):567-571. [Italian]

17. Vliet, E. L. 1995. *Screaming to Be Heard*. New York: M. Evans and Co.

18. Sundstrom I., D. Ashbrook, and T. Backstrom. 1997. Reduced benzodiazepine sensitivity in patients with premenstrual syndrome: a pilot study. *Psychoneuroendocrinology* 22(1):25-38.

19. Vliet, E. L. 1995. *Op. cit.*

20. Sarrel, P. M. 2000. Effects of hormone replacement therapy on sexual psychophysiology and behavior in postmenopause. *J Women's Health Gend Based Med* 9(Suppl 1):S25-S32.

21. Grumbach, M. M., and R. J. Auchus. 1999. Estrogen: consequences and implications of human mutations in synthesis and action. *Clin Endocrinol Metab* 84(12):4677-4694.

22. Fink, G., B. Sumner, R. Rosie, H. Wilson, and J. McQueen. 1999. Androgen actions on central serotonin neurotransmission: relevance for mood, mental state and memory. *Behav Brain Res* 105(1):53-68.

23. Sherwin, B. B. 1997. Estrogen's effects on cognition in menopausal women. *Neurology* 48(5 Suppl 7):A21-26.

24. Hapidou, E. G., and G. B. Rollman. 1998. Menstrual cycle modulation of tender points. *Pain* 77(2):151-161

25. Anderberg, U. M., I. Marteinsdottir, J. Hallman, and T. Backstrom. 1998. Variablility in cyclicity affects pain and other symptoms in female fibromyalgia syndrome patients. *J Musculoskel Pain* 6(4):5-22.

26. Vliet. 1995. *Op. cit.*

27. Sears, B. 1999. *The Anti-Aging Zone*. New York: HarperCollins.

28. Weinstock, M. 1997. Does prenatal stress impair coping and regulation of hypothalamic-pituitary-adrenal axis? *Neurosci Biobehav Rev* 21(1):1-10.

29. Shanks, N., R. J. Windle, P. Perks, S. Wood, C. D. Ingram, and S. L. Lightman. 1999. The hypothalamic-pituitary-adrenal axis response to endotoxin is attenuated during lactation. *J Neuroendocrinol* 11(11):857-865.

30. Homko, C. J., E. Sivan, E. A. Reece, and G. Boden. 1999. Fuel metabolism during pregnancy. *Semin Reprod Endocrinol* 17(2):119-125.

31. Sola, A. E. 1985. Trigger point therapy. In: *Chemical Procedures in Emergency Medicine*. J. Roberts and J. Hedges, eds. Philadelphia: W. B. Saunders.

32. Davison, J. M. 1997. Edema in pregnancy. *Kidney Int Suppl* 59:S90-6.

33. Innes, K. E., and J. H. Wimsatt. 1999. Pregnancy-induced hypertension and insulin resistance: evidence for a connection. *Acta Obstet Gynecol Scand* 78(4):263-284.

34. Calder, A. A. 1994. Prostaglandins and biological control of cervical function. *Aust N Z Obstet Gynaecol* 34(3):347-351.

35. Egoscue, P., and R. Gittines. 1998. *Pain Relief*. New York: Bantam.

36. Tsen, L. C., and W. R. Camann. 1997. Trigger point injections for myofascial pain during epidural analgesia for labor. *Reg Anesth* 22(5):466-468.

37. Hubbell, S. L., and M. Thomas. 1985. Postpartum cervical myofascial pain syndrome: review of four patients. *Obstet Gynecol* 65(3 Suppl):56S-57S.

38. Berggren-Clive, K. 1998. Out of the darkness and into the light: women's experiences with depression after childbirth. *Can J Commun Ment Health* 17(1):103-120.

39. Wisner, K. L., and Z. N. Stowe. 1997. Psychology of postpartum mood disorders. *Semin Reprod Endocrinol* 15(1):77-89.

40. Thomas, S. A., and R. D. Palmiter. 1997. Impaired maternal behavior in mice lacking norepinephrine and epinephrine. *Cell* 91(5):583-592.

41. Vliet, E. L. 1995. *Op. cit.*

42. Guttuso, Jr., T. J. 2000. Gabapentin's effects on hot flashes and hypothermia. *Neurology* 54(11):2161-2163.

43. Stearns, V., C. Isaacs, J. Rowland, J. Crawford, M. J. Ellis, R. Kramer, et al. 2000. A pilot trial assessing the efficacy of paroxetine hydrochloride (Paxil) in controlling hot flashes in breast cancer survivors. *Ann Oncol* 11(1):17-22.

44. Davis, S. R. 1999. Androgen treatment in women. *Med J Aust* 170(11):545-549.

45. Yunus, M. B., F. Inanici, J. C. Aldag, and R. F. Mangold. 2000. Fibromyalgia in men: comparison of clinical features with women. *J Rheumatol* 27(2):485-490.

46. Thomas, T. J. 1988. Fibrositis in men. *West Virginia Med J* 84:235-236.

47. Southwick, S. M., C. A. Morgan III, D. S. Charney, and J. R. High. 1999. Yohimbine use in a natural setting: effects on posttraumatic stress disorder. *Biol Psychiatry* 46(3):442-444.

48. Camargo, Jr., J. N., and A. Nucci. 1997. Saphenous nerve entrapment manifested as proximal cruralgia. *Rev Paul Med* 115(5):1553-1534.

49. Sears, B. 1999. *Op. cit.*

50. Travell, J. G., and Simons, D. G. 1992. *Myofascial Pain and Dysfunction: The Trigger Point Manual, Vol. II.* Baltimore: Williams and Wilkins.

51. *Ibid.*, p. 118.

52. *Ibid.*, p. 121.

53. *Ibid.*, p. 121.

54. *Ibid.*, p. 187.

55. *Ibid.* p. 191.

56. *Ibid.* p. 197.

57. *Ibid.* p. 194.

58. *Ibid.* p. 203.

CHAPTER 12

Age-Related Issues:
Infants to Seniors

Most adults who receive a diagnosis of fibromyalgia (FMS) and/or chronic myofascial pain (CMP) believe that their problems started fairly recently, but when they are questioned closely, they often remember childhood symptoms. Perhaps their first sign of FMS was difficulty sleeping. Their first trigger points (TrPs) could have been seen as growing pains. Fibromyalgia may have a genetic component, and both FMS and CMP have perpetuating factors that may run in families. If you have FMS, watch your children for possible signs. No one is helped by denial, and you may be able to save them a lot of pain and grief. You can give your children the tools to deal with the reality of these conditions, so that they can move through life as effortlessly as possible.

Juvenile primary FMS is common.[1] In children, FMS is characterized by diffuse pain and sleep disturbance, and there may be fewer than eleven tender points.[2] It is very important to ensure that your child gets deep, refreshing sleep. In this study, most patients (median age thirteen years old) improved over two to three years. Trigger points can cause considerable pain in a rapidly growing child. They can often be treated effectively, rapidly, and relatively painlessly by using vapocoolant Spray and Stretch therapy, moist heat, and a continuing stretching program.[3]

Prenatal and Infant Care

Human infants and experimental animals that experience stress in the womb exhibit attentional deficits, hyperanxiety, and disturbed social behavior when they are born.[4] Maternal stress response during pregnancy may cause the child to have a greater chance of impaired ability to cope in stressful situations, as well as possible hypothalamic-pituitary-adrenal (HPA) axis dysregulation (see chapter 1). Can maternal stress response cause FMS in children who have the genetic tendency? Perhaps. Other studies indicate that this is a possibility.

Infants need to be cuddled and touched. Current research indicates that massage and touch can stabilize your infant's cardiovascular responses and enhance immunity, as well as help to develop healthier sleep patterns.[5] Massage can be very helpful and your infant may enjoy it. When your child was in the womb, s/he was constantly receiving the sensation of touch. Then there was the trauma of birth, and the separation from that touch. Your baby has been introduced to this *big*, alien world out here; full of strange sights, sounds, and smells. It has to be overwhelming.

I was a very sensitive child and I remember being very hurt when I was laughed at, because I could be so sick and tired one day and by the afternoon of the next day, I would recover. I had bouts of losing my strength. Many times I would find a spot and fall asleep during the day. Very early in life, I learned not to complain about the way I felt, because I was not taken seriously.

I suffered terribly from nasal stuffiness when I would lie down. I carried a Vick's inhaler constantly. I also suffered from severe headaches, especially on hot, sunny days. I remember having blurred vision. I had a lot of colds. I used to get terrible cramps in my stomach. I would have diarrhea without warning. Every cut or scrape meant infection. When I would run and play, if I did not twist my ankle, I would get a stitch in my sides. When I swam, I would get leg cramps. Once after a high school dance, I was in bed all weekend because my legs were so weak and sore. When I participated in sports, I would have pains in my legs and could not understand why nobody else playing the sport felt the way I did. I learned to live with muscle pains as just being a normal part of life. I believe I would have had a much better quality of life if I had only known that something was physically wrong with me.[15]

Infants need careful support and protection for their heads and necks. There is a little-recognized condition of suboccipital strain in newborns that may add to the normal stress of life for many babies. The suboccipital muscles are the muscles located in the base of the neck. They emerge in a "V" shape from the center of the spine, and help to provide mobility and stability. They are used in rocking and tilting the head.

KISS syndrome (kinematic imbalances due to suboccipital strain) was the subject of a talk presented by Dr. Jeff Rockwell,[6] a teacher at Parker Chiropractic College. KISS can cause the following problems: head tilting to one side (*torticollis*); scoliosis; asymmetric muscle development; slow development of the hip joints; and asymmetrical, slow development of motor skills. Some other common symptoms that were identified were restless sleep, and not eating or drinking well. Common factors causing this suboccipital strain include the position of the fetus in the womb, the use of forceps or vacuum extraction during the birth, prolonged labor, and multiple fetuses.

Too often, asymmetric posture in infants and young children is disregarded. It is important to have this assessed as soon as possible, so that it can be remedied. Perhaps all you need to do is pay gentle attention to the child's muscles and encourage gentle stretches. Make sure that those tiny bones are aligned properly. There is gentle bodywork that can be performed on infants, and there are even bodyworkers who specialize in this.

Pain control is important for infants, too. Infants can feel pain as newborns, although conscious memory does not develop until later. Imagine going through teething with the pain amplification of FMS. Also, pain and stress caused by medical procedures can cause permanent structural and functional changes.[7]

During birth, or shortly thereafter, trigger points (TrPs) can form in the rectus abdominis muscle (see chapter 8) in the area of the navel, and cause cramping or colic. These symptoms can be quickly and dramatically relieved by vapocoolant spray or by a cool, brief sweep with an ice cube along the sides of the navel.[8] If your child should develop explosive diarrhea or projectile vomiting, check for TrPs. Trigger points can start with a flu or other infection, and continue after the instigator has gone, until they are treated appropriately. Many cases of infant colic might be remedied more quickly if pediatricians and parents were instructed in the correct use of vapocoolant spray.

Infants take time to learn how to digest food. It is a complex task. Gastroesophageal reflux in infants can be a frustrating experience for both infant and caregiver. Craniosacral therapy is an effective, nontraditional treatment that is gentle and noninvasive. It should be explored before considering more invasive treatment.[9] Avoid the use of an infant seat if your infant has reflux, as it may worsen the condition.[10] Once your child begins eating solid food, if the food continues to come up right after it has gone down, try thickening the feeding.[11]

Communications in a Toddlin' Town

For children, the outcome of FM is more favorable than it is for adults,[12] *if* these children are diagnosed, and their needs are met. Talk to your children as much as possible, and encourage them to talk to you. Also, if you suspect they may be developing FMS or CMP, talk to your pediatrician about your suspicions.

Don't keep the diagnosis from them when they are old enough to understand. Explain matters as simply as possible. Tell them there are a lot of things that they can do to help how they feel. Give them "children's words" to describe their pain. Let them know you will understand when they say they feel all "fuzzy," or "foggy," or they have a "really big owie all over." How do they feel when they wake up? Do they look and act rested? Are they confused during the day? Do they have problems following directions? Observe, take notes, and talk about it with them. Include your other children in these conversations. It is important for them to understand as well.

It can help your child, and you, to end each day with a routine. Start from infancy. Make the choices quiet ones. This may include a bath, teeth brushing, story time (but not action-adventure stories), and prayer or meditation, or at least quiet reflection on the past day. Emphasize positive events of the day and what your child has learned.

Teach Your Child How to Cope

Your children may be feeling miserable, but may not be communicating this. Children don't know what being a child is supposed to feel like. In one study, of 338 "healthy" school children checked, 6.2 percent had fibromyalgia.[13] Children may recognize the symptoms when they are described to them, and they need to know that what they are feeling is not their fault. They also need to know that something can be done about the way they feel. Ask your pediatrician for advice on ways to talk about chronic illness in an emotionally supportive manner.

Teach your children about simple perpetuating factors, such as repetitive movements. Emphasize the importance of good sleep and good food. Let them know that the sooner they start preventative care such as simple stretching, the sooner they will feel better. There is a marvelous chapter about children and FMS in *What Your Doctor May Not Tell You About Fibromyalgia*.[14]

Children with FMS and CMP have a right to be validated. Listen to what they say. Be sure that their teachers know that when tiny hands let things fall, it is due to grip failure; not to naughtiness. Make sure the teachers understand that your child's pain and limitations are real. Be sure that your child understands that s/he can participate in just about any school activity if the appropriate care is taken.

Young Children

The symptoms of FMS in children are similar to those in adults.[16] In one study of eighty-one children with musculoskeletal pain, thirty-five fulfilled the criteria for FMS.[17] FMS in younger

> I remember having horrible pain in my hips and legs when I was a child. There was a doctor who made a house call when I was about eight, who said he wanted to "try something." He pressed an area in my hip, and suddenly the pain vanished.
>
> This experience made me want to become a doctor and to learn how that doctor could relieve pain so fast and with so little effort. Unfortunately, I found out that they weren't teaching that brand of magic in medical school. It was only later, when I saw the Trigger Point Manuals, that I understood what had been missing in my education.

people may also cause discomfort after minimal exercise, low-grade fever or below-normal temperature, and skin sensitivity.[18]

Restless leg syndrome can occur in childhood and adolescence and may be more common than is recognized.[19] Also, there is a strong association between joint hypermobility and FMS in schoolchildren.[20] In older children, active TrPs in the lower side of the abdominal wall can cause bedwetting.[21] One study indicated that dizziness and lack of balance in children with FMS are not caused by central (brainstem) and peripheral vestibular (inner ear) mechanisms, and that these symptoms are probably caused by proprioceptive orientation.[22] This may be due to FMS, but it may also be due to TrPs (see chapter 8), and TrPs can be treated.

When kids have FMS and CMP, they miss a lot of school, and teachers and classmates may misunderstand this. There also may be some cognitive confusion and other symptoms that are not properly recognized for what they are. Educate the parents of your children's friends, and educate their teachers. For example, your child may be on a different biological clock, and his/her study hours may have to be adjusted. If needed, check into an Individualized Education Plan at your school. FMS and CMP kids need resources, too. Check the Internet for children's support groups, start clubs, and get a connection going for them. They need to know that they aren't alone.

The Child's Point of View

FMS and CMP can confront an adult with a seemingly unending obstacle course. Adults have more leeway in charting their course in life, and they get more respect. Too many adults forget that children are people, too. It's time for kids to become empowered and enabled.

Children in pain (and children of parents in pain) can be at risk for mental health problems. Children don't understand why chronic illness occurs. If your child exhibits poor concentration, big changes in habits or functioning at home or school, difficulty relating to other children, lasting feelings of hopelessness, sadness, fear, or anger, or destructive or aggressive behavior, it may be time for some counseling. Or, if not counseling a talk with your child's doctor about your observations, and the presence of possible neurotransmitter dysfunction may be in order. If love is there, everything else can be worked out.

> I didn't have parents, just guardians. I had to learn how to be independent, and how to cope, at an early age. I made friends with the snakes under my bed, and they kept the monsters away. Try it, kids. It worked for me.

At School

Fibrofog and other cognitive deficits can combine with TrPs to cause slurred words, stuttering, and other verbal difficulties. This can easily be misunderstood. Your child may not be able to concentrate enough to pay attention to the teacher's words. It may be necessary for teachers to hand out lists of homework assignments to ensure that they will be remembered. Make sure that your child has adequate sleep and a good meal, before s/he heads off to school. Note that a breakfast heavy in carbohydrates (the typical American breakfast) may leave you son or daughter in the fog.

Encourage your child to get sufficient exercise. If your child doesn't get outside much and is overweight, that could be the first sign of insulin resistance.[23] Watch what your teen eats. You may want to put the brakes on the potatoes, breads, and sweets and encourage balanced meals with plenty of protein.

Check for unintentional weight lifting. One study done found that 34.8 percent of school children carry more than 30 percent of their bodyweight at least once a week in backpacks. Back pain in adolescents is common, recurs, and increases with age.[24]

Some adult artists with CMP can do calligraphy and elaborate drawings, yet they can't handle cursive writing. This can be hard to explain to a teacher who doesn't understand that a homework assignment involving lengthy writing can be painful to a child with upper body TrPs. Go back to chapter 8, and reread it from your child's point of view. Think about the effect these symptoms might have on your child. No wonder that the FMS or CMP child sometimes becomes the class clown, or withdraws entirely, just trying to cope.

The Sleep Issue

Once you understand how much sleep your child needs, establish a pattern and stick to it. Do your best to ensure that your child has a room and bed that are comfortable for sleep. Avoid disturbing TV shows before bedtime. Observe and listen. Do your children wake up alert and refreshed? Are they in school and yet still need a nap every day? Many behavioral problems can be traced to the lack of restorative sleep.

Children should not take melatonin. Melatonin helps to regulate the biological clock. A drop in melatonin levels signals the body to begin puberty.[25] Benadryl is often a safe medication to consider if your child has sleep problems, but discuss this with your child's doctor first. Your child may not need it every night.

Some children do well on guaifenesin therapy (see chapter 15). For specific information on pediatric guaifenesin therapy, you can download an electronic book on pediatric guaifenesin therapy (see Appendix B).

Pain

A child has no reason to believe that other children aren't dealing with the same obstacles. When raising an arm in class can become extremely painful, school days can be extremely difficult. It is bad enough to enter the human race with a handicap, but to have it undiagnosed is doubly cruel. Guilt is piled on top of sometimes insurmountable pain and dysfunction. When children can't cope and don't know why, they often think that all of their difficulties are of their own making. This can be a recipe for disaster. Children vary tremendously in their pain perceptions and pain management. FMS children, like adults, respond in individual ways to different medications. Pay close attention to the effects of any medications your child is taking.

The Turbulent Teens

Puberty magnifies the problems of life. Young girls must wrestle with menstruation and may be stricken with severe cramps and premenstrual syndrome (PMS). Often they are effectively disabled by their menstrual periods. Depression can set in due to the inability to keep up with the other teenagers in school or to take part in extracurricular activities.

The Transition Years

With the first rush of hormones, the brain begins to rewire itself.[26] Teens begin to see the world differently. They may experience enormous growth spurts, and the lack of restorative sleep can constrain their growth. During puberty, some sex hormones also have a close relationship with the sleep cycle.

Adolescents are even more impaired by sleep loss than are the rest of us. Sleep loss affects how students learn and, once they start driving, it increases the chance that they will have automobile accidents. Bad sleep habits may make it more likely that your son or daughter will develop chronic sleep disorders. Adolescents often have a biological clock that kicks them into becoming classic night owls, staying up late and sleeping in late. Most teenagers don't get tired until much later in the evening than adults do.

The teenage years are difficult at best. It may be hard to keep the communication channels open. Work at it. Older children with chronic pain conditions are at a high risk of suicide. Make sure that they know that someone understands, and that they always have a place they can go to for help—a place where someone will listen to them.

Senior Citizens

My friend and correspondent Clarissa Badger calls old age "the year after tomorrow." Lynn Johnson, in one of my favorite comic strips, "For Better or for Worse," has one of her characters say, "We are the only products that tend to improve while the packaging deteriorates." But some of that deterioration may be unnecessary. "The stiffness and the relatively painless but progressive restriction of movement that characterize decrepitude of advancing age are often due largely to latent TrPs."[27] This is often reversible with proper treatment and a stretching program.

Many doctors miss the symptoms of FMS and CMP and view them as characteristic of advancing age or arthritis.[28] Because of that mind-set, these doctors may dismiss declines in physical ability, muscle strength, or cognitive skills. *Don't let them!* I strongly believe that many "symptoms of old age" can be eased by treating coexisting FMS and CMP. Often, circulation can be improved and cognitive impairments diminished.

Many older people are already taking many medications and fear the need for yet another one. But new medications may not be needed. For example, if you have "arthritic fingers," review the section on interosseus TrPs in chapter 8. "Inactivating the related myofascial TrPs and the *elimination of their perpetuating factors* appear to be important parts of early therapy to delay or abort the progression of some kinds of osteoarthritis."[29]

Speak Up

Older people may be less likely to report pain, because they assume that pain is a natural part of aging. It is not. Or they may fear that the pain they feel signifies approaching disability and the beginning of a long slide toward death. But we know that the percentage of TrPs increases with age,[30] and we also know that TrPs are treatable. And although fibromyalgia is common in seniors,[31] chronic pain is *not* a normal part of growing older. It profoundly affects the quality of your life, and it is only logical that you try to discover what is its cause. It is a source of unending joy to me that my myotherapist has relieved so many seniors of their aches and pains and has even helped some recover the use of functions they had thought were lost forever. For example, you should never think of incontinence as just a part of growing old. It is not (see chapter 8).

Pain management for the elderly is often inadequate.[32] If one part of your body hurts, tell your doctor, and don't allow him or her to dismiss your complaints as "old age." The other parts of your body are just as old! Once a diagnosis has been established that explains what is causing your pain, ask what your options are for treatment, pharmaceutical and nonpharmaceutical. Treatment may not restore the vigor of youth, but it might enable you to cut down on your medication and improve the quality of your life. There are many gentle techniques, such as Spray and Stretch, myofascial release, and craniosacral release that can work wonders, although you still need to work on those perpetuating factors.

Some of the falls and fractures so common among seniors might be avoided if TrPs and the proprioceptive disruption they may cause were removed from the picture. If you are a senior, you may need to address insulin resistance and reactive hypoglycemia with diet. You might also need to address neurally mediated hypotension and other coexisting conditions you might have. For example, an altered cortisol response to acute and/or chronic stress is often a part of FMS. This could have detrimental effects on memory, and could be an important factor if you have experienced memory loss.[33]

Senior Sexuality

Sexuality is an important part of life for adults, no less for seniors. Romance can reach its peak in the senior years. Broaden your concept of romance and fall in love all over again. For men and women, regular sexual activity helps to preserve sexual ability. Sexual dysfunction is not an inevitable consequence of old age, but is rather the result of an illness, an imbalance, a medicinal side effect, or an emotional problem or other specific cause, and it requires medical attention. You may want your doctor to run an endocrine evaluation for you. That's the only way to find out if your hormones need boosting. Don't be shy about discussing this with your doctor.

If you have had a heart attack, and are concerned that sexual activity may bring on angina or another attack, be sure that your doctor understands that TrPs in the sternalis and pectoralis muscles can cause or add to arrythmias and chest pain. Vapocoolant spray (see chapter 21) may help stop the pain of these TrPs, but you need the attention of a TrP myotherapist or myofascial release specialist to get rid of them.

Medications

In addition to hormonal changes, coexisting illness and medications may negatively affect sexuality. Your doctor needs to take into consideration the side effects of your medications, both alone and in combination, on the total quality of your life.[34]

It's a good idea to have your medications evaluated every year. Too often another medication is just tacked on when a new symptom appears. Over-the-counter (OTC) medications including herbals can cause problems. Even commonly used NSAIDS (nonsteroidal anti-inflammatories), can interact with many other medications. This effect can be worse in seniors. Some studies indicate that physicians should avoid prescribing NSAIDS because of their side effects and suggest alternative pain medications and bodywork[35] for pain relief in seniors.

Many seniors metabolize medications more slowly than other adults do, and need smaller amounts. Use only one pharmacy for all of your medications, especially if you are taking many medications prescribed by many different doctors, so that you can be alerted to prevent harmful drug interactions. If you have a tendency to keep adding medications, you might want to ask yourself whether a better, more balanced diet or adding more exercise to your life might be what you need.

There are many things to take into consideration when a medication is prescribed. For example, ask your doctor if many of your medications are metabolized by your liver. If so, perhaps there is a medication you can switch to that is metabolized by your kidneys. It is a good idea to try and spread the metabolic work around as a way of being kind to your organs. They work for you. Treat them well and they'll do the same.

Make sure you take your medications correctly. Written informational sheets are fine if you understand them, but the instructions may have to be modified for your specific needs. You may need to have some things explained.

If you have difficulty swallowing pills, let your doctor know. Your medication may not work the same way if it is crushed, especially if it is in a timed-release form. There may be another oral form of medication you can use instead. Be sure that you drink a lot of water with any oral medication, because you don't want the pills to become caught in your esophagus and dissolve there. Medication is not designed to dissolve in the esophagus and could cause severe irritation.

Ask your doctor or pharmacist about any possible side effects your medications may have, and about what you can do to handle the minor ones. For example, a dry mouth from one medication may mean you can't dissolve a nitroglycerine tablet under your tongue. If you put a few drops of water under your tongue, that will relieve the problem. There is also a nitroglycerine spray available. Explore your options.

Your diet is also an important factor in how well your medications work, (as well as any other medications you may take, such as diuretics). For example, it is important for your doctor to know how often you eat, and what types of foods, because this may have some effect on your medications.

Often elderly patients have problems with sleep organization just like the sleep problems that those with FMS have. These can include difficulty falling asleep, less time spent in the deeper stages of sleep, early-morning awakening, and less total sleep time.[36] There is also a high prevalence of sleep apnea and nocturnal myoclonus in elderly people.[37] Sleep apnea can be life-threatening and must be addressed.

Periodic leg movements and restless leg syndrome are more common in the elderly than in other adults. Trigger points should be promptly treated and perpetuating factors addressed. If you soak your legs and feet in a warm Epsom salts and ginger bath, get a good TrP myotherapist or myofascial release therapist, and take up regular exercise, you may get quite a bit of relief. Talk to your doctor about having a vitamin and mineral profile done on your blood. You may have to beef up (forgive me, vegetarians, but "veg up" doesn't work) your nutrients.

Adapt your house to your particular needs. Talk to your myotherapist or see an occupational therapist that knows TrPs. If you need help with the ordinary tasks of life like getting in and out of the tub, using the toilet, and managing in the kitchen, you can find it. Look into the use of adaptive equipment. Talk with your local librarian and pharmacist about this. There are long-handled sponges; mechanical "arms" that can help you cleanse yourself after a bowel movement if your movement is restricted, but check out those quadratus lumborum and paraspinal TrPs first. You may be able to regain that range of motion. You may need railings in some areas of your house and they can be decorative as well as useful. Eliminate area rugs or put non-skid matting under them. Use lighter-weight dishes and cookware. Try before you buy. I found the "special" plastic ware containers for arthritics too hard for me to open.

Fibromyalgia and CMP can come at anytime in a life. Dealing with perpetuating factors promptly and effectively may make "anytime" a more pleasant time. The key is to realize what you are dealing with, and then to deal with it. If you don't deal with it, or if life throws too much at you, you may experience a life crisis. That is what we will look at next.

Endnotes

1. Romano, T. J. 1991. Fibromyalgia in children: diagnosis and treatment. *W V Med J* 87 (3):112-114.

2. Siegel, D. M., D. Janeway, and J. Baum. 1998. Fibromyalgia syndrome in children and adolescents: clinical features at presentation and status at follow-up. *Pediatr* 101(3 pt 1):377-382.

3. Aftimos, S. 1989. Myofascial pain in children. *N Z Med J* 102(874):440-441.

4. Weinstock, M. 1997. Does prenatal stress impair coping and regulation of hypothalamic-pituitary-adrenal axis? *Neurosci Biobehav Rev* 21(1):1-10.

5. Hayes, J. A. 1998. TAC-TIC therapy: a non-pharmacological stroking intervention for premature infants. *Complement Ther Nurs Midwifery* 4(1):25-27.

6. Rockwell J. 1995. The 1995 Convention of the National Association of Myofascial Trigger Point Therapists: Parker Chiropractic College, Dallas, Texas. September.

7. Porter, F. L., R. E. Grunau, and K. J. Anand. 1999. Long-term effects of pain in infants. *J Dev Behav Pediatr* 20(4):253-261.

8. Simons, D., J. Travell, and L. S. Simons. 1999. *Myofascial Pain and Dysfunction: The Trigger Point Manual*. Second edition. Baltimore: Williams and Wilkins.

9. Joyce, P., and C. Clark. 1996. The use of craniosacral therapy to treat gastroesophageal reflux in infants. *Inf Young Children* 9(2):51-58.

10. Orenstein, S. R., P. F. Whitington, and D. M. Orenstein. 1983. The infant seat as treatment for gastro-esophageal reflux. *N Engl J Med* 309(13):760-763.

11. Orenstein, S. R., H. H. Magill, and P. Brooks. 1987. Thickening of infant feedings for therapy of gastro-esophageal reflux. *J Pediatr* 110(2):181-186.

12. Buskila, D., L. Neumann, E. Hershman, A. Gedalia, J. Press, and S. Sukenik. 1995. Fibromyalgia syndrome in children—an outcome study. *J Rheumatol* 22(3):525-528.

13. Buskila, D., J. Press, A. Gedalia, M. Klein, L. Newman, R. Boehm, et al. 1993. Assessment of nonarticular tenderness and prevalence of fibromyalgia in children. *J Rheumatol* 20(2):368-370.

14. St. Amand, R. P., and C. C. Marek. 1999. *What Your Doctor May Not Tell You About Fibromyalgia*. New York: Warner Books.

15. Day, J. M. No date. Unpublished paper. 3 Inglis Place, St. Johns, Newfoundland A1A 4L7 Canada.

16. Calabro, J. J. 1986. Fibromyalgia (fibrositis) in children. *Am J Med* 81(3A):57-59.

17. Malleson, P. N., M. al-Matar, and R. E. Petty. 1992. Idiopathic musculoskeletal pain syndromes in children. *J Rheumatol* 19(11):1786-1789.

18. Reiffenberger, D. H., and L. H. Amundson. 1996. Fibromyalgia syndrome: a review. *Am Fam Phys* 53(5):1698-1712.

19. Walters, A. S., D. L. Picchietti, B. L. Ehrenberg, and M. L. Wagner. 1994. Restless legs syndrome in childhood and adolescence. *Pediatr Neurol* 11(3):241-245.

20. Gedalia, A., J. Press, M. Klein, and D. Buskila. 1993. Joint hypermobility and fibromyalgia in schoolchildren. *Ann Rheum Dis* 52(7):494-496.

21. Travell, J., and D. Simons. 1992. *Myofascial Pain and Dysfunction: The Trigger Point Manual*. First edition. Baltimore: Williams and Wilkins.

22. Rusy, L. M., S. A. Harvey, and D. J. Beste. 1999. Pediatric fibromyalgia and dizziness: evaluation of vestibular function. *J Dev Behav Pediatr* 20(4):211-215.

23. Vanhala, M. 1999. Childhood weight and metabolic syndrome in adults. *Ann Med* 31(4):236-239.

24. Negrini, S., R. Carabalona, and P. Sibilla. 1999. Backpack as a daily load for children. *Lancet* 354(9194):1974.

25. Dement, W. C., and C. Vaughan. 1999. *The Promise of Sleep*. New York: Delacorte Press.

26. *Ibid.*

27. Simons, Travell, and Simons. 1999. *Op. cit.*, p. 113.

28. Holland, N. W., and E. B. Gonzalez. 1998. Soft tissue problems in older adults. *Clin Geriatr Med* 14(3):601-611.

29. Simons, Travell, and Simons. 1999. *Op cit.*, p. 792.

30. *Ibid.*

31. Wolfe, F., K. Ross., J. Anderson, I. J. Russell, and L. Hebert. 1995. The prevalence and characteristics of fibromyalgia in the general population. *Arth Rheum* 38(1):19-28.

32. Monti, D. A., and E. J. S. Kunkel. 1998. Management of chronic pain among elderly patients. *Psychiatr Serv* 49(12):1537-1539.

33. Lupien, S. J., S. Gaudreau, B. M. Tchiteya, F. Maheu, S. Sharma, N. P. Nair, et al. 1997. Stress-induced declarative memory impairment in healthy elderly subjects: relationship to cortisol reactivity. *J Clin Endocrinol Metab* 82(7):2070-2075.

34. Gelfand, M. M. 2000. Sexuality among older women. *J Womens Health Gend Based Med* Suppl 1:S15-S20.

35. Chawla, P. S., and M. S. Kochar. 1999. Effect of pain and nonsteroidal analgesics on blood pressure. *WMJ* 98(5):22-5, 29.

36. Neubauer, D. N. 1999. Sleep problems in the elderly. *Am Fam Physician* 59(9):2551-8, 2559-2560.

37. Gentili, A., and J. D. Edinger. 1999. Sleep disorders in older people. *Aging (Milano)* 11(3):137-141.

CHAPTER 13

Life Crises: Preparation, Prevention, and Management

Flare

Fibromyalgia (FMS) and chronic myofascial pain (CMP) symptoms vary from day to day, and hour to hour. This changeable nature of our symptoms can be the most difficult aspect of the two disorders for others to understand and accept. Even changing weather can affect the nature of pain we feel.[1] Sometimes, symptoms may be almost in remission. Other times they are very active. And then there is *flare*.

Flare is a time of high-intensity pain and grief; an overwhelming episode of symptom intensity that can either creep up slowly or hit like an express train barreling down on you. Flare, like a flash fire, is all consuming. FMS is a disorder of sensory perception, not just pain. Your entire body is hypersensitive, like a raw nerve,[2] and when you are in flare, that nerve is dragged over hot coals. Your whole body screams for attention. When you are in flare, you may experience new symptoms and the old ones may worsen

What Causes Flare?

Usually, one or more activities or stressors trigger flares. The stressor could be a virus, a severe yeast infection, or a traffic accident. It might be as complex as a divorce or as simple as a game of volleyball. It can be triggered by a menstrual period, a dip in a swimming pool that is just a little too cold, a draft or a sudden temperature change, or the onset of allergy season. Any one of these events, alone or in concert, could cause a flare. Some people can go into flare because of a major argument, or even a sudden very loud noise. It isn't unusual for someone with FMS and CMP to suffer a severe flare after an upper-respiratory infection or an allergy attack. None of us can live in an isolation chamber, nor should we wish to, although, at times, an Antarctic research station sounds very appealing to me.

Anything that interrupts or disrupts sleep can be a flare instigator, such as an injury, a new baby, visitors, holidays, a time change, jet lag, travel, vacations, or shift work. In general, the more sensitive you are to stimuli, the more your perpetuating factors are out of control. When you gain some measure of control over your perpetuating factors, you gain some measure of control over your life. Still, life happens, and life means change. What seems to be most important is the way in which we respond to stress. We need to identify our common stressors and find out

There was a robot in the old *Lost In Space* program that went crazy whenever it was confronted with a crisis. Its arms, which resembled flexible dryer ducting, would flail about wildly as it shouted, "Danger! Warning!" endlessly. When I listen to some people planning activities for *my* trips, I sometimes feel like imitating that robot. It is important to set boundaries, understand your limits, and not allow inappropriate behavior, as a matter of self-preservation.

why they afflict us so strongly. The material below describes how to manage one stressor that can be a frequent cause of flare.

Identify the stressor: With FMS and CMP as constant companions, travel, even for a vacation, can be a major stressor. I was often asked to speak at seminars, and relatives expected me to visit as well. I was in denial and permitted the "good sport syndrome" to take over. Until I was willing to tackle this flare factor, even a brief trip resulted in months of agonizing and expensive rehabilitation. Getting away from "it all" can be a trial if "it all" includes your carefully built support structure. Identifying problems is the first step in dealing with flares.

Communications flow: Involve your hosts in your travel preparations. Let them know what you will need when you arrive, such as time to decompress, or a bath and/or a nap, a nearby place for bodywork, time to relax during your visit, or a hotel with a hot tub. Be especially clear about your dietary needs, including meal frequency and timing. It is especially difficult to plan trips over holidays. This is already a time of high stress. If your hosts consider your visit "party time," you may go into sensory overload and flare. When you say "no" to afternoon wine and cheese, late night dinners and heavy desserts, you are not being antisocial. You are practicing self-preservation. Help others to understand.

Travel tips: If you are traveling all or part of the way by car, get out and stretch *at least* every half hour. Walk around the car. Stoop. Stretch your legs and arms. You needn't take a lot of time, but use the time you have wisely. If you are driving (sometimes it is more comfortable driving because the seat is more adjustable), use cruise control and automatic everything, if possible. Adjust your seat to your maximum benefit. If you have bucket seats, try a pad in back under your butt to counter the bucket effect.

If you are traveling somewhere you have never gone before, plan your travel carefully. Decide what you want to see beforehand. Check out books and videos from your library. Talk to friends. Send away for information packets. Read the travel section of your Sunday paper. There are tours for people with limited mobility. Ask your travel agent about them. Some hotel chains have rooms designed for people with disabilities. Find out exactly what each hotel means by this. It may not fit *your* needs. *Get written confirmation* of verbal promises from hotels and other travel providers. Ask about:

- Walking distance and number of stairs to the room, eating facilities, pool, and shops

- Tours and transportation available from the hotel

- Temperature of the pool and hot tub

- Availability of room service and laundry service (you can carry less if you can wash clothes)

- Types of beds available

- Health spa accommodations

Crisis management: I have learned how to travel when I must, but I space my trips carefully, pace myself, and take precautions. I carry an inflatable mattress, my own pillow, and extra medications. I always have enough books or working material with me, in case of delays. If I am going on a long or difficult trip, I have a planning session with my doctor to figure out survival strategies beforehand. I plan to stretch as often as I can during any trip. I now take Valium for the immobile parts of the trip (e.g., a long plane ride) and I no longer have as many lasting muscle aches. (You may need to find another medication that relaxes your muscles without side effects.) I set up myotherapy and chiropractic visits before and after the trip. If flying, I avoid the overhead bin, and take one small bag to stow under the seat. I carry an ice pack that can be filled and refilled as needed during the flight, and both a tennis ball and lacrosse ball (see chapter 19). I carry balanced food bars because I can't depend on finding healthy things to eat. I *always* carry earplugs in my pocketbook. I try to anticipate possible difficulties *before* I travel, to minimize their impact *when* I travel.

I keep a long checklist to minimize the chance of forgetting important things. It is vitally important to stay as mobile as possible during the trip itself, and during the visit. I try to make business travel fun, and see something I want to see. I always allow time to "decompress," from the stress of travel. Whenever possible, I travel with my main life support, my husband, Rick.

What are your stressors? What contributing factors add to them? Do you go into flare whenever cousin Elmo visits? Have you been putting up with inappropriate behavior, and do you need better boundaries? Is someone in your office a flare instigator? It may be time to draw some boundary lines. Does the stress of paying taxes or bills set off your symptoms? Get some help. Take a close look at your stressors and decide what you can do to diffuse their negative impact.

The yeast beast: If you take antiyeast medication, such as Diflucan (see chapter 21), you can expect a yeast die-off phenomenon. You are improving your health by killing the yeast, but your symptoms may temporarily worsen as the yeasts die and release toxic chemicals. This can precipitate flare. You may think the medication isn't working, and stop taking it. Then, the yeast begin to multiply once again, adding to your misery. If you are already in a flare due to yeast infection, especially if your diet is high in carbohydrates, the yeast die-off side effects can be extreme and difficult to endure. If you understand what is happening and take it very easy, you can ride it out. Make sure you are as prepared as possible before you start the medication. A good diet and bodywork regimen is a great start. Have a supply of food and other necessities at home, so that you don't have to drive. Arrange to have friends drop in and help, if necessary.

Flare warnings: Flare has a way of creeping up on you when you aren't expecting it. As you learn to listen to your body, it will give you clues if you are approaching flare. For example, even at the best of times, some of us with FMS cannot tolerate the sound of a child crying, or of phones ringing. You may be sensitive to noise of a certain frequency. Some people can't take bass sounds, and hearing them can cause dizziness or nausea. I don't do well with the sound my phone makes when I punch in a number. Each tone feels like a knife in my eardrum. Some of us have to avoid parties or department stores because of the confusion and noise. Others can't abide the frantic pace and sounds of cartoons. Any staccato repetitive sound, like rap music, may be an intense stressor. If you suddenly have much less tolerance to these kinds of stimuli and they irritate you way out of proportion to what is your usual tolerance, your body may be telling you that a flare is approaching.

If a flare is approaching, you may experience slurred speech, and stuttering. This may make you sound stupid, drugged, or drunk. Some of this *may* be due to increased medications, which may be due to increasing symptoms. It may also be due to TrPs in your throat area, or disconnects in your brain. Your body is warning you to cut down on stimuli because it is having difficulty functioning. Your muscle strength may become unreliable, and you may drop things more often than usual.

For example, you may become aware of weakness during certain movements, such as when pouring liquids, turning a doorknob, or opening a can of pet food. (If it is dog food, your dog will be patient and understanding until you can get help. If it is cat food, cats generally have lawyers on retainer, and there *will* be repercussions.) Or you might be enjoying music, and suddenly you can't stand to listen to another note. This tolerance limit can be reached with conversation, too, and the shutoff can come abruptly. It is as if you have reached your absolute limit, and your mind needs time to process what you have heard. You may need to lie down in a quiet, dark room for a bit, or go for a quiet walk.

You may experience a feeling of disconnectedness. This can come after trauma, physical or emotional, as your body/mind system shuts down in response to sensory overload. In the first edition, we wrote, "When people have been traumatized in some way, they often report that they feel disconnected from everyone else." We have received several letters from people who had had this feeling and had never recognized it until they read that sentence. Then their tears came and they began to heal old wounds.

Spatial disorientation is another symptom of an approaching flare. You can bump into walls and fall over curbs. You may need to restrict yourself to one floor. Along with or instead of this symptoms you may have disturbed weight perception. *All* food becomes finger food when you are in or approaching flare, as nothing will stay on your fork. You may need to use a straw to raise a drink to your mouth without spilling it.

Fibrofog, the inability to think clearly, may become extreme. The fog may creep up along with the flare and become so thick that you are unaware of being in flare. Depression caused by chronic pain may worsen, as may the pain itself. You may not want to admit to yourself that you're in a flare. It's still hard for me, though I rarely go into flare nowadays, and it doesn't last long.

My goal was to write this book without going into a flare. That didn't happen. There were far too many *other* traumas that struck during this period. I was able to cope, had my support structure in hand, and got back on track pretty fast. Mary Ellen Copeland's Wellness Recovery Action Plan (WRAP) helped (see chapter 16).

It helps to analyze actions or processes that have sent you into flare previously. Then, if you find you're on an express train to Flare City, you can grab your WRAP and read your flare-prevention strategy. If you seem to be in a permanent state of flare, you have one or more perpetuating factors that you haven't addressed. You and your medical team need to do some detective work. People with chronic invisible illness live on the edge and, sometimes, the seatbelt is strengthened by survival skills like humor.

Humor: Paws to Refresh

Writing this book was a labor of love, but it was also heavy-duty work. Dealing with countless medical journal references and books required a very disciplined focus. For someone with FMS and CMP, this was hard to accomplish because my mind usually runs along more tracks than a multilevel freeway overpass system. Keystrokes are repetitive, causing muscle strain, and the steady work took its toll. Just when I was drowning in research, a friend with the skills I needed became available to help. One day this assistant sent me a "forgotten" reference item to add to my text.* There followed a brief paragraph that paralleled my usual medical notation, although I didn't remember including the *Journal of Feline Management* in my research!

> Observation of two subjects in a double-blind study indicates subjects' RTM (rapid tail movement) during sleep shows significant and continued awareness of nocturnal environment. Known genetic proclivity to require and demand nourishment and attention at all hours of the day, combined with genetic and societal programming to find sport and nutritional supplements by attacking and consuming small, noxious or potentially threatening life forms, is shown to lead subjects to adopt behavior aggravating to humans. Since feline subjects may be intractable, long-term training for humans is essential.

The laughter this brought was a much-needed break in my work routine. My friend was reminding me that I needed some relief from the work load.

When a cat came to call by my computer, it was often to lure me to a ten-minute playtime. However, I didn't take enough of them. I put in some very long days, and even with structured stretching breaks, scheduled bodywork, and a lot of social support, I knew I was pushing beyond my limits. I kept my emergency plan close by. I was prepared.

If, in spite of all your precautions, flare comes your way, don't look at it as a "defeat." Life happens. Flare is a temporary condition. It's a sign that you have perpetuating factors that have gotten out of control. Be aware that when you are stressed by flare, you may be tempted to reach for high-carbohydrate "comfort food." This food may cause you to feel better temporarily because it will send more glucose to your brain. But eventually you will get a rise in insulin, which suppresses glucagon and increases cortisol which will stress your body and mind even more.[3] This spiral can continue unless and until you interrupt it, so remember, *carbohydrate-rich foods will lengthen your stay in Flare City.* Decide whether you want to set up permanent residence there, or find a way out as fast as possible.

People in severe health crises may reach for anyone who can throw them a lifeline, and then they may cling to that person for dear life. When we are under severe stress, it is normal to attach ourselves to someone who can provide what we need. A strong swimmer sometimes can save someone else who is drowning. But if ten drowning people climb on top of that swimmer, they will all go down. There are millions of people with FMS and CMP. Trying to cope with the correspondence overload that resulted from the publication of the first edition of this book used to put me into flare. People would call, email, write, and fax, or even show up at my door. Today, I try to set firmer boundaries and pace myself, putting what I know into books, videos, and on my Web site. I can't expect people who are in survival mode to understand the words, "I can't do any more." But overwork will push me into survival mode, too, and that helps no one. I can't take each person in need and lead him or her by the hand through the fire. That is not empowerment, nor is it effective. I *can* lead the way.

To avoid flare, learn to pick your battles. Decide what is most important to you. Simplify your tasks and save your energy for what must be done. You may have to revise your idea of "what must be done." Learn to ask for help. Write helpful strategies in your journal so that the next time you are feeling low, you won't have to relearn these lessons. FMS and CMP are high maintenance illnesses. They use up a lot of time and energy. If you want to optimize your quality of life, learn how to deal with your illnesses in the most effective ways you can. Take the time. You are worth the effort.

---

* Katzpajamas, A., L. Gatogrande, and I. Pusskinski. 2000. Nocturnal eating syndrome in felines as directed toward and influenced by human response to loud, repetitive vocalizations and/or by covert activity of rodentia in culinary area of domicile. *J Feline Manage* 1(1):1-100.

Endnotes

1. Jamison, R. N., K. O. Anderson, and M. A. Slater. 1995. Weather changes and pain: perceived influence of local climate on pain complaint in chronic pain patients. *Pain* 61(2):309-315.

2. Dohrenbusch, R., H. Sodhi, J. Lamprecht, and E. Genth. 1997. Fibromyalgia as a disorder of perceptual organization? An analysis of acoustic stimulus processing in patients with widespread pain. *Z Rheumatol* 56(6):334-341.

3. Sears, Barry. 1999. *The Anti-Aging Zone.* New York: HarperCollins.

CHAPTER 14

Taking Control: Dancing with Dragons

Some days it seems that frustration is the guiding force in our lives. Why does everything seem to go wrong at such times? It's the rules. You know, the rules that tell the little thingie in the sink drain to plug up whenever you try to run water through it, but not to hold water when you want it to. Don't allow those "rules" to get your down. It is often our emotional responses to these frustrating but normal events, and our fibromyalgia (FMS) amplification of these responses, that cause us to lose control.

As I mentioned in the last chapter, FMS is a disorder of sensory perception, as well as pain perception. Emotional amplification can be a part of this. Emotional responses are controlled by neurotransmitters, hormones, and other informational substances, and different informational substances can be out of balance in different patients with FMS. No two of us are alike. Most of us are conscious of the pain amplification, but we may be unaware that some of our other sensory responses may be similarly distorted.

This chapter requires you to use a little imagination. If you look at your life carefully, you will find that dragons have crept in, one at a time, and are simply waiting for you to identify and deal with them. If you don't deal with them, they will push you as far as they can, and take whatever liberties you allow them.

Identifying Dragons

Dragons come in many forms and it may not be easy to identify them, because many are masters of disguise. One key identifier is that dragons often seem like obstacles or roadblocks that keep you from your path. Many dragons have to do with emotions and attitudes, such as the dragons of confusion, intolerance, negativity, manipulation, and denial. There are many of these kinds of dragons. Then there are dragons that appear in the form of people and their attitudes or mind-sets. Dragons also may come in the form of events in your life that continue to affect your attitude. They may be things that you do, like smoking, or that you fail to do (like take your medications).

Too often, we try to meet these obstacles with a frontal assault, and succeed only in frustrating ourselves and angering the dragons. Then we may feel defeated and frustrated. Dragons can be very stubborn. But I have found that even the most resistant dragons sometimes can be persuaded to dance with you if you change your interaction pattern. Then you may be able to continue on your path. The trick is to learn how to dance with the dragon. Each dragon is different, and requires an individualized approach, depending on its nature and the circumstances of your interaction.

How you react to events is more important than the events themselves. Your biochemistry may dictate the intensity of your feelings, but it is within your power to modify your response to them. You can be in control, if you develop the right tools to do so. It's important that you learn to take responsibility for your actions. You can't blame chance, or luck, or God, for the way things are. If there is a gulf between what you expect out of life and what happens, you can modify your reaction to this difference. This modification is called resilience. This change can profoundly affect your life.

One of my elderly friends died recently. She had FMS and chronic myofascial pain (CMP), as well as many other ailments. On the warm, humid, summer day of her memorial service, as her favorite Christmas hymn drifted over the perspiring congregation, I knew that even after death, Arlene was still in control. She taught me a lot about empowerment. She knew what she wanted and, whenever possible, she got it. How about you? How much does your schedule reflect your priorities? Are you *leading* your life, or are you allowing dragons to steer you in a direction not of your own choosing?

One obstacle to taking control is identifying which dragons are preventing you from doing just that. You may have been in denial of FMS and CMP, but by this stage of the book you can pretty much tell if they are your companions. So do you gear up to do battle with FMS and CMP, or do you learn to identify and accept your individual limits, and gently, with time and improvements in your health, push those barriers back? Are FMS and CMP really the dragons we face, or are they teachers in disguise? If they are the teachers, what are the dragons? I've learned about this process by studying t'ai chi, and one thing I have learned is that direct resistance is not the most effective way to manage most dragons. Sometimes it's more logical to work with what you've got, if you can do this in a positive manner.

You have needs. The dragons crowding you have needs, too. Dragons need to be fed and encouraged. For example, the smoking dragon needs to be fed cigarettes, and needs you to be in situations where your desire to smoke is enhanced. The negativity dragon needs you to be around emotionally draining people, and wants you to focus your mental energy on misfortunes and bad news. The people who are dragons need you to tolerate their actions and attitudes. Successful dragon dancers learned to work on their own training before they could dance with dragons. This means self-empowerment, which requires self-reflection. Your education will be a continuously ongoing process, for life itself is an educational process.

Self-Empowerment

To be self-empowered, you must educate yourself and learn to talk to your caregivers as peers and to think about them as equals. By so doing, you will reduce the pain and frustration of not communicating effectively and increase your probability of being understood. Good communication can help to avoid patient and caregiver burnout and hostility. You may need to brush up on communications skills. One book I have found of great help in this regard is *The Tao of Conversation*, by Michael Kahn.[1] I have read many books on communications skills, but this is the most compact, comprehensive, and understandable. It helps me to identify my dragons. I am getting better at not tolerating inappropriate behavior, and because of it, I am much better at expressing myself and my own needs and desires.

Working with Your Health Care Team

One of the first rules in choosing your health care team is to avoid situations in which you allow your care providers to become dragons. You don't want to work with people who cause you to doubt yourself, and who whittle away your self-esteem. For example, some caregivers want you to keep quiet and just take orders, and they resent any educating and/or questioning from you. That is inappropriate. You can communicate with your health care providers more effectively by following these steps:

1. Tell your team members that you want copies of all of their reports for your own records.

2. Learn to write everything down. Take detailed notes, or carry a tape recorder to your doctor's office and to therapy sessions. That way, you won't forget anything, and your doctor or therapist may be a little more focused when they speak to you if they see that you are recording everything.

3. Keep a daily journal. When you write in a journal every day, and read through your entries every few weeks, you will be able to chart patterns and see relationships that might otherwise escape your attention.

4. Doctors, nurses, and therapists who are doing their job properly will not feel threatened by your interest and involvement in your own treatment. If they start blowing smoke and belching flame in your direction, don't tolerate it. Identify your needs, express them simply, and if your health care provider does not respond appropriately, identify your needs in writing and mail your letter to the appropriate person. All of us have bad days, but you should not accept abusive behavior from anyone, including your insurance company.

Remember, when you can precisely *identify* your needs, you have a much better chance of *fulfilling* those needs. Confusion is a dragon that works by blowing smoke. Let the wind blow the smoke away. When something gets you down, or blocks your enjoyment of life, look hard at what is happening, and how you are reacting to it. What is it that bothers you so much? Can you identify the dragon? How would you like it to change? You may find that there are some people who have become dragons, and you don't need them in your life at all.

You need a primary care doctor who not only believes that FMS and CMP exist, but who is also willing to stay current on new therapies and research, and to share that information with you. You need a doctor who understands chronic pain management, and a pharmacist to match. There's absolutely no reason you should be denied adequate medication for pain control. Taking medication to control pain does not turn you into a drug addict. If you are in pain, there is no reason to compound it by adding guilt.

Take Responsibility for Your Own Health

Taking responsibility for managing your own health care doesn't mean assuming blame for your illness; it means orchestrating the progress you make toward achieving an optimum quality of life. You deserve to feel the best you possibly can. It has been shown repeatedly that those who take charge of their own health care and reach out to others for advice, assistance, and support, are those who achieve the highest levels of health.[2]

It's important to have a complete physical evaluation and to address any problems that might be causing or aggravating your symptoms, such as hypothyroidism or anemia. FMS and CMP symptoms can be triggered by other physical problems, which your physician can detect and treat. Learn all you can about FMS and CMP. This will help you to make decisions and solve

One reader said our first edition of this book was too heavy for her. She cut the binding off with a paint scraper, and punched holes in the pages. Then she put it in a looseleaf notebook so she could lay it flat on the bed, or take out a chapter that she wanted to read. Others have gotten around the heavy book problem by putting a pillow on their laps to hold the book. Janet Travell recommended a semicircular board to use as a desk in an armchair. It has a cutout for your body in the middle. Then you prop pillows around to support your arms. There are always options.

problems. If you are well-informed, you can ask your health care professionals the right questions. Use your supersensitive FMS creativity to find solutions to everyday problems.

Take Inventory of Your Resources

There are resources available to help you gain control of your life. Locate the medical libraries in your area. You may not be permitted to check out books, but you may be able to review information in the library. Find out what your local reference librarian can do for you. If you have access to a computer, connect to the Internet for up-to-date information from all over the country. If you don't have a computer, your local librarian may be able to help you with such a connection. Check to see that the sources are reliable. Decide for yourself what constitutes reliability. Some "experts" who have spent a great deal of time in respected medical schools remain uneducated about FMS and CMP. They have a lot of letters after their names, but they don't "believe in" FMS and CMP. Then there are the graduates of the Academy for Myofascial Trigger Point Therapy in Pittsburgh who are often able to take a patient with FMS and CMP out of a wheelchair within weeks. It may be the lack of information on the part of their health care providers that was responsible for the need of the wheelchair in the first place.

Consult with a variety of health care professionals who have expertise in FMS and CMP. Ask for advice on treatment scenarios. Explore these options thoroughly. Then, based on what you learn, begin whatever treatment you decide is in your best interest. Know which treatments you would want to begin if your symptoms get much worse. Attend related support groups, workshops, and conferences. Join national organizations so you can receive their newsletters and discover other informational resources. (See Resources.) Find local heroes. I have a compounding pharmacist who sheds brilliant ideas like cut corduroy sheds lint. When I talk with him, I need to keep a tape recorder on, because I can never remember all of his ideas. There are similar people in your community. Make an effort to find them.

Understand and Respect Your Limits and Yourself

When you talk to yourself in times of frustration, what do you say? Pay attention, and make sure that you are giving yourself *positive* feedback. Emotions are stored in your body at the cellular level. When you give those cells food for thought, make sure it is healthy food. Keep positive. Pay attention to your feelings and how they affect the state of your health. It may be hard at first to separate your feelings from what is actually happening around you to cause those feelings, but doing this will help you to regain some measure of control. It is part of leaning how to manage the frustration dragon.

Every time you catch yourself saying, "How could I be so stupid!" or "I can't do anything right," stop. Just stop. Substitute phrases like, "I can learn from this," or "Let me stop a minute and think what I should do next." Give yourself the time and space to maneuver, so that you don't trip over the dragons. Taking control means nurturing your inner child. Remember, children with FMS are hypersensitive. Treat your inner child with love and respect. People with FMS are especially sensitive, and this is not always a bad thing. In her book *The Highly Sensitive Person*[3] Elaine Aron explains that sensitive people are often portrayed as victims by the media. We can't afford to take on those negative thought patterns.

Be specific when you ask for help. Don't allow others to give you inappropriate help. This can come in the form of interference, or by others giving you things you don't want or need. Giving you things you don't want or need may fill some need for the giver, but if it is not your own need, you don't have to accept it. This can be a subtle form of the manipulation dragon that may turn nasty when you no longer are willing to play the game. It's always good to take the high road, but don't allow these dragons to leave ill-smelling piles in your path.

Set Realistic Goals

Are you your own worst dragon? I know I am, but I am working hard on changing that. The denial dragon causes you to think that you can get away with pushing your limits too far. You can keep your goals realistic by educating yourself, accepting your diagnosis and symptoms, becoming involved, and knowing what your priorities are. Of course, one of the marvelous aspects of human nature is to reach for the stars, and we all should have dreams. Logically, however, you have a much better chance of success if you set out to pick a tomato from your garden. You may never ride the dragons, but you may be able to stop them from blocking your path. You may even be able to teach them to dance with you in a way that you both enjoy. When you dance with a dragon, don't let the dragon lead. You have basic rights. Don't give them up.

Don't Overtax Yourself

Some days, people will want you to do too much. At such times, give them a choice; for example, you can say, "I can either go shopping or cook dinner. Which do you want?" This is a perfectly sensible response when you know that too much exertion will drain your energy, cause stress, and possibly aggravate your symptoms.

If you are a grandmother or grandfather, it can be heartbreaking when you cannot pick up your little grandchildren. In such a situation, be honest. Say, "I'm hurting today and can't pick you up. Come over to the sofa and you can sit in my lap. I'll tell you a story." This can save the day, as well as your back.

Avoid Digging Deeper Holes

Don't dig your hole any deeper than it already is. Smoking is a deadly habit, not only for you, but also for those around you. Smoking is particularly bad for FMS and CMP patients. The nicotine in cigarettes causes your blood vessels to constrict and decreases the flow of blood, oxygen, and nutrients to your muscles. This increases pain and muscle tension. The carbon monoxide that enters your bloodstream via the smoke binds to the hemoglobin in your blood and decreases the amount of oxygen available to your muscles. Less oxygen means more pain. It's as simple as that.

Everyone has many bad habits. Do you seem to be getting in deeper and deeper to yours? Review chapter 7 on perpetuating factors. Then check your hands to see if you are carrying a "shovel." You may be doing something, consciously or unconsciously, that is causing the hole you are in to become deeper. The first step to getting out of the hole is to stop digging. Mind your perpetuating factors and you will be better able to see obstacles in your path and avoid them. Take the time to plan some good things, so that your "path" has a bubbling well, gleaming waterfall, or some blooming flowers to anticipate.

Begin attending an FMS and CMP support group. Make sure it is an emotionally positive group. You don't need extra negativity. Everyone needs to vent now and then, but a gathering focused on negativity will not do you any good, and may do you some harm (see chapter 16). You don't need extra negativity. You are supposed to be at a *support* group.

Say no to negativity dragons, and form your own group if necessary. Set up a support network of family members and friends who can help you out if and when the going gets tough. The best antidote to negativity is to have a clear picture of yourself and to value who you are. A strong self-image will enable you to judge for yourself whether there is any validity to what someone else says about you. You may find that your life improves more by what, and who, you delete than from anything you add to it. "Clean out the clutter, let go of the obligations that make you feel resentful, and challenge people who drain your energy to stop."[4]

Set Reasonable Boundaries

One of the best ways to take control is to learn to set reasonable boundaries. Establishing good boundaries has decreased the amount of sensory overload in my life. One book that helped me with this issue is called *Boundary Power*.[5] It is a difficult discipline to let in only what you want and to keep out what you don't, but it is necessary to reclaim a measure of control over your life. It takes a lot of practice.

Many of us find that when we articulate positive thoughts about ourselves, it brings up a great deal of emotion that requires an emotional release, usually crying. That may be an indication of unresolved past issues. John Barnes has a good audiotape that may help you deal with these (see Resources under Myofascial Release). Myofascial unwinding can also be very therapeutic in this regard (see chapter 19).

One of my t'ai chi sisters, Mary Wright, told me a good dragon story. She had been discussing one of her dragons with a counselor. The counselor smiled and said, "You know, we have a dragon parking lot outside." The first words that popped into Mary's head were, "Not *my* dragon!" Most of us resist parking our own dragons, or at least, setting them out to graze. Are you willing to let go of your dragon? Make that your intent, and a dragon parking lot will appear.

Measuring Success

How can you measure your success at controlling the dragons in your life? One measure is how closely you live in tune with your ideals. This year I've fallen flat on this measure, but my prime goal has been to get this edition and some articles for medical journals finished. When I write, the computer constantly malfunctions, and the printer doesn't work, and they both do better than my body and mind. That's the way it goes. No matter what kind of equipment I am using, it doesn't like the electromagnetic (EM) forces my body generates when I am tied up with it hour after hour. It's a trade-off. I know I won't be doing it forever, so I add all the support mechanisms I can to get me through. I must be very careful not to allow other people to fill up my time after my work is finished. I will need to reassess my priorities. It's that boundary issue again.

Tasso Spanos, the founder of the Academy for Myofascial Trigger Point Therapy, says, "When you have multiple trigger points, life often consists of hurting yourself. You must choose *how* you hurt yourself. Are you going to hurt yourself playing the flute, or putting the dishes away? Are you going to hurt yourself scrubbing the floor, or taking a walk?" Learn to accept trade-offs. Learn to decide how to use the tolerances and limits you have in the way that provides what is most important for you. These decisions will allow you to dance with dragons, without allowing them to lead. Like most learning processes, educating yourself about FMS and CMP is an ongoing project. The more you know about your own health issues and the more control you can exercise, the more your health care practitioners will be able to help you. This will result in a happier, healthier life, and a better arrangement with your dragons.

Endnotes

1. Kahn, M. 1995. *The Tao of Conversation*. Oakland, CA: New Harbinger Publications.

2. Laurent, D. D., and H. R. Holman. 1999. Evidence suggesting that a chronic disease self-management program can improve health status while reducing hospitalization: a randomized trial. *Med Care* 37(1):5-14.

3. Aron, E. *The Highly Sensitive Person*. New York: Broadway Books.

4. Richardson, C. 1998. *Take Time for Your Life: A Personal Coach's 7-Step Program for Creating the Life You Want*. New York: Random House.

5. O'Neil, M. S., and C. E. Newbold. 1994. *Boundary Power*. Antioch, TN: Sonlight Publishing, Inc. 4809 Honey Grove Drive, Antioch, TN 37013.

CHAPTER 15

New Research

There are an overwhelming number of clinical studies published every year relevant to fibromyalgia (FMS), chronic myofascial pain (CMP), and their perpetuating factors. These studies are written in medical language, and care must be taken when they are interpreted. Medical studies described in popular newspapers and magazines are frequently misinterpreted, both by the authors and the readers. The studies described are frequently chosen on the basis of popular appeal and marketability. Research on transfatty acids (see chapter 23) won't sell as many magazines as a story on Viagra™ will. Significant research findings may never be picked up by the popular press, or even by the general medical press.

We live in a world of information overload, without a way to filter the information. There is a shortage of writers like Carl Sagan or Isaac Asimov who can understand multispecialty research, grasp its significance and potential ramifications, and then translate the results into clear language for the average nonscientist. Such skilled writing not only takes rare abilities, it also takes a great deal of time.

As a rule, a single study doesn't prove something absolutely works or does not work. All that an individual study can do is to indicate that, in the group of patients studied, something happened that may be significant. Some studies even contradict other studies. There are many variables in each study that affected the conclusions drawn. You may not see the variables if you read only the abstracts or summaries available from online indexes like PubMed or Medline. A "finding," i.e., something that occurred in the test subjects during the testing, may be coincidental and not caused by the therapy or medication being tested. You must read the whole article.

Screening Research

It was quite frustrating to research papers on FMS and CMP. For example, many studies that claim to be about FMS patients did not eliminate those with CMP. If such a study tests a therapy or medication that helps to alleviate FMS symptoms and doesn't help CMP, but the study focuses on symptoms caused by CMP, the conclusions reached may be totally inaccurate, or only partly true. To reach valid conclusions, researchers need to understand the difference between these conditions. We do need studies on patients with *both* FMS and CMP, but the researchers must be aware that these two conditions exist, that they are different, and must know what those differences are.

Some research papers are based on the erroneous assumption that all widespread pain is caused by FMS, and don't state the methods by which the researchers determined that the patients in the study actually had FMS (such as the American College of Rheumatology criteria), so the researchers' conclusions are suspect. I read a paper on patients with "FMS/CFS" (the title assumed that both of these conditions were the same), yet it was about the symptoms of myofascial trigger points (TrPs), and not about FMS or Chronic Fatigue Immune Deficiency Syndrome (CFIDS) at all! These patients *may* have had FMS and chronic fatigue, but the paper described nodules and ropy taut bands, localized referred pain, and other phenomena associated with TrPs. Other researchers will base their research on the conclusions of this paper, which was based on the possibly false assumption that all patients who took part in this study had FMS. This error was common. As Jan Dommerholt noted at the Travell Focus on Pain Seminar 2000 (Mesa City, AZ, March 9–12), "Faulty research leads to more faulty research."

Some medical studies are done only on men or only on women, and the conclusions reached may not apply to the opposite sex. There are also age, dietary, and perpetuating-factor variables that may not be taken into consideration. Neuroendocrine differences in the subsets of those with FMS may make a big difference in studies. Once researchers understand how common reactive hypoglycemia is in both FMS and CMP patients, a lot of research may need to be redone or reinterpreted. Vitamin and mineral inadequacies also affect many research results and are rarely taken into account. Even the time of the menstrual cycle can influence women's reactions to medications and therapies. So, with all of these caveats in mind, here is some information about current research projects that you might find interesting and/or useful.

FMS and the Thyroid Connection

You read earlier that the hypothalamus-pituitary-adrenal (HPA) axis is dysfunctional in FMS (see chapter 1). This dysfunction affects many of the body's regulatory systems, including the hypothalamus-pituitary-*thyroid* axis, which further imbalances the HPA axis. Dr. John Lowe, Director of the Fibromyalgia Research Foundation, believes that many of the symptoms of FMS are due to inadequate thyroid hormone regulation.

What the Thyroid Does

The thyroid is a butterfly-shaped gland located in the front of the throat near the windpipe. It controls metabolism (the rate at which the body turns food and oxygen into energy) by producing a hormone called thyroxine (T4). The body turns T4 into another, more powerful and rapidly acting hormone called triiodothyronine (T3). The levels of these hormones in the blood affect heart rate, body temperature, alertness, mood, and many other functions. T3 increases the flow of blood. This enhances ATP (and energy) production.[1] The thyroid is controlled by the pituitary gland, which does that by releasing or withholding thryoid-stimulating hormone (TSH), depending on the levels of T4 and T3 in the blood. Studies indicate that chronic stress will change thyroid axis function, and that this will change the immune response.[2]

Your thyroid gland may be producing enough T4 and T3, but your tissues may not be able to use them properly. According to Dr. Lowe's research,[3] the T3 uptake thyroid test is useful because it can distinguish how well your thyroid gland is actually functioning. This test separates FMS patients into two categories: (1) *hypothyroid* patients who have poorly functioning thyroid glands and need a T4-T3 combination supplement; and (2) *hypometabolism* patients who have thyroid glands that function, but who have a problem *metabolizing* thyroid hormones and who respond better to T3 supplementation. He found that FMS patients with hypometabolism and a percentage of FMS patients with hypothyroid do not benefit from treatment with synthetic T4 or desiccated thyroid.

Hypometabolism doesn't show up on common thyroid tests. Hypothyroidism is a condition due to a deficiency of thyroid hormone. Tissue hypometabolism is different. Your body may be *making* sufficient thyroid hormones, but it may not be able to *metabolize* them normally. Dr. Lowe's research team found that FMS patients who test within the normal or low normal range for hypothyroidism may have partial peripheral tissue resistance to thyroid hormone.[4] You could have "normal" thyroid test results, and still have the symptoms of low thyroid, due to thyroid inefficiency at the cellular level.

Thyroid hormone is a major regulator of cell metabolism. It regulates vital biochemicals that take part in converting the food you eat to adenosine triphosphate (ATP), the energy source in the mitochondria, which are the energy-producing cells. Thyroid hormones increase the size and activity of mitochondria as well as their oxygen consumption and their ATP production. But even if your thyroid gland produces the proper amount of hormones needed for metabolism, that doesn't necessarily mean that the hormones are metabolized properly, or used correctly in the cells.[5]

John Lowe has found that thyroid function tests are of *no value* for patients who have hypometabolism.[6] There are no common, cheap, specific and reliable tests for thyroid metabolism in peripheral tissue. Dr. Lowe discovered that most FMS patients who test low or low normal on thyroid tests have many of their FMS symptoms relieved by a combination of T3 and T4 (available as Armour Thyroid™ or Thyrolar™). J. B. Eisinger, one of the leading researchers in the field of FMS and metabolism, has confirmed this in France.[7]

Fibromyalgia patients whose tests show that they are producing normal amount of thyroid hormones respond better to T3 supplementation. Fibromyalgia patients treated according to Dr. Lowe's thyroid protocol showed significant improvement, and this improvement was not maintained when thyroid treatment was withdrawn.[8]

Once testing has determined what type of thyroid hormone may best help your FMS symptoms, you are started on thyroid supplementation. In Dr. Lowe's clinical and research experience, FMS patients with hypometabolism may require a much higher level of T3 than a healthy thyroid gland produces, because the body isn't using it efficiently.

He has found the safe and effective dosage range to be between 75 mcg and 162.5 mcg orally. He has found that T3 taken at this level is a safe and significantly effective treatment for FMS patients who test *normal* in common thyroid testing. Thyroid supplements are started at a low level and increased gradually until you reach the dose that provides optimum FMS symptom relief. Adverse affects should be remedied by adjusting the dose. These doses did produce thyroid function test results that indicated hyperthyroidism, i.e., an excess of thyroid hormone, but short-term and long-term testing of these patients revealed *no clinically significant adverse target tissue effects*, in spite of those test results.[9]

Doctors must learn to treat the *patients* in these cases, and not treat the blood tests. Your doctor should be familiar with the total Lowe protocol as specified in his book. Thyroid supplementation is only *one* facet of the Lowe thyroid protocol for FMS. Patients must exercise to tolerance, eat wholesome foods, use nutritional supplements, and receive appropriate bodywork. They must also address all perpetuating factors and coexisting conditions, such as myofascial TrPs.

Contraindications for this type of treatment: Patients diagnosed with osteoporosis before beginning thyroid supplementation may be at greater risk for fractures. Elderly patients with low cardiovascular conditioning *are* at risk, especially if they take large increases of thyroid hormones.

Indications of thyroid overstimulation include: increased appetite, fatigue, heat intolerance, increased perspiration, nervousness, weakness and weight loss, tachycardia, cardiac arrythmias, palpitations, faster pulse rate, frequent bowel movements, hair loss, anxiety, acne, and bladder leakage. Dr. Lowe can be reached at www.drlowe.com

FMS, CMP, and the Geloid Mass: A Modern Mystery

This segment will provide you some insight into how research can develop. One day my myotherapist, Justine Jeffrey, called my attention to what she called a "myoblob." *Myoblobs* are areas of dense, geloid, or hardened tissue sometimes found over trigger points (TrPs). These TrPs were resistant to standard therapies. I had observed them, too, in people with both FMS and CMP. Myoblobs covered a substantial portion of my own body. When my myotherapist worked on these areas with conventional forms of myotherapy, I felt extreme pain of a different nature than typical FMS and CMP pains. Even gentle pressure on them activated many TrPs on the same side of my body. This was devastating, as I have head-to-toe TrPs, and also have some perpetuating factors beyond my control. We tried many forms of bodywork without being able to substantially reduce these masses. They seemed to add to my general pain level and to my underlying TrPs' resistance to treatment.

I sent queries to care providers with palpation skills, asking if they had observed these myoblobs. Some providers recognized them and made some suggestions for treatment. Others had never noticed what we described. Whatever myoblobs were, they were real, but elusive.

My mentor, David Simons, provided key clues. His first reply was a politely worded inquiry wondering what was I getting into now. This was followed by an email saying that he remembered articles mentioning a similar phenomenon. His next message included specific references to two clinical studies done before FMS and CMP were shown to be separate conditions, and before the mechanisms of how TrPs develop were discovered.[10, 11] They also included carefully described biopsies of "fibrositic nodules." The descriptions were clear, concise, and closely matched what we had observed. These papers contained the results of thorough microscopic studies of these areas. The masses that had been biopsied consisted of large molecules now called glycosaminoglycans (GAGs). I suspected they had biopsied *myoblobs*. Then, I did a literature search on the Internet. (Research is, in part, a paper chase for clues.) Here is some of what I found.

Clues

Elevated plasma hyaluronic acid (HA), the most common GAG, was high in patients with arthritis.[12] An Israeli study found HA levels are even higher in women with FMS.[13] Hyaluronic acid forms a gelatinous material in the ground substance (part of the myofascia). It absorbs water and can change the ability of the tissue to stretch and conform to its surroundings, and may be involved in interstitial edema.[14] I have observed that interstitial edema is common in patients with both FMS and CMP.

Hyaluronic acid is found all over the body, and can be synthesized by most cells.[15] It is injected into joints to stop arthritis pain because it creates a gelatinous cushion. Perhaps the same effect can cause geloid swelling. Glucosamine sulfate acts as a foundation for GAGs.[16] I have observed there is a subset of patients with FMS and CMP whose symptoms worsen when they take glucosamine. Is this caused by high levels of hyaluronic acid?

One form of tissue overgrowth is associated with high levels of GAGs.[17] I had observed tissue overgrowth in patients with both FMS and CMP, ranging from ingrown hairs and overgrown cuticles to fibroids. Dr. Chang-Zern Hong, prominent myofascial pain researcher and clinician, told me that he had observed such tissue overgrowth only in his CMP patients who also had FMS. I received that email years ago, but it stayed in my mind as an important clue.

One old term for FMS or myofascial pain was *myegelosis*, especially in Germany. Some of these myoblobs felt geloid, like silicone. One study on myegelosis found a microscopically significant narrowing of the spaces between the individual muscle fibers in myogelotic areas.[18]

Skin Rolling

A recent study discussed the "skin rolling technique" as a possible diagnostic test for FMS.[19] Skin rolling is a form of bodywork in which the skin is lifted between the thumb and forefingers and rolled with the thumb pushing and the fingers pulling. This action can be useful to separate the skin from the fascia lying directly beneath it. I had observed that patients with both FMS and CMP may have skin so stuck to underlying layers that skin rolling is prohibitively painful or impossible. Others agreed. What caused this? I had discussed the combination of FMS and CMP with researchers and clinicians all over the world. Some, like J. B. Eisinger in France, also suspected that FMS and CMP together are more than the simple sum of the two. Perhaps we were on the trail of one of the reasons this is so.

I assembled more than fifty references that implied excess HA *might* be causing changes in some patients with both FMS and CMP that could lead to myoblobs forming near TrPs. I started looking at hyaluronidase (H-ase), a group of several enzymes that break up HA. It is used as a medication to increase the ability of local anesthetics to penetrate the pores, or to reduce traumatic or postoperative edema.

My local compounding pharmacist and wizard, George Roentsch, formulated a topical HA cream, as well as a matching blank (placebo). He didn't tell me which was which, but just labeled them "A" and "B." One week I put some of the contents of A on the worst myoblobs, and the next week I used B, and then I switched again. Many of the myoblobs started to diminish. The TrPs underneath them were becoming more available for treatment. Something significant was happening, but the symptom relief didn't match up with the change of the formulations.

H-ase

Later, I found that there was about a seven-day lag time on the therapeutic effect, which had confused the issue of which tube caused the symptom relief. H-ase was also very expensive and hard to get. Isaac Asimov once said that the person who learned to make a nutritious and tasty soup out of common ingredients would be more successful than the person who made it out of peacock tongues. Was there an easily available substance that was relatively cheap and had been already shown to be safe in patients with FMS or CMP?

The formation of H-ase can be triggered by the use of T3 (triiodothyronine), a naturally occurring thyroid hormone discussed in the previous section. George made up a formulation, and I started using the T3 cream on myself, keeping careful records. It wasn't as dramatic as H-ase, but in combination with my usual bodywork and self-care, the masses were becoming smaller and less dense. We planned a clinical study to test the formulation on patients with FMS, CMP, and myoblobs, using a topical cream. Oral medications often lose potency during the metabolic pass through the liver. We could probably use less T3 than would be needed orally to get the same effect. By this time, Dr. Simons had renamed the "myoblob" the "geloid mass."

I wrote to Dr. Lowe, who has been a friend for some time, as well as to Dr. Garrison, another friend who had worked with Dr. Lowe. They both expressed extreme interest and support, and Dr. Garrison helped me draft a paper on the topical T3 preparation. Dr. Simons had followed the whole process, and supplied an incredible amount of time, guidance, and insight. He also closely mentored my case study, our first paper on the geloid mass phenomenon.

The participants in the study had FMS, CMP, and geloid masses. They were taught the methods of application, how to keep daily charts, and potential side effects. The Israeli study had been done on women. We included three men in our study. None of these patients had ever exhibited low thyroid function in any tests. None were on thyroid medication. The purpose of the study was to see if the geloid masses would soften/become more pliable/reduce in size, and/or the symptom load diminish, with the topical T3 therapy.

The preliminary results are very promising. Most of the study participants improved significantly (some dramatically reduced their pain medications). I have been able to put only a few hundred hours into correlating the data, and must wait until this edition is finished before the article is written and submitted to a peer-reviewed medical journal. By the time this book goes to press, the initial case study on the presence of the geloid mass will have been published.[20] The complete details of the T3 formulation have been sent to the Professional Compounding Centers of America (see Resources). They will help you find a local compounding pharmacist. If your insurance will not cover the transdermal form, there is an oral form of T3, Cytomel, but you may require a higher dose.

One interesting note: A new study[21] contradicts the Israeli study. This research team used exactly the same HA assay. What does this mean? The H-ase and the T3 seemed to work on the geloid masses. Is there another variable, like a coexisting condition such as insulin resistance, that might be involved? We don't know. We do know that more research is needed.

Calcium Channel Blockers

I don't plan on doing any more research studies. I *am* intrigued by the new understanding of TrP mechanisms. If a key to TrP formation is excess calcium release at the motor endplate, a topical calcium channel blocker might be effective on resistant myofascial TrPs. I know that Dr. Hong is researching the effect of a systemic calcium channel blocker. George formulated some topical creams to use on resistant TrPs without geloid masses. The preliminary results inspire hope, but we don't know what the safety issues might be. One study on two patients[22] found that their TrP injections were no longer effective when they were put on systemic calcium channel blockers. Was this due to the changes in balance of inter- and intracellular calcium? There is much we don't know. I hope more research is done, and soon.

Fibromyalgia and the Vitamin Connection

Dr. J. B. Eisinger, metabolic researcher and clinician, believes that vitamin B1 abnormalities found in people with FMS are caused by a nutritional deficiency. People with FMS may have a problem converting thiamine into cocarboxylase, also called thiamine pyrophosphate (TPP). Cocarboxylase is required for cellular energy generation. This metabolic deficit could be one reason why we lack adequate ATP (adenosine triphosphate).[23] Thiamine and its derivatives have been prescribed for years to treat neurotransmitter dysfunction and chronic pain.

Dr. Eisinger has found that cocarboxylase works better than thiamine, alone or in combination with magnesium, to relieve FMS symptoms. He urges further research into other B vitamins, minerals, amino acids, and other biochemicals that stimulate this metabolic pathway. Compounding pharmacists can create cocarboxylase in sublingual forms (medications that dissolve under the tongue). This medication is also available in IM (injectable) form. Dr. Eisinger can be reached at Service de Rheumatologie, Center Hospitalier Toulon-La Seyne, BP 1412, 83056 Toulon, France.

Electrical Galvanic Glove Stimulation

Dr. Carolyn McMakin has developed a unique method to deliver electrical stimulation to her patients. She believes that the microcurrent therapy she has developed, delivered through vinyl graphite gloves worn by trained therapists, can restore tissues to a more balanced state and allow healing to take place.[24] She has been able to successfully treat areas of fibrotic tissue often found in patients with both FMS and CMP.

Your body can use very small amounts of current to stimulate critical protein production and enhance the available ATP to promote cellular healing. Dr. McMakin has been able to separate FMS into several subsets associated with: (1) prolonged emotional or physical stress and resulting adrenal exhaustion; (2) organic chemical, heavy metal, or pesticide exposure; (3) genetic tendency, with frequent allergy or dysfunction in liver metabolism; (4) viral or immunization onset; and (5) neck trauma or surgery. These five subsets respond to different frequencies and types of current.

Dr. McMakin has found that patients with head and neck trauma experience nerve-generated symptom intensity not present in her other FMS patients. Even these patients respond to specific microcurrent treatment. She has taught them to maintain pain relief with a home unit. She also uses nutritional supplements. These patients have greatly reduced or eliminated their pain medication.

During the treatment the patients feel only warmth and tissue softening. After an average of about eleven treatments, her patients had a lasting reduction of pain even after more traditional treatments had failed. There is a posttreatment "detox" that starts about ninety minutes after the treatment, which can last for twenty-four hours. This includes a flulike ache, nausea, and a temporary increase in pain. For more information, contact Dr. McMakin at 17214 Division Suite 2, Portland, OR 97236. Phone: 503-762-0805; fax: 503-760-1015.

Cellular Acidity and FMS

Jim Clements believes that FMS is the result of an overacid situation. Glucose requires a lot of processing to turn it into ATP, and more processing is needed to turn ATP into usable energy. He thinks that the mitochondria process ATP incompletely in those who have FMS. Each cell generates far less than the maximum amount of ATP it could produce if it were healthy. One reason for this may be lower than normal available oxygen at the cellular level due a more acidic state. The pH range (the way of measuring acidity) of the blood is about 7.30 to 7.45. When blood is at 7.45 pH, it can carry almost 50 percent more oxygen than blood at 7.3 pH. Mitochondria need the oxygen to generate ATP and energy, just as fire needs oxygen to burn fuel.

Changes in pH can also affect the cytoskeleton, the structural matrix of the cell. That can affect cell shape or movement. When cellular pH is low, cells can stick together, forming clumps that obstruct normal function.[25] Low pH may also cause the formation of a type of phosphate that can weaken muscular force if those muscles become fatigued. Because myofascial TrPs also weaken muscles, this could be another reason why FMS and CMP are mutually aggravating. Jim Clements has found a way to process water so that consuming it creates a less acidic cellular environment in the body. If you wish to learn more, contact Jim Clements at Total Health Marketing P.O. Box 521739, Salt Lake City, UT 84152, or write to him at info@thmi.com

Myofascial TrPs and Botulinum Toxin Injection

Botulinum toxin inhibits muscle contraction, and appears to be effective in treating myofascial pain such as chronic head and neck pain after whiplash, and also some low-back pain.[26] It blocks the release of acetylcholine. Remember that myofascial TrPs form due to an excess of the neurotransmitter, acetylcholine, which causes the release of excess calcium (see chapter 3).

Dr. Robert Gerwin restricts the use of botulinum toxin to the treatment of TrPs that are resistant to other therapies but which affect his patients' quality of life. The TrPs must have responded temporarily to standard TrP injection. If the TrPs keep coming back in spite of standard therapies, he puts the patient into his botulinum study. It must be used carefully, according to specific procedures, in minute amounts. Following botulinum toxin injection, there may be problems with temporary muscle weakness lasting several hours, and this must be taken into consideration when injecting load-bearing muscles.

Myofascial TrPs are often a treatable contributor to many chronic pain states, even when the underlying cause of pain or structural abnormality cannot be remedied. Dr. Gerwin and Jan Dommerholt found that 100 percent of the patients they treated for chronic pain caused by whiplash over a period of six months had chronic myofascial TrPs relevant to their pain. **Note:** *Fibromyalgia does not respond to botulinum toxin.* We need more research data to support the use of botulinum toxin in CMP. Dr. Gerwin can be reached at Pain and Rehabilitation Medicine, 7830 Old Georgetown Road, Suite C-15, Bethesda, MD 20814-2432. Phone: 301-656-0220; fax: 301-654-0333.

The Impact of Pain

Researchers are studying the effects of pain at the molecular level. We are discovering the mechanisms involved in how and why we feel pain. Dr. Tony Yaksh reported at the Travell Seminar held in 2000 that after a trauma, an excess amount of hydrogen ions has been observed in the involved tissue, which causes it to become acidic.[27]

This changes the way the tissue responds to biochemical processes. Pain affects clotting time, wound healing, immune function, muscle tone, cardiovascular stability, sleep, gastrointestinal motility, and our emotions. Inadequately treated acute pain can lead to processes that result in a sensitized state, such as the allodynia and hyperalgesia of FMS. Currently, researchers are separating and identifying pain receptors and cellular mechanisms and pinpointing their roles as links in the chain of pain.

More selective and safer delivery systems for analgesics are being developed. We are finding ways to slip molecules past cell membrane barriers and to target areas of dysfunction more selectively. We are also finding ways to move medications safely through the *blood-brain barrier*. This barrier safeguards the brain from chemical and biological toxins and other agents that may be circulating in the bloodstream, but it also prevents some medications from accessing the brain. Dr. Yaksh expects that the massive amount of current research in neurobiology will result in breakthroughs in chronic pain relief. Dr. Yaksh is Professor of Anesthesiology and Pharmacology at UC San Diego, working on a NIH research grant studying adenosine receptors. He can be reached at UCSD, Anesthesiology 0818, 9500 Gilman Drive, La Jolla, CA 92093-0818.

Fibromyalgia and Guaifenesin

Excess calcium and inorganic phosphate can cause mitochondrial hyperpermeability.[28] This will allow excess fluids, ions and other substances into the mitochondria that don't belong there, producing swelling and interfering with normal function. This may be part of what happens in FMS. Dr. R. Paul St. Amand believes FMS is caused by an abnormality in phosphate excretion, which may be due to a genetic defect. Retention of phosphates eventually interferes with energy production in the affected cells.

One study[29] found a 20 percent reduction in the level of ATP in muscle biopsies taken from people with FMS. Excess inorganic phosphate in the mitochondria, your energy-generating cells, slows formation of ATP. Muscle pain after exercise is also linked with an increase in inorganic phosphate.[30]

Calcium is the main buffer for phosphate. A buffer is a substance that diminishes a pH change that would otherwise take place when acid is added. In this case, the calcium ions, which are alkaline in nature, balance the phosphate ions, which are acid in nature.

Guaifenesin is usually an ingredient in cold preparations. In its original form, as a tree bark extract called guaiacum, it was used to treat rheumatism in the year 1530. In the new *PDR for Herbal Medicines*[31] guaiacum officinale is again indicated for rheumatism. Over twenty years ago it was synthesized, named guaifenesin, and pressed into tablets. Guaifenesin is totally absorbed by the intestinal tract within two hours after taking it.

Using guaifenesin therapy, Dr. St. Amand found a 60 percent increase in phosphate excretion and a 30 percent increase in oxalate in his patients' urine. I believe that these phosphoric and oxalic acids (also excreted in sweat) carry with them other excess acids that may be significant. We don't know.

About 20 percent of Dr. St. Amand's patients go through FMS reversal relatively quickly, taking 300 mg of guaifenesin twice a day. St. Amand believes that FMS develops in a cyclical process. At first, as FMS develops, there are times when we experience symptoms interspersed with periods when we feel fine. Then, the periods without symptoms become shorter, the symptomatic episodes become more frequent, and the symptoms worsen. This is what St. Amand calls "cycling." He believes that guaifenesin therapy causes a reversal of this process.

Your most recent symptoms will fade first. When enough of these substances are eliminated, every once in a while you will have a period where your symptoms ease. You may then begin to experience whole days where you feel well. It is important not to overdo on these days. Your body is struggling to regain balance. Don't overtax it. When you get to the point where there are clusters of good days, the contrast can be remarkable. Knowing what is happening helps you to deal with the reversal symptoms. The bad days are still bad, but you know why, and you know you are on a path to better health.

If the cyclic process described below hasn't begun after two weeks, patients are raised to 600 mg twice a day. Seventy percent of all patients experience FMS reversal at that dose. Another 20 percent of his patients need 1800 mg a day. The final 10 percent require 2400 mg or more per day.

The Cycling Process

The body works hard to process chemical toxins and excess materials so that they can be excreted. When the first cycle begins, as stored toxins and excess phosphates start releasing, there is usually a period of flulike fatigue. For the first few months of guaifenesin therapy, you can expect to spit out a lot of mucus that has been clogging your airways. Headaches are very common during this process. You may have other symptoms, including strong smelling perspiration and urine and burning on urination. Your urine *may* become very dark. Also, the crease between your buttocks and the perineal area may become sore and need protective cream.

It is important to follow the guaifenesin protocol. If severe and unusual side effects appear after beginning guaifenesin therapy, discontinue use at once and check with your doctor. You may need to go on the hypoglycemia diet for a while, or decrease your exposure to toxic chemicals. Something else may be happening. Your liver may not be able to handle the wastes and chemical toxic by-products that are coming out, for example. You may decide to resume guaifenesin therapy at a later time. Do so very slowly, starting with 100 mg a day and working up in increments of 100 mg at a time. For a list of products with salicylates, consult Dr. St. Amand's book (see Reading List) or the Guaifenesin Internet Support Group (see Resources). *Do not change your dosage of guaifenesin or any other medication without checking it with your doctor.* Keep track of what happens. Start by taking 300 mg of guaifenesin twice a day. Take 300 mg twice a day for one week. *If your symptoms become distinctly worse, you have found the dosage right for you.* The symptoms in reversal are not side effects of taking guaifenesin. They are from the chemical toxins and wastes being released by the guaifenesin, and are good signs, although they don't feel like it at the time. Do not use any medications or herbal products containing salicylates. They can block the action of guaifenesin.

Map your areas of pain and symptoms carefully before you start therapy. I have seen some people start gentle guaifenesin therapy on 200 mg a day. The correct dosage varies from patient to patient. If, after one week, no obvious change occurs, increase the dose to 600 mg twice a day for about a month. Check your initial map, and draw a new one periodically, saving them as a record of your treatment.

Each person seems to have a different sensitivity to the guaifenesin blocking effect of certain salicylates. If you've found your proper dosage and suddenly the cycling stops and your symptoms worsen, check out secondary sources such as camphor, almond oil, coconut oil, lauric acid, and so forth. This has happened to me and to others, and we've always been able to track down the offending salicylate and eliminate it, with a subsequent return to improvement. These setbacks and subsequent resolutions are yet another indication to me that guaifenesin is doing something important.

We don't know for sure why guaifenesin works in so many people with FMS. It could even be that it is affecting a common perpetuating factor, such as insulin resistance or cellular pH. We just don't know. I see it working, Dr. St. Amand sees it working, and countless other doctors have seen it working. Only phosphate is known to decrease ATP formation when it accumulates in the mitochondrial matrix. ATP is essential to almost all cellular functions.

Guaifenesin therapy for FMS is not simple. Doctors can't just prescribe a standard dose and expect to see symptom remission. St. Amand begins by taking a careful medical history of the patient. He examines the patient's body for swollen areas, which he maps. As patients progress, the symptoms tend to disappear in the reverse order in which they first appeared. For the reversal to become evident in patients with reactive hypoglycemia, they *must* be on a balanced diet. This means *no excess carbohydrates.* I have found that the Sears' Zone-type diet works well (see Reading List), although it must be tailored to individual needs. For many people, guaifenesin therapy seems to result in remission of symptoms. There may be coexisting conditions, like myofascial TrPs, that also need attention, and you may have other perpetuating factors that must be identified and addressed.

The only double-blind study on FMS guaifenesin therapy was done at the University of Oregon.[32] This study of twenty women showed guaifenesin equal to placebo. The study was flawed, through no fault of the researchers, because of the following reasons:

1. The study was started before we knew the signs of reversal are not obvious if uncontrolled reactive hypoglycemia is present. At that time, no one knew how common reactive hypoglycemia/ insulin resistance was.

2. All the patients in the study were given 600 mg of guaifenesin twice a day. Only about 50 percent of patients respond at this dosage; and even in these patients, the reversal won't be

evident if they have reactive hypoglycemia and are eating excess carbohydrates. The dosage must be individually tailored.

3. Dr. St. Amand did not know about the blockage of guaifenesin by some salicylate-containing herbs until September 1995. The study ended in June 1995. Each person seems to have different sensitivity to various products.

4. Some people say Dr. St. Amand's patients feel better because he's charismatic. He *is*. I love the guy. He is charming and has a superb wit. But how can these positive attributes cause me to have dark, smelly, acidic urine that cleans the iron stains from my toilet bowl? Toilet bowls *do not* respond to the placebo effect.

There is another study currently underway on guaifenesin using the *exact same* flawed protocols that were used in the previous study, in spite of St. Amand's explanations on the parameter requirements. Dr. St. Amand contacted the head of the study, offering to fly there at his own expense, but his letters were ignored.

Dr. St. Amand and I agree to disagree on some issues. Respectful controversy is healthy. We both believe that phosphate retention is a common perpetuating factor of FMS, and that guaifenesin is not a *cure* for FMS. Please understand that symptom reversal is not the same as a cure. Right now, there is no cure for FMS. With guaifenesin therapy, some patients have been able to get rid of many or all of their symptoms, or at least ease them considerably. They still have FMS. If they don't keep their perpetuating factors (overwork, poor diet, lack of sleep) under control, the symptoms will return. Taking guaifenesin will not change the metabolic conditions that caused you to need it in the first place. As soon as you stop taking it, as far as we know, the biochemicals will begin to build up in your body again.

I have seen many people given a new lease on life with guaifenesin, and I have experienced it myself. If you wish to learn more, read St. Amand's *What Your Doctor May Not Tell You About Fibromyalgia* (see Reading List). Some of the data for this section has been adapted from this book, with permission from the authors. There is a guaifenesin Internet support group, and Web site. Guaifenesin may be purchased over the counter through Hyrex Pharmaceuticals (see Resources), and they will ship to other countries. Nevertheless, both Dr. St. Amand and I feel that guaifenesin therapy should take place only under a doctor's supervision.

Relaxin and FMS

Many FMS patients have reported remission of symptoms during pregnancy, and the return of symptoms one to two months after delivery. These observations started Dr. Samuel Yue's search for a biochemical that changes in availability during this time span. He found the hormone relaxin. Relaxin's effects include an increase in elasticity and relaxation of muscles, tendons, and ligaments during pregnancy, particularly in the pelvis. Dr. Yue believes FMS is related to a systemic deficit of relaxin, or an inability to use the existing hormone.

Dr. Yue thinks that FMS is a form of *dysautonomia*. Dysautonomia describes a delayed, inappropriate, and exaggerated response of the autonomic nervous system (ANS) to an external or internal stimulus. The ANS consists of the sympathetic and the parasympathetic systems. The sympathetic system of the ANS is responsible for many functions, including increase in heart rate and bowel smooth muscle tone, decrease in blood flow, and increase in blood pressure. The parasympathetic system controls opposing effects, such as increasing blood flow and decreasing blood pressure. These balancing systems maintain function. This system of balances is disrupted in FMS.

The leaky gut syndrome (see chapter 23) affects how your body absorbs nutrients. The bowel lining acts as a filter to allow necessary nutrients into the bloodstream so that they can be used. The closing and opening of the filter to allow the passage of nutrients is directly related to the ANS balance (sympathetic versus parasympathetic systems). Poorly digested foods can get into the bloodstream, and needed nutrients can be blocked from entry. When undigested small foreign proteins are allowed into the bloodstream, allergic-type reactions begin. The degree of reaction depends on the amount of foreign proteins absorbed.

Dr. Yue utilizes a comprehensive program of treatment for both FMS and CMP. He has been one of the pioneers of botulinum injection for myofascial TrPs. His program includes the use of supplements, exercise, digestive enzymes, and guaifenesin. He has found that patients with irritable bowel syndrome (IBS) sometimes have difficulty with the timed-release forms of guaifenesin. For these patients, he uses short-acting forms.[33] Dr. Yue is Clinical Director of HealthEast Pain Clinic, HealthEast Bethesda Lutheran Hospital and Rehab Center, 559 Capitol Blvd, St. Paul MN 55103. Phone: 800-442-3200; 612-232-2319; fax: 612-232-2328.

SyNAPs Neurotherapy and Fibromyalgia

Dr. Mary Lee Esty believes fibromyalgia (FMS) is misnamed because the dysfunction is in the brain, not in the muscle fibers. Trauma-induced changes in the central nervous system (CNS) perpetuate FMS symptoms. The CNS ability to filter and process signals is modified, leaving increased perception of pain. Dr. Esty has found that most FMS patients seen in her clinic have a history of mild or moderate brain trauma. When brain cells are damaged by physical or biochemical trauma, imbalances appear, regardless of the cause of damage. The first two grades of concussion do not involve loss of consciousness and many people remain unaware that they have sustained a concussion. Brain trauma is cumulative. Minor brain traumas through life can culminate in a variety of major dysfunctions. The majority of FMS patients have had brain trauma that is sufficient to affect functioning.

Improvements and enhancements to older equipment and treatment protocols have resulted in SyNAPs (Synergistic Neurotherapy Adjustment Process System). SyNAPs is a painless, noninvasive procedure guided by monitoring and analyzing EEG signals from the patient's brain once or twice a week. The signals are recorded through surface electrodes held on the scalp with a conductive paste. SyNAPs uses an invisible and imperceptible electromagnetic signal radiating from equipment that is FDA approved. Signal power is approximately the same as normal brain-wave activity (a trillionth of a watt). During treatment the exposure length of stimulation is modified according to the specific needs and responses of the individual patient.

The initial evaluation includes a brain map and a treatment. The quantitative EEG (QEEG) and the SyNAPs maps are painless measures of brain function. The EEG patterns reveal imbalances, and are predictors of treatment response. In a healthy person, brain waves are regular and relatively smooth. When healthy adults are awake, the slower brain waves (1-2 cycles/second) should be relatively equal in energy and smoothness. EEG activity in FMS patients is excessive in the front of the head, indicating an imbalance consistent with energy, mood, restless mind, sleep, cognitive, loss of libido, dysautonomia, and pain problems. This inefficient energy state reflects the very real life problems of people with FMS.

As the electroencephalogram (EEG) amplitudes begin to lower, FMS patients experience a reduction of symptoms. Dr. Esty has found that patients with FMS are able to delete or reduce medications substantially. As FMS "fibrofog" lifts, some patients become aware of sharper, localized myofascial TrP pain. These TrPs are then treated with appropriate bodywork, and localized symptoms are relieved. The majority of people without chronic infection who complete SyNAPs treatment have achieved virtual remission of FMS symptoms. The researchers found that some FMS patients concentrate with their eyes closed because this cuts down on sensory stimuli. This may be useful for us to remember in times of fibrofog.

SyNAPs is effective for traumatic brain injuries. Gentle stimulation "tickles" the brain, and is thought to activate symptomatic change by enhancing neural plasticity, the capacity of the brain to change. Mechanisms that may be activated by this stimulation include increased blood flow, changes in glucose metabolism, stimulation of neuron healing, and a change in cell inhibitory/excitatory potentials. For information contact Mary Lee Esty, Ph.D., LCSW-C, President of the Neurotherapy Center of Washington and Washington DC, 5480 Wisconsin Avenue, Suite 221, Chevy Chase, MD 301-652-7175, www.neurotherapycenters.com. For video information, see www.fm-research.com.

The Mechanism of Muscular Contraction

Dr. Kuan Wang and his colleagues discovered five proteins (*filamin, nebulin, nebulette, talin,* and *titin*) involved in muscle structure that may provide clues as to why our muscles can become so tight they hurt. Dr. Leepo Yu studies how muscles produce force from energy at the molecular level. Their discoveries may explain some of what happens when myofascial TrPs form.

When a healthy muscle is at rest, it is supple and elastic. When it's at work, it contracts and then returns to its original size and shape. This all takes place because of changes that occur at the molecular level. These changes affect the *sarcomeres*, which are the basic units of contraction in the muscle. Changes in the shape of the sarcomeres are important in TrP formation.

Inside each sarcomere, there is a cytoskeleton. This is a structural matrix built of elastic titin and nebulin protein strands. These provide structural connection to the muscle cells. Titin is a giant molecular protein spring.[34] Titin allows the sarcomeres to return to their former length after they contract.

Titin holds the sarcomeres together. It is important for the integrity of muscle structure. It is a complex, information-rich molecule, like DNA. Titin is present in striated muscle, and is also found in smooth muscle cells like heart cells. The discoveries of the mechanisms of these molecules have relevance to conditions other than myofascial TrPs, like congestive heart failure. In congestive heart failure these proteins are significantly decreased.[35] This may be part of the interstitial edema/myofascial connection (see chapter 5). The possibility of developing congestive heart failure may be another reason why some of us, those with carbohydrate cravings, reactive hypoglycemia, or insulin resistance need to monitor our diets carefully. We need more research on nonstriated muscle in both FMS and CMP.

We should all take hope that the functioning of the muscle structure at the molecular level is being thoroughly studied. Drs. Kuan Wang and Leepo C. Yu may be reached at the National Institutes of Arthritis, Muscular and Skin Diseases, NIH, Bldg 6, Room 408, 6 Center Drive, Bethesda MD, 20892-2755.

So Much More

In the first edition of the *Survival Manual*, I wrote that I believed glial cells were more than just scaffolding. Glial cells function in the central nervous system similar to the way the myofascia functions in the musculoskeletal system. Both FMS and CMP researchers should be studying glial cells. Since the first edition, we have learned that some glial cells affect mineral ion concentrations. We have also learned recently that nerve cells can regenerate, and that glials are a key to this nervous system renewal. Glial cells may control the number of synapses that develop between nerve cells, as well as the stability and function of those synapses.[36] They are also important in nerve cell development and activity.[37] Recent research indicates that T3 (triiodothyronine) is involved in the regulation of glial cell development.[38] Glial research is still in its infancy, and is linked with cytoskeleton research. It promises to offer new hope in the understanding of both FMS and CMP.

Some of us have rising cholesterol levels that don't seem to reflect our dietary habits. As I worked on this edition, I became acquainted with a number of researchers. One such researcher is Dr. Salih Ozgocmen in Turkey.[39] In his well written study, which compares patients with FMS, patients with myofascial pain, and healthy controls, those with myofascial pain had significantly higher total cholesterol, triglycerides, low-density lipoprotein cholesterol, and very low-level density cholesterol than both the control group and the FMS group. The study factored into consideration exercise and many other variables. We don't know whether these differences help to cause myofascial TrPs, are a result of TrPs, or are simply coexisting phenomena. What the study does indicate is that there is a relationship between lipids (fats) and TrPs. More research needs to be done in this area.

Another study links HPA axis abnormalities (found in FMS) with abdominal obesity and insulin resistance.[40] Overreaction to environmental stressors may be one of the HPA dysfunctions leading to abdominal obesity.

Some of the information in this chapter is from the Focus on Pain Seminar. Was your doctor there? For information ON these seminars, contact The Janet G. Travell MD Seminar Series, 7830 Old Georgetown Road, Suite C-15, Bethesda, MD 20814-2432. Phone: 301-656-0220; fax: 301-654-0333. The research profiled here is but a tiny sample of work going on all over the globe. Always remember that even though some doctors try to deny the existence of FMS and CMP, there are many doctors who know better, and they are working to understand all aspects of these illnesses. They are also working on symptom relief methods. They are the light at the end of the tunnel, and it beckons us brightly. You only need to look in the right direction.

Endnotes

1. Wrutniak-Cabello, C., F. Casas, and G. Cabello. 2001. Thyroid hormone action in mitochondria. *J Mol Endocrinol* 26(1):67-77.

2. Cremaschi, G. A., G. Gorelik, A. J. Klecha, A. E. Lysionek, and A. M. Genaro. 2000. Chronic stress influences the immune system through the thyroid axis. *Life Sci* 67(26):3171-3179.

3. Lowe, J. 2000. *The Metabolic Treatment of Fibromyalgia.* Boulder, CO: McDowell Publishing Company.

4. Lowe, J. C., R. L. Garrison, A. L. Reichman, J. Yellin, M. Thompson, and D. Kaufman. 1997. Effectiveness and safety of T3 (triiodothyronine) therapy for euthyroid fibromyalgia: a double-blind placebo-controlled response-driven crossover study. *Clin Bull Myofas Ther* 2(2/3):31

5. Lowe. 2000. *Op. cit.*

6. *Ibid.*

7. Eisinger J. 1998. Place du syndrome polymyalgies-hypothyroidie instable dans le cadre des manifestations musculaires des hypothyroidiens traits. *Lyons Med* 35(2):37-40. [French]

8. Lowe, J. C., A. J. Reichman, and J. Yellin. 1997. The process of change during T3 treatment for euthyroid fibromyalgia: A double-blind placebo-controlled crossover study. *Clin Bul Myo Ther* 2(2/3):91-124.

9. *Ibid.*

10. Awad, E. A. 1973. Interstitial myofibrositis: hypothesis of the mechanism. *Arch Phys Med Rehabil* 54(10): 449-453.

11. Brendstrup P., K. Jesperson, and G. Asboe-Hansen. 1957. Morphological and chemical connective tissue changes in fibrositis muscles. *Ann Rheum Dis* 16:438-440.

12. Goldberg, R. L., J. P. Huff, M. E. Lenz, P. Glickman, R. Katz, and E. J. Thonar. 1991. Elevated plasma levels of hyaluronate in patients with osteoarthritis and rheumatoid arthritis. *Arthritis Rheum* 34(7):799-807.

13. Yaron, I., D. Buskila, I. Shirazi, I. Neumann, O. Elkayam, D. Parran, et al. 1997. Elevated levels of hyaluronic acid in the sera of women with fibromyalgia. *J Rheumatol* 24(11):2221-2224.

14. Liu, N. F., and L. R. Zhang. 1998. Changes of tissue fluid hyaluronan (hyaluronic acid) in peripheral lymphedema. *Lymphology* 31:173-179.

15. Chen, W. Y. J., and G. Abatangelo. 1999. Functions of hyaluronan in wound repair. *Wound Rep Reg* 7:79-89.

16. Kelly, G. S. 1998. The role of glucosamine sulfate and chondroitin sulfates in the treatment of degenerative joint disease. *Altern Med Rev* 3(1):27-39.

17. Mariani, G., C. Calastrini, F. Carinci, L. Bergamini, F. Calastrini, and G. Stabellini. 1996. Ultrastructural and histochemical features of the ground substance in cyclosporin A-induced gingival overgrowth. *J Periodontol* 67(1):21-27.

18. Windisch, A., A. Reitinger, H. Traxler, H. Radner, C. Neumayer, W. Feigl, et al. 1999. Morphology and histochemistry of myegelosis. *Clin Anat* 12(4):266-271.

19. Zohn, D., and D. Clauw. 1999. Skin rolling as a diagnostic test for fibromyalgia. *J Musculoskel Pain* 7(3):127-136.

20. Starlanyl, D. J., and J. L. Jeffrey. 2001. Geloid masses in a patient with both fibromyalgia and chronic myofascial pain. *Phys Ther Case Rep* 4(1):22-31.

21. Bliddal, H., H. J. Moller, M. Schaadt, and B. Danneskiold-Samsoe. 2000. Patients with fibromyalgia have normal serum levels of hyaluronic acid. *J Rheumatol* 27(11):2658-2659.

22. Simons, D. G., J. G. Travell, and L. S. Simons. 1999. *Travell and Simons' Myofascial Pain and Dysfunction: The Trigger Point Manual.* Second edition. Baltimore: Williams and Wilkins, p.75.

23. Eisinger, J. B. 1998. Alcohol, thiamin and fibromyalgia. *J Am Col Nutri* 17(3):300-303.

24. McMakin, C. 1998. Microtreatment of myofascial pain in the head, neck and face. *Top Clin Chiro* 5(1):29-35.

25. Sperelakis, N., ed. 1998. *Cell Physiology Source Book.* San Diego: Academic Press.

26. Cheshire, W. P., S. W. Abashian, and J. D. Mann. 1994. Botulinum toxin in the treatment of myofascial pain syndrome. *Pain* 59(1):65-69.

27. Yaksh, Tony. 2000. New developments in the pharmacologic management of pain. Paper presented at the Focus on Pain Seminar, Mesa City, AZ.

28. Savage, M. K., and D. J. Reed. 1994. Oxidation of pyridine nucleotides and depletion of ATP and ADP during calcium- and inorganic phosphate-induced mitochondrial permeability transition. *Biochem Biophys Res Communications* 200(3):1615-1620.

29. Bengtsson A., K. G. Henriksson, and J. Larsson. 1986. Reduced high-energy phosphate levels in the painful muscles of patients with primary fibromyalgia. *Arthritis Rheum.* 29:817-821.

30. Aldridge, R., E. B. Cady, D. A. Jones, and G. Obletter. 1986. Muscle pain after exercise is linked with an inorganic phosphate increase as shown by 31P NMR. *Biosci Rep* 6(7):663-667.

31. Medical Economics Staff. 1998. *PDR for Herbal Medicines.* Montvale, NJ: Medical Economics.

32. Bennett, R. M., P. De Garmo, and S. R. Clark. 1996. A 1 year double-blind placebo-controlled study of guaifenesin in fibromyalgia. *Arth Rheum* 39: S212.

33. Personal communication. June 29, 2000.

34. Horowits, R. 1999. The physiological role of titin in striated muscle. *Rev Physiol Biochem Pharmacol* 138:57-96.

35. Hein, S., S. Kostin, A. Heling, Y. Maeno, and J. Schaper. 2000. The role of the cytoskeleton in heart failure. *Cardiovas Res* 45(2):273-278.

36. Ullian, E. M. , S. K. Sapperstein, K. S. Christopherson, and B. A. Barres. 2001. Control of Synapse Number by Glia. *Science* 291:657-661.

37. Barres, B. A., and Y-A Barde. 2000 *Curr Opin Neurobiol* 10:642-648.

38. Lima, F. R., A. Gervais, C. Colin, M. Izembart, V. M. Neto, and M. Mallat. 2001. Regulation of microglial development: a novel role for thyroid hormone. *J Neurosci* 21(6):2028-2038.

39. Ozgocmen, S., and O. Ardicoglu. 2000. Lipid profile in patients with fibromyalgia and myofascial pain syndromes. *Yonsei Med J* 41(5):541-545.

40. Vicennati, V., and R. Pasquali. 2000. Abnormalities of the hypothalamic-pituitary-adrenal axis in nondepressed women with abdominal obesity and relations with insulin resistance: evidence for a central and a peripheral alteration. *J Clin Endocrinol Metab* 85(11):4093-4098.

CHAPTER 16

Wellness Recovery Action Planning

Fibromyalgia (FMS) brings change to your life. It profoundly affects your ability to manage your life on a day-to-day basis. Fibromyalgia is a chronic condition that can affect every aspect of your life, for the rest of your life,[1] so it is important to develop long-term strategies to deal with it.

Managing the chronic symptoms of a complex illness can be a daunting task. After reading all the suggestions in previous chapters about what you can do to help prevent flares and to relieve and recover from symptoms, you may literally not know what to do next. Developing a Wellness Recovery Action Plan (WRAP) for yourself and using this plan on a daily basis will help to relieve your anxiety, and also help you to feel as well as you possibly can.

A Wellness Recovery Action Plan is a structured system for doing the following:

1. Monitoring uncomfortable or distressing symptoms, unhealthy habits, or behavior patterns;

2. Reducing, modifying, or eliminating those symptoms or habits through planned responses;

3. Creating the life change you want;

4. Planning an advanced directive that instructs others on how to make decisions for you, take care of you, and support you in case your symptoms escalate to the point where it is impossible for you to take care of yourself.

Anecdotal reports from people who are using this system indicate that their level of wellness increases and their overall quality of life improves significantly when they follow the plan. Following it means to take ongoing preventive actions by responding to symptoms when they first appear rather than when they become severe, and by responding in ways that help to reduce, relieve, or eliminate the symptoms.

This monitoring and response system was developed by people who have been dealing with a variety of chronic conditions for many years and who work hard to feel better and get on with their lives. It is not a replacement for working with a caring team of health care providers. *WRAP is a safe and wise addition to any chosen course of treatment.* You can use it effectively to deal with fibromyalgia, chronic myofascial pain (CMP), and any perpetuating factors, co-occurring illnesses, or distressing lifestyle issues. You can also use it to work on personal goals and priorities. For instance, one woman uses this plan to deal with fibromyalgia, recurring chronic depression, and carbohydrate addiction.

You need to develop a plan for yourself. You are the only person who can make it work for you. No one else can develop a Wellness Recovery Action Plan that will work for you as well as you can.

These are the supplies you will need to develop your own recovery monitoring system:

1. A three-ring binder, one-inch thick. I prefer the kind that has pockets for inserting papers inside the front and back covers. You can use these pockets to keep copies of medical records, information about medications, "generic daily plans," lists of supporters, and lists of enjoyable diversionary activities, or any other important papers you want to keep within easy reach.

2. A set of five divider sheets or tabs.

3. Three-ring filler paper.

4. A writing instrument of some kind.

5. And, if possible, a friend or other supporter to give you assistance and feedback.

You may prefer to use a computer to develop your Wellness Recovery Action Plan. Then, you can refer to the plan on your computer, or you could print it out on three-ring paper for a binder.

Developing a Wellness Toolbox

The first step in developing your own Wellness Recovery Action Plan is to develop a Wellness Toolbox—a listing of "tools" you will use to develop your WRAP. This list should include things you have done in the past to help yourself feel better, and new things you would like to try. Your tools may have been learned from the first edition of this book, from health care providers, or other resources. As you learn to use new tools, you can add them to this list and integrate them into your plan wherever you think they will be helpful. You can also list those activities, people, or thoughts that you want to avoid.

The following list of tools and avoidances comes from other parts of this book. Write out your own list of activities, behaviors, ideas, or people that you think might be helpful to you, along with those you want to avoid. Later on, you can modify your list to meet your specific needs more closely.

Lifestyle

• reduce the clutter in your home • simplify your life • get help with chores • ask others to take over household responsibilities • take personal time for activities that bring you pleasure • make lists of tasks and chores • break up larger tasks into smaller units

Physical Activity and Comfort

• wear loose clothing • stand and stretch regularly • use back, arm, or wrist rests that are adjusted to fit you ergonomically • use a speaker phone or headset • use a footstool • sit in a chair that supports good posture • wear Hand-eze gloves (see Dome Company in Appendix A) • use an alternative to a computer mouse • drive with cruise control • get plenty of exposure to outdoor light.

Physical Therapies

• ultrasound with stimulation • electrostimulation • neuromuscular electronic stimulation • trigger point myotherapy • myofascial release • chiropractic care • massage • craniosacral release • Alexander technique • Bowen therapy • Feldenkrais • Reiki • vapocoolant spray and stretching • strain-counterstrain • manual lymphatic drainage • proprioceptor neuromuscular facilitation (PNF).

Self-Help Strategies

• self-massage • exercise • gentle stretching • breathing exercises • cold packs • hot packs • tennis ball acupressure • Yoga • Jin Shin Do (with Taoist breathing) • Shiatsu • Qi Gong • T'ai Chi Chuan • mentholated rub • elevate your feet • acupressure

Life Enrichment

• read something enjoyable • work in your garden • work with clay, wood, paints, etc. • play with children, pets, friends • play board games • visit art galleries and museums • watch videos • cook • gaze at a pleasant view • have a pet • listen to or make music • write in a journal • wear colors that please you.

Health Care

• get a complete physical evaluation • medications • vitamins and other food supplements • acupuncture • alternative or complementary medicine • reflexology.

Relaxation and Stress Reduction

• subliminal tapes • focusing exercises • hypnotherapy • pet therapy • biofeedback • polarity therapy • relaxation exercises • breathing exercises

Spiritual Resources

• visualization • meditation • prayer • guided imagery • mindfulness

Support

• professional counseling • reach out to a friend for emotional and/or physical support • reach out for physical assistance • peer counseling • attend a support group • ask for what you need • ask for help

I found that there were activities I had stopped doing long ago, such as playing the piano and sewing, that really make me feel good. In the "busyness" of life, including raising children and developing a career, those activities had been forgotten. Now they are part of my wellness toolbox. If I am sad or stressed, perhaps experiencing early warning signs of an approaching flare, I make sure to spend some time involved in such an activity. It makes me feel better and my life feels enriched.

M.E.C.

Whenever I see a comic strip that provokes a good laugh, I cut it out. I have a huge notebook of comics and jokes, waiting for me whenever I'm feeling down. I make it a point to watch several British comedies on television. I get at least several good laughs out of them. The comic strips *For Better or Worse* and *Doonesbury* tickle my laughter palate.

D.J.S.

> Since I have come to realize that every aspect of my existence affects my physical and mental vitality, and my ability to deal with my limits, the positive changes in my life have been amazing.
>
> M.E.C.

Managing Your Symptoms

- educate yourself   • use your Wellness Recovery Action Plan

Personal Care

- take a warm shower or bath   • take an Epsom salt soak
- wear support hose   • eat a balanced diet   • drink lots of water   • eat frequent, small portions of food   • wear comfortable shoes

Feel Better About Yourself

- cognitive therapy/thought stopping   • list your strengths and talents   • list your achievements   • give yourself rewards   • take very good care of yourself

Activities to Avoid

- staying in the same position for long periods   • traveling extensively without a break   • performing repetitive movements   • exercising too much   • immersing yourself in water less than 88 degrees Fahrenheit   • becoming overtired   • going without food   • wearing high-heeled shoes   • wearing tight clothing   • doing heavy work •   exposing yourself to electromagnetic fields for extended periods of time   • smoking nicotine, or ingesting alcohol, salty food, junk food, or caffeine   • spending time with people who treat you badly

Keep this list of tools handy as you work on the rest of your plan. Add new tools to your list whenever you learn about them. Keep your Wellness Toolbox list in the front of your binder.

Daily Maintenance List

Now, on the first of your five divider sheets or tabs, write "Daily Maintenance List," and insert it in the binder followed by several sheets of filler paper.

On the first page, describe yourself when you are feeling all right so that you have a reference point. You may have been sick for so long that you hardly remember what it's like to feel well. Do the best you can. You might even write what you would *like* to feel like. Keep it simple. Do it in list form using descriptive words. Some descriptive words that others have found useful are these:

a fast learner	active	athletic
breathe easily	calm	capable
competent	contemplative	content
coordinated	curious	easy to get along with
energetic	flamboyant	flexible
happy	industrious	minimal pain
move easily	optimistic	outgoing
peaceful	quick	quiet
reasonable	responsible	sleep soundly
supportive		

When you are not feeling well, this list will help you to remember what "being well" feels like.

You may have discovered that there are certain things you need to do *every day* to maintain your wellness or to keep yourself from going into flare. Writing these things down and reminding yourself to do them every day is an important step toward keeping yourself as healthy and pain-free as possible. A daily maintenance plan helps you to acknowledge and recognize those activities you need to do to remain healthy, and to plan your time accordingly. Also, when things have been going well for a while and if you notice you are starting to feel worse, it's important to have a reminder of what you did to feel better previously. When you start to feel out of sorts, often you can trace it back to not doing something on your Daily Maintenance List.

On the second page, make a list of activities you know you need to do for yourself every day to keep yourself feeling as well as possible. Refer to your Wellness Toolbox for ideas. Don't put so many things on your list that you couldn't possibly get them done in one day. You may also want to add a list of avoidances. This list is different for everyone.

The following is a sample daily plan for a woman with both fibromyalgia and chronic myofascial pain.

Sample Daily Maintenance List

- Eat three healthy meals and three healthy snacks. • Drink at least six 8-ounce glasses of water. • Do fifteen minutes of stretching in the morning and fifteen minutes in the evening. • Use hot packs for one half hour. • Do fifteen minutes of tennis ball trigger point release. • Get exposure to outdoor light for at least half an hour. • Take medications and food supplements. • Do a relaxation exercise each morning and evening. • Write in my journal for at least fifteen minutes. • Spend at least one half hour doing something I enjoy. • Talk to someone with whom I can be real.

Avoid

- caffeine, sugar, junk foods, alcohol • repetitive motion activities • sitting or standing still for long periods of time • people who treat me badly

On the next blank page (or pages), make a reminder list for things you *might* need to do. This will be a reminder to consider whether or when you need to do any of the "sometimes" activities on this list. They may be things you want to remember to do once a week or once a month. Reading this list on a daily basis will help keep you on track and will alleviate the stress you would feel if you forgot to do something you need to do to stay as well as you can.

For instance, you could include the following on this list:

- Get a massage. • Set up an appointment with a health care provider. • Arrange for a physical examination. • Do some peer counseling. • Explore a new treatment option. • Learn more about fibromyalgia. • Take a nap. • Go to a support group. • Take a day off from responsibilities.

That's the first section of your Wellness Recovery Action Plan binder. You can change it whenever you want or need to. You can write whole new lists. You may not think so just reading these instructions, but you will be surprised at how much better you will feel after taking just these first few positive steps on your own behalf.

Triggers

Triggers are external events or circumstances that may cause or worsen your pain and other symptoms. If you don't respond to a trigger by dealing properly with it, it may continue to worsen your symptoms until you do respond. Being aware of your susceptibility to certain triggers, and developing plans to deal with triggering events when they arise, will increase your ability to cope and will keep your condition from worsening. *Do not project a catastrophic possibility, such as a very serious illness or a huge personal loss. If those things were to occur, you would simply use the actions you describe in your Triggers Action Plan more often and increase the length of time you use them.* When listing your triggers, write those that are more likely to occur, or those which may already be present in your life. (See the sample triggers below.)

Now, on the second divider sheet or tab, write "Triggers" and add several sheets of binder paper. On the first page, write down those events that, if they took place, might cause an increase in your discomfort and pain. These things may have triggered or increased your symptoms in the past. Following is a list of some possible triggers:

Possible Triggers

- being overtired • staying in one position too long • overworking • too much exercise • family friction • stress • physical illness • hearing bad news

On the next page, develop a plan for what to do if your triggers are activated to keep them from causing serious symptoms. Include activities that have worked for you in the past and ideas you have learned from others. Refer to your Wellness Toolbox for more ideas.

Sample Daily Triggers Action Plan

- do a relaxation exercise or meditate • give myself a massage, or get a massage;
- take a nap • do T'ai Chi for fifteen minutes • take a warm bath • pray

It's a good idea to have a list of effective generalized responses to triggers. You may also want to develop plans for specific responses to triggers. Here are some examples of possible responses to specific triggers:

- If my teenager and I start to argue, I will

    — Tell her that I am going to take a short walk to cool down.

    — Take a short walk.

    — Remind myself to breathe.

    — Pray.

    — Return, tell her I love her, and try to work out the problem calmly.

- If a rainstorm is due, I know my symptoms will increase, so I will

    — Check the weather report daily.

    — Take my medication in advance of a storm.

    — Cancel my appointments if a big storm is due.

    — Lie down to rest fifteen minutes of every hour during low-pressure weather.

Early Warning Signs

Early warning signs are internal signals and may be completely unrelated to reactions to stressful situations. In spite of your best efforts at reducing or relieving your symptoms, you may begin to experience early warning signs, subtle, internal signs of change that indicate you might need to take some further action. These are the kind of signs that are often overlooked. Reviewing early warning signs regularly will help you to become more aware of them, and encourage you to take action before they worsen.

On the third divider sheet, or tab write "Early Warning Signs." Follow that tab with several sheets of lined paper. On the first page, make a list of early warning signs you have noticed. Some early warning signs that others report include the following:

fatigue	anxiety and nervousness
forgetfulness	aches and pains
numbness and tingling	increased irritability
feeling slowed down or speeded up	poor motor coordination
dizziness	muscle cramping
excessive sweating	feelings of tightness in the body
morning stiffness	bladder irritability
eyes constantly watering	skin mottling
very cold skin	cold spots on the skin
feeling compelled to take too much pain medication	increase in number of painful trigger points
increase in postnasal drip	stuffy sinuses
increased craving for sweets	yeast infection
itchiness	shakiness
bruising	clumsiness
reflux	intestinal cramping
nausea	

When you notice your early symptoms, you will want to take action before they get worse. Using the ideas in your Wellness Toolbox, develop a plan you can follow that will help reduce your early warning signs and keep yourself from going into a *crisis*.

Sample "Relieve Early Warning Signs" Action Plan

- Ask others to take over my household responsibilities for a day.
- Check in with my physician or other health care professional.
- Arrange an acupuncture appointment.
- Take a warm bath.
- Do a guided imagery exercise.
- Spend an hour listening to favorite music.

When Things Are Getting Worse

In spite of your best efforts, your symptoms may progress to the point where you are in a lot of pain, but you may still able to do some things to help yourself and perhaps even relieve some of your symptoms. It is helpful to identify in advance those symptoms that indicate to you that things are getting worse. Then you can develop a very specific plan, more specific than your previous plans, about what you can do if you have one or several of these symptoms.

On the fourth divider, or tab write "When Things Are Getting Worse." Then make a list of the symptoms which, for you, mean that your pain and other symptoms are much worse and that a strong response is critical for preventing a crisis.

Others have noted that the following symptoms indicate to them that "things are getting worse." Remember that symptoms vary from person to person.

acute abdominal pain	acute or severe diarrhea
avoiding eating	being touched hurts
chest tightness	chest pain
difficulty swallowing	ear pain
increase in the pain	excessive weight loss
extreme fatigue	headaches
increased coughing	increase in referred pain
increased reflux	pain in new places
pain that "feels different"	poor motor coordination
reduced tolerance level for noise	sensitive to light
severe itchiness	severe sweats
shortness of breath	stiff neck
tempted to drink alcohol	unable to sleep for (specify for how long)
unable to exercise	weak grasp

On the next page, write a plan of what you need to do if you have one, several, or many of the symptoms that indicate things are getting much worse. Now, your plan needs to be very directive with fewer choices and very clear instructions.

Sample "Things Are Getting Worse" Action Plan

If these symptoms come up I need to do *all* of the following:

- Call my doctor or another of my health care team members; ask for and follow their instructions.

- Call and talk for as long as I need to my supporters.

- Arrange for one or several supporters to stay with me and take care of me until my symptoms subside.

- Arrange for and take at least three days off from any responsibilities.

- Do three deep breathing relaxation exercises of at least thirty minutes length each.

- Do very mild stretching every hour.

- Spend an hour involved in an activity that makes me laugh.

- Arrange for a session of craniosacral release as soon as possible.

- Take at least two warm baths every day.

Crisis Plan

Some people like to have a plan in place that others can use to help them if they become unable to care for themselves. Such a plan can keep you in control even when it feels like everything is out of your control—when you have so much pain, and your symptoms are so severe that you can't think well enough to make decisions and are too debilitated to take any form of action. If you have depression from time to time, or other co-occurring illnesses, to having a crisis plan can be especially valuable. It will keep your family members and friends from wasting time trying to figure out what to do for you. A crisis plan helps relieve the worry and guilt felt by family members and other caregivers, who may wonder whether they are taking the right action. It also ensures that your needs will be met and that you will get better as quickly as possible. You can decide if you need such a plan.

A crisis plan needs to be developed when you are feeling well. However, you cannot do it quickly. Decisions like these take time, thought, and often collaboration with health care team members, family members, and other supporters.

The crisis plan differs from the other action plans in that it will be used by others. The four earlier sections of this Wellness Recovery Action Plan process are implemented by you alone and need not be shared with anyone else; therefore you can write them using shorthand language that only you need to understand. But when writing a crisis plan, *you need to make it clear, easy to understand, and legible.*

If you decide that a crisis plan would be of benefit to you, write "Crisis Plan" on the fifth divider sheet, or tab and insert it into your binder with a good supply of paper. *Don't rush the process.* Work at it for a while, then leave it for several days and keep coming back to it until you develop a crisis plan that you feel has the best chance of working for you. Collaborate with health care team members and other supporters when developing your crisis plan. Once you have completed it, give copies to the people you name on this plan as your supporters.

The most helpful crisis plans include lists of the following kinds of information:

- How you feel when you are well (you can copy this from the first section of your book) so that health care providers who may not have known you previously can get an idea of what you are like when you are well.

- Those symptoms that would indicate to others that you are in a crisis, things like difficulty breathing, severe pain, inability to move, severe diarrhea, or acute abdominal pain.

- Who your supporters are, including family members, friends, and your health team members, how they help you, and their phone numbers. Include as many family members and friends as possible, as they are usually much more accessible than health team members. Depending on your situation, you may also want to include a list of people you do not want involved in providing you with support and care.

- The names and phone numbers of your physician(s), pharmacy, and insurance company.

- Any allergies you may have and any other things or circumstances that need to be avoided.

- Medications you are currently using and why you are using them; also make a list of medications you would prefer to take if additional medications are deemed necessary, and make a separate list of medications that should be avoided, along with the reasons for avoiding them.

- Treatments that would be helpful to you and those you would want to avoid.

- Activities your supporters could do for you that would be helpful. You can also list things they might tend to do that you would not want done or that might be harmful. Include a list of tasks that need to be done and who you would want to do them, such as cleaning the house, getting the groceries, paying the bills, and feeding the pets.

- Indicators that you have recovered enough to take responsibility for your own care again, such as "when I have been able to reduce my medication to [list the dosage]" and "when I can speak coherently."

Think about whether you want to give someone the authority to make legal decisions in your name if you were to become severely disabled.

Using Your WRAP

To use this plan most effectively, you will need to spend up to fifteen or twenty minutes daily reviewing the pages you have written and be willing to take the prescribed actions if they are indicated. Most people report that in the morning, either before or after breakfast, is the best time to review the materials in the binder. As you become familiar with your symptoms and plans, you will find that the review process takes less time and that you will know how to respond to certain symptoms without even referring to the binder.

Begin with the first page in section 1, the Daily Maintenance Plan. Review the list of how you are if you are all right. If you are all right, do the things on your list of things you need to do every day to keep yourself well. Also refer to the page of things you *may* need to do to see whether there is anything specific you need to do on this day. If you need to do something on that list, make a note to yourself to include it in your day.

If you are not feeling well, review the other sections to see where on the spectrum the symptoms you are experiencing fit. Then, follow the action plan you have designed.

For instance, if you feel very anxious because you got a big bill in the mail or had an argument with your spouse, follow the plan in the Triggers section. If you noticed some early warning signs (subtle signs that your symptoms might be worsening), such as increased numbness and tingling, muscle cramping, and a craving for sweets, then follow the plan you designed for the Early Warning Signs section. If you notice symptoms that indicate things are seriously worsening, such as extreme fatigue, an increase in pain, sweatiness and chest tightness, follow the plan you developed for When Things Are Getting Worse.

If you are in a crisis situation, the materials in the binder will help you to understand that, so you can get in touch with your supporters and let them know they need to take over. However, in certain crisis situations, you may not be aware of the severity of the situation, or you may not be willing to admit that you are in crisis. This is why having a strong team of supporters is so important. They will observe the symptoms you have reported and take over responsibility for your care, whether or not you are willing to admit you are in a crisis at that particular time. Distributing your crisis plan to your supporters and discussing it when you are feeling well is a great aid in facilitating this process.

A Personal Example of How WRAP Works

I have fibromyalgia and chronic myofascial pain along with recurring episodes of major depression. Having and using a Wellness Recovery Action Plan would have helped me to avoid the following very difficult set of circumstances. In May and June of 2000 I set myself up for a major health disaster.

As part of my work I had to travel extensively all around the country. Consequently, I was seated for many hours in cramped positions in airline seats, unable to move. I also traveled by car to Washington, D.C., about ten hours each way. I gave numerous presentations, many that lasted all day long, that required me to stand at a podium. If I wasn't standing on my feet, I was sitting for hours in an uncomfortable chair. Sometimes, I wore my medium-height, but nevertheless high-heeled shoes for an entire day. I tried to eat properly, but it was often difficult to find healthy food, get plenty of water to drink, or take the time to exercise. It was also difficult to get a sound night's sleep in an unfamiliar hotel. Appointments with my medical team were deferred.

By July, I began having severe pain all over my body along with numbness and tingling. Moving became a big challenge. In addition, I was depressed. Getting through each day was a struggle. I fell behind in my work and my family members had to take over more and more of my home responsibilities. Along with seeing my doctor and a physical therapist, I began to use a variety of self-help techniques to get back on the right track. The question for me became: "How can I avoid this problem in the future?" Examining that question gave me the clues for developing my Wellness Recovery Action Plan.

In retrospect, the points that became very clear to me were that I need to:

1. Make adjustments to my schedule so that I avoid so much travel in such a short period. I should limit myself to one, and occasionally two, airline trips per month.

2. Avoid traveling by car for more than an hour and a half without taking at least a ten-minute break. I should avoid all car trips more than four hours total traveling time. Traveling by train or air are preferable options.

3. Avoid wearing high-heeled shoes under any circumstance. Comfortable but fashionable flat shoes will have to suffice.

4. Request a high stool (preferably a padded bar stool with a back rest) for presentations rather than standing on my feel all day, so that I can alternate sitting and standing.

5. Avoid sitting in uncomfortable chairs for more than an hour at a stretch. I can get up and stand in the back of the room and/or bring a pillow so that I can sit on the floor for part of the time.

6. Carry healthy foods and bottled water with me so I don't have to eat and drink whatever is available.

7. Make sure the hotel I stay at has exercise facilities, so I don't have to resort to walking on concrete sidewalks.

8. Pack some familiar items like family pictures and buy myself some flowers to decorate my hotel room to make it more "homey."

9. Avoid deferring appointments with my health care team. Being unable to fit them in is a sign that I have overscheduled myself and that I am courting trouble.

I asked myself, "What can I do to move myself back to feeling well again?" What follows are the answers to that question.

1. Take a break from traveling for three weeks. Toward the end of June, when I was beginning to notice early warning signs of impending trouble, I canceled several trips.

2. Ask family members to help me with, or take over, many of my household responsibilities.

3. Arrange an appointment with each of the people on my health care team. I trust them so I will ask for, *and follow*, their advice.

4. Eat well (my husband is providing me with a supply of fresh vegetables from the garden and fresh fruit from the farmers' market). Drink plenty of spring water. Get at least a half hour of mild exercise each day. Stay home and sleep in my own comfortable bed.

5. Spend at least an hour each day doing something I really enjoy, puttering in the garden, reading a good book, writing in my journal, painting a picture, listening to good music, or going out to a movie or community event.

6. Spend time each day talking about my situation with a supportive friend or family member. It helps me to keep things in perspective.

For further information on developing a Wellness Recovery Action Plan, consult: *Winning Against Relapse*.[2]

Keeping a Journal

There are many good reasons why it is helpful for a person who has fibromyalgia and/or chronic myofascial pain to keep a journal. At this point, you may be saying to yourself, "This is just one more thing I need to do. And keeping a journal will be really hard on my hands. I have a hard time writing already." You may have trigger points (TrPs) (see chapter 3) that make writing painful and/or difficult. However, there are several things you can do to address this problem. They include the following:

- Talk to your physical therapist and doctor about ways of relieving this problem.

- Tape record your journal.

- Use a felt tip marker or a soft (No. 2) pencil that is easy to write with and a spiral notebook.

- Keep your writings brief, a few minutes a day is plenty. Make lists and use phrases rather than writing complete sentences.

Why Keep a Journal?

Many people who struggle with chronic pain have found it very helpful to keep a journal.

- Keeping a journal provides a record of your daily life that can be useful when you want to search for things you may have done or behavior patterns that may have contributed to an increase in your symptoms, or treatments and medications that have been helpful. You may often overlook things you do that worsen your symptoms. By keeping a record of what you do and how you feel, you can identify patterns that exacerbate your symptoms and create change that helps you to feel better. Include in your journal information things like records of your symptoms, medications, therapies, and both the stressful and good things that are going on in your life. These records may be of great value to you at some later time.

- Once you have written out what you are thinking, you can more easily arrive at new and more positive conclusions. The deep inner exploration and evaluation that keeping a journal encourages can be an invaluable asset for coping with FMS or FMS coupled with chronic myofascial pain.

- You may find that solutions for problems that once seemed insoluble will present themselves to you in the course of keeping a journal.

- Too often, people with chronic invisible illnesses are misunderstood and/or not believed by others. This failure of communication is invalidating. This causes low self-esteem as well as a loss of our sense of self. Because of this invalidation people find it difficult to talk to others. Keeping a journal begins the process of reconnecting by creating a dialogue with the self. You may find that when you begin putting your thoughts down on paper, that communication of other kinds becomes easier.

- When you are experiencing a lot of pain, your life can become very chaotic and confused. Writing your thoughts and organizing them can bring order out of this confusion and chaos.

> Writing is very painful for me. Using the computer is somewhat better. It isn't that much less painful, but it is much more legible. I find that both are made easier by the use of Hand-eze hand supports and frequent breaks.
>
> I use a notebook for passing thoughts and impressions and the computer for longer journal entries—like the letters I write that I don't intend to mail. I have written to God, long-dead relatives and friends, and to famous people (living or dead) with whom I will never have an opportunity to converse. I get a chance to tell my story, and everyone needs that.
>
> D.J.S.

- When your thoughts are constantly racing around in your head and the same negative ideas are repeating over and over, like a record stuck in the same groove, you get the most devastating type of negative reinforcement. You become your own worst enemy. You will find that putting your thoughts down on paper will enable you to sort and examine your ideas and feelings. Doing this can help silence the inner negative dialogue that can be so harmful to your self-esteem and sense of self.

- A journal is a safe place to deal with negative emotions. Think of it as a completely trusted friend. It can be like a drain in an infected wound, allowing the negative emotions of the past to seep away, so that true healing can begin. The pain, rage, or fear that you might be unable to express to another human being can be safely expressed on paper. When you have finished writing, the negative emotions may have lost some of their intensity and some of their ability to make you unhappy may be diminished. You may be able to think more clearly, or to think new thoughts, and you may gain a broader perspective.

- A journal can be used to record your hopes, dreams, and ambitions. Ideas that might seem too silly, daring, or ambitious to speak out loud can all be entered safely in a journal and, sometimes, when they are written down, they begin to seem possible. Then ways to turn them into reality may occur to you, and you can begin to make plans for turning your dreams into realities.

It is a good idea to reread your journal entries often so you can detect any patterns that indicate a need for change, give yourself credit for progress you have made. and perhaps gain a new perspective that only the passage of time allows.

Getting Started

If you haven't already started a journal, you may want to start one soon. If you are unsure where to start, you can begin with a simple record of symptoms, medications, treatments, and therapies. Write down what works for you, and what doesn't. Tell your journal which treatment elements affect which symptoms. It is also a good place to record and store any notes that you might take at your support groups.

All you need to do is get some paper and a writing tool (or a tape recorder) and start to write. Write anything you want, anything you feel. It doesn't have to make sense. It doesn't even have to be real. It doesn't need to be interesting. It's all right to repeat yourself over and over. Whatever is written is for your eyes and your use only. This is yours. This is your private kingdom.

One person said about keeping a journal, "It's the cheapest kind of therapy. All you need is paper and something to write with, and a place to keep your journal (a safe, private space like the bottom of your underwear drawer or a high shelf that is inaccessible to others in your household)."

Tips for Getting Started

If you are still having a hard time starting to keep a journal, some of these suggestions may help you:

1. Write a letter to yourself, pretending you are your own best friend, and tell yourself why you like yourself so much. Mention how your day went, and what tomorrow holds for you.

2. List the best things that have happened this day (month, year) in your life.

3. Describe the worst thing that ever happened to you.

4. Make a list of all the reasons that you to want to be alive. Include the little things, as well as the larger ones, that make your life worth living.

5. Write your own prayer.

6. Describe yourself.

7. Describe a special moment.

8. Write a dialogue with another person, or describe an event, a part of your body, or a famous person.

9. Make lists of the following: activities you want to do in your life, why you like yourself, why you like someone else, why you feel stressed, what you fear, reasons to stay with your partner, things to do when in flare, things you would never do again, what makes you laugh, what makes you cry, what makes you happy, what makes you sad, your favorite people.

Guidelines for Journal Keeping

1. Say anything you want to say, however you want to say it. You will not be criticized or judged. Avoid being critical yourself. You can rant, rave, and carry on like a two-year-old

child having a tantrum if you feel like it, or you can express hopes and desires that you wouldn't dare share with anyone else. You can write poems, paragraphs, comic verses, novels, novellas, political rants, your autobiography, someone else's biography, wishes, letters, fantasies, dreams, beliefs, loves, and hates. Your entries can be similar each time, or they can be very different. You can draw or paste pictures or words into your journal. You can doodle. Don't think too much about what you are writing; just let the writing flow.

2. You don't have to worry about punctuation, grammar, spelling, penmanship, neatness, or staying on the lines. (You don't even have to used lined paper if you don't want to.) You can scribble all over the page if that makes you feel better. (Ferocious scribbling can be a wonderful way to get rid of tension.) You can write at any speed you want, fast or slow. You can write as much or as little as you want.

3. The privacy of the journal should not be violated. Choosing to share your writing is a personal choice. You don't have to share what you have written with anyone unless you want to. Some people find it helpful and feel comfortable sharing some of their journal entries with family members, friends, or health care professionals. Other people never let anyone see a line they have written. Again, this is your personal choice. You have the right to change your mind anytime you wish. Other people in your household should respect your right to a private journal and not read your entries unless you tell them it is okay. If the privacy of your journal cannot be assured, you may want a trusted friend to keep your journal for you. If it is stored elsewhere, a three-ring binder might work best. Keep a supply of paper on hand and write when you feel like it; then take the pages to your friend at another time. Write your name, address, and phone number inside the front cover if you plan to carry your journal with you. Add a statement, something like this, "This contains private information. Please do not read it without my permission. Thank you!"

4. You may want to set aside a time every day for journal keeping, for instance, early in the morning or before going to sleep at night, but it is not necessary. Spend as little or as much time writing as you want. Some people even like to set a timer. It is easy to get lost in your journal, but that's okay, too. You can make entries in your journal at any time, daily, several times a day, weekly, before you go to bed, when you wake up, after supper, whenever you feel like it—the choice is yours.

5. You don't have to make a commitment to keeping a journal for the rest of your life—just when you feel like it.

6. Some people like to take a quiet moment to ground themselves before starting to write. You can do this by taking several deep breaths and then focusing on something pleasant for a moment or two, such as a flower, a pet, or the view outside your window. You might want to take a warm bath or go for a short walk, whatever quiets you down. You might wish to note what you use for centering, or have a page in the beginning of the journal that lists your favorite methods of grounding or centering before you begin to write in your journal.

7. Claim a quiet space to do your journal writing. Turn off the phone, and ask others to respect your need for quiet and privacy. Parents may choose to make journal entries when the baby is napping, the children are in school, or after the children have gone to bed.

8. Date your entries if you wish. Dated entries do help to keep things in perspective when you review what you have written over time, and they also help to pinpoint patterns if you are looking for them.

9. Don't fix your mistakes. Just keep writing. Remember, spelling, grammar, handwriting, and style do not matter.

Your journal can take any form you wish and there are no limits to what you can record there. If you define some goals before starting a journal, they will guide you along the way.

It may be that you already keep a journal. If so, examining your past experiences in journal keeping can help you decide what kinds of things you should record. You may want to change its focus, or modify it to include more of your impressions. You may want to keep two journals. One could be more like a daybook to record medications and symptoms, and the other could be more like a diary of feelings.

Endnotes

1. Henriksson, C. M. 1994. Long-term effects of fibromyalgia on everyday life. A study of 56 patients. *Scand J Rheumatol* 23(1):36-41.

2. Copeland, M. E. 1999. *Winning Against Relapse*. Oakland, CA: New Harbinger Publications.

CHAPTER 17

Fibrofog and Other Cognitive Deficits

Fibromyalgia (FMS) has been described as the "Irritable Everything Syndrome." Some of the most frustrating, and at times the most disabling, symptom of FMS may be the cognitive deficit (something missing from normal brain function) that we aptly, but not affectionately, call fibrofog.

What Is Fibrofog?

Perhaps you psych yourself up to go to the grocery and arrive only to discover you've forgotten your wallet. You return home, retrieve the wallet, and set out again. After you reach the store the second time, you realize you've left your shopping list and coupons at home. Once again, you return home, all the while berating yourself for your forgetfulness and stupidity. You search and search, but the list can't be found. By then, you're too exhausted to shop. Later, you may find the list under the car seat, or used as a bookmark. That's fibrofog at work.

You may spend hours every day trying to find various items, like your keys. (After a while, you may feel as though your mind is one of those misplaced items.) You may not recognize things when they are right in front of you but are not in their accustomed place, or when it's in a different package or form.

Some FMS patients become very confused in large malls, or even in small crowds. They have to leave because they can't process all the sensory input. John Lowe believes that some of this is due to the brain having a higher metabolic rate than other tissues and, with FMS, there is insufficient delivery of oxygen, glucose, and other substances that the brain cells need to function. When your brain cells are thinking, their metabolic rate and the flow of blood to those cells increase. Lowe also believes that some fog is caused by inadequate thyroid hormone regulation of these processes (see chapter 15).[1]

The Wheel Is Turning, But the Hamster Left Town

When you are in fibrofog, steam irons are stored in the refrigerator. Freshly made milk drinks go on a shelf, where they silently turn into a dismal green mold. You transpose letters

> Fibromyalgia may cause you to forget key pieces of information, such as the names of your relatives. Needless to say, this can cause embarrassment. I often talk to my cats at home, and when I go out into the world, I may see a dog in town and say in greeting, "What a good kitty."

when you write, and you do the same with numbers when you try to balance your checkbook. Some days, you can't even put a coherent sentence together. The words rattle around in your mouth and don't seem to connect coherently to the ideas in your head. This state of utter confusion can last for hours, weeks, or, in the period of magnified symptoms called flare, for months. Fibrofog can go way beyond any normally confused state of mind or, for that matter, way beyond any other cognitive impairments. Many people have lost their jobs or have had to drop out of school because of the extreme nature of the flare/fibrofog combination. It is one of the least recognized and most serious symptoms of FMS.

People with fibrofog seem to sense things as patterns and series of patterns. Trying to establish a new pattern can cause a short circuit. You can reach for the light switch on the wall by the door, but it won't be there. That's because the light switch was in that location in an apartment you had thirty years ago.

Some researchers have found that FMS causes slowed psychomotor speed for tasks that require sustained effort.[2] Our minds and muscles don't speak the same languages, or at least they use different dialects. Sometimes, just getting up in the morning is the first obstacle of the day. It's not unusual for people with FMS and chronic myofascial pain (CMP) to fall down when trying to take their first steps out of bed.

If the dizziness doesn't get you, the foot pain, buckling knee, weak ankle, or something else will. All of these symptoms can be compounded by fibrofog. The worst indignity of all is when you forget to do the things you normally do to minimize your physical symptoms. Or when it takes you so much longer to do the tasks you must do (earning your livelihood, preparing meals, etc.), that you have no time or energy to do needed bodywork, like stretching, or mindwork, like meditating. People with FMS and/or CMP have high maintenance bodies and minds. The lack of maintenance, plus the additional stress brought about by fibrofog, can lead to a flare.

Fibrofog frustration is compounded when you're experiencing it, because you can't express yourself well. However eloquent you are at other times, you may be incapable of putting together a coherent sentence when you are in a fog. You may even stutter as you vainly grasp for the right words. You are left vulnerable by your scrambled psyche, and the slings and arrows of an uncaring world zip right through your crumbling defenses. You have lost control, and you can't explain why.

People experiencing fibrofog take a hefty amount of abuse from those who are unaware of the reason for their confused state of mind. For example, when you fumble at the grocery checkout counter, trying to get your change from your purse, people glare at you for holding up the line. To others, we often sound and look stupid, and the great tragedy is that often we feel stupid, when, in actuality, we are struggling to function in the face of sometimes overwhelming, but invisible, odds. The miracle is, we often succeed.

One of the Internet FMily described fibrofog this way:

It's like I'm walking down the hall of my mind, on my way to retrieve a piece of information. I know I have to go to a certain room in the house of my mind. But when I get into the room, either the box with the information is not there or I have forgotten which box I was looking for. So I wander around looking for it, until I get tired and give up.

When You're Finally Holding All the Cards, Why Is Everyone Playing Chess?

When you are suffering from fibrofog, you're in a game where the rules keep changing, and no one tells you what they are. The scientific part of my brain calls it the time when all constants become variables. Life passes you by. You stand with your nose pressed to the window and you look in with longing, but you are unable to join in the action. Of all your symptoms, you may find that the mental aspects of FMS are the most disruptive, and the hardest to explain. Perhaps you can deal with the pain, but you want your brain back. One person wrote, "Sometimes I feel like my body is just a shell, and I'm only dust inside. And I can't get out." That's heavy-duty fibrofog.

Fibrofog often drifts in slowly. It creeps up on little cat feet, and you may be too fog-benumbed to be aware of it. (That also happens with flare. It sneaks up on you.) Fibrofog can also cause depression, because you don't know what to do about it and you feel helpless in its grasp. Depression can add to the cognitive confusion, and you may not even be aware that you are depressed, or that the depression is affecting your performance.[3]

Fog Formation

There are probably many factors that contribute to the symptoms of fibrofog. SPECT (single photon emission tomography) scans show that people with FMS have decreased blood flow in the right caudate nucleus of the brain, as well as in the left and right thalami.[4] This decreased blood flow could be caused by neurotransmitter dysfunction, or by a problem in the equivalent of myofascia in those areas of the brain. This equivalent is called the *glial cell*.

Glial Cells

For a long time, the world of medicine thought of glial cells only as neural scaffolding, just as it dismissed myofascia as structural framework only (see chapter 15). Now we see that glial cells are active in brain cell permeability.[5] This permeability is crucial in allowing molecules like electrical ions, to move in and out of the cells, thus affecting how well the brain functions. There is a bioelectric connection between glia, ion exchange, and cellular swelling in the brain.[6] If too much fluid is allowed into the cell due to increased permeability, cellular contents come under increased pressure. I believe that some fibrofog may be due to this form of water retention. Your whole brain can feel swollen. Perhaps it is.

In many chronic pain states, cognitive complaints are common. Some researchers feel that these complaints may be due to interference between ongoing pain and mental tasks, as they share common and limited attentional resources.[7] Research indicates that glial cells are involved in preventing and reversing sensory abnormalities that may develop in some altered pain states.[8]

In one study, researchers found that some chronic pain patients performed some tests more poorly than patients with head injuries. This study suggests that pain can disrupt cognitive performances that depend on intact speed and storage capacity for information processing.[9] Processing pain occupies most or all of our thought processing networks, thereby interfering with concurrent cognitive tasks such as thinking, reasoning, and remembering.[10] For example, you may not be able to decide what clothes to wear after you get up in the morning. (This mind-boggling task could be simplified by taking time the night before to put out your clothes for the next day.) Trying to make a decision, even a simple one, may keep you from living your life. This lack of decisiveness may be caused by an adrenaline/noradrenaline imbalance.

Other Causes of Fibrofog

Other substances may also play a role in causing fibrofog. For example, an overabundance of histamine can lead to permeable membranes and interstitial edema along with the uncoordinated firing of nerve cells. The neurotransmitter serotonin can affect perception and awareness, and can slow thought processes. We know that serotonin depletion, which is a common affliction among people with FMS, can lead to learning dysfunction in rats.[11] Whether human beings are similarly affected by serotonin depletion is not yet known.

Specific changes in the human brain have been documented in patients after hypoglycemic (i.e., sugar deficiencies in the blood) injury. One study found that after hypoglycemic episodes, an MRI (magnetic resonance imaging) scan revealed specific lesions in some areas of the brain. These localized lesions might represent tissue degeneration.[12] We don't know why, but this is yet another reason to avoid excess sweets and starches. Carbohydrates can also feed yeast, which may add to the fog.

Bodywork can indirectly cause fog. This is actually a promising sign. As the myofascial constrictions are broken up, wastes and chemical toxins are freed into your circulatory system. Then they travel to your detoxification units, your liver and kidneys, so that they can be processed and excreted. What a relief to have these toxins gone from your life! But your body takes time to process these biochemicals. There is no telling how long it took them to accumulate. Use the amount of fog and residual soreness you feel to judge the time you need between therapy sessions to recover. It is important not to overload your body's chemical detoxification factories.

Cognitive Function and FMS

Research at the University of Michigan has validated the reality of fibrofog.[13] These researchers had observed a similarity between neuroendocrine dysfunction in patients with FMS and older but otherwise healthy people. They wanted to see if there was a matching similarity in the decline of cognitive functions, specifically, of memory functions.

They compared three groups of people. One group had FMS. One control group was composed of similar, healthy people of the same age and educational background. The third control group was made up of healthy people who were twenty years older than the other two groups, but also had the same educational background. These three groups were given a variety of age-sensitive neuropsychological testing, resulting in two separate but interrelated studies. Cognitive function begins to decrease, even in healthy people, as soon as adulthood is reached. The purpose of the tests was to compare cognitive dysfunction caused by FMS with normal cognitive loss caused by aging.

For those with FMS, memory loss and other complaints about mental function were similar to those losses experienced during the normal aging process. (Standard psychological tests for depression showed that these FMS patients didn't meet the criteria even for mild depression, so any cognitive dysfunction was not due to depression.) As expected, the older control (healthy) group did perform worse than the younger controls.

When it came to speed of cognitive function and recognition memory, the FMS group tested equal to healthy people of the same age, which was a relief and a surprise. When it came to working memory (how much information you can actually use, manipulate, and store at one time), the FMS group had the same capabilities as those in the *older* control group. This was also true for verbal fluency and long-term memory.

People with fibromyalgia do *not* have the same mental agility as healthy people of the same age. They performed even worse when it came to vocabulary, a cognitive function that normally doesn't decline with age. Fibromyalgia patients scored even lower than the older group, with a significant vocabulary deficit. We honestly have trouble finding the right worms! Er, words. This study has significance besides validating cognitive deficits in FMS. Clearly, whatever is occurring in FMS to cause cognitive deficits, it isn't the same as that which occurs with normal aging.

In a companion study,[14] the researchers investigated *metamemory*. This is our ability to accurately assess our own memory skills. These FMS patients were also tested to eliminate major depression as a possible contributing cause of cognitive dysfunction. They were asked about difficulties dialing a telephone, concentrating on a task, or shopping for items without a list.

The FMS patients reported lower memory capacity, less control over memory function, more cognitive deficits, and greater memory deterioration than even the older control group. *The study found that they were accurate in their assessments.* Their memory problems were not due to poor motivation, as some insurance doctors would like us to believe. Fibromyalgia patients used more memory improvement strategies, such as lists and calendars, and were more highly motivated as to the importance of a good memory, and had more anxiety about memory function than the other groups.

These patients were trying to make the most of what they have in every way they knew how. They reported a greater perception of loss than the older control group did, even though their memory loss was similar. The study notes that this is an accurate perception, since *the cognitive function of the FMS patients is not age-appropriate.*

Your health care team should be informed about these studies. Fibromyalgia patients often feel that the cognitive deficits of FMS are more disabling than the other symptoms (which can be disabling on their own). We struggle to do the best we can in spite of these invisible handicaps, but we often meet with disbelief and even ridicule from our companions and our medical care providers. These studies indicate the need for more research in this area, as well as the need for more support to find ways in which we can cope with and minimize these cognitive deficits.

These studies verify what many of us have felt all along. The cognitive dysfunction we are dealing with hasn't changed because of the studies. It is only the perception of "what we are dealing with" that *should* change in the eyes of others. Now we have a greater chance to receive support and understanding for our cognitive deficits. These researchers are continuing in their efforts to document our problems and to find clues as to the origin and nature of these deficits. When we know why and how they occur, we have a greater chance to find ways to remedy or prevent them. The authors of these studies hope to do more research, focusing on multitasking. Many of us have difficulty with series of tasks, as well as completion of several tasks at once. It is vitally important that we support the FMS- and CMP-related charities that fund this kind of research.

If you keep a journal, it may give you some clues to the origin of *your* fibrofog. If you are undergoing a period of extreme stress, for example, your confusion may be caused by that stress, depression, lack of sleep, or approaching flare. One study suggests that daytime sleepiness causing fatigue, coupled with the distracting effects of persistent pain, contribute to impaired mental function in FMS.[15] Other studies indicate that sleep quality is an important factor in memory.[16]

Cutting Through the Fog

It is very easy to lose your focus at even the best of times. When the fog rolls in, any distraction can cause you to feel fragmented. Your brain is wired differently, and you begin to realize that it would never pass any electrical code. Try creating a greater degree of organization in your life; it won't clear the air, but may help you navigate through the fog. Train yourself to stop and review what you have to do and where you have to go before you leave home. That way you sometimes can remember things you might have forgotten. Go through files, drawers, and closets regularly to get rid of unneeded clutter. Keep things simple and pared down to essentials.

I have severe FMS and CMP, with many perpetuating factors. I have trouble dialing a phone number. I must keep my finger on the number and check each number as I punch it in. I still make mistakes. I find cognitive deficits frustrating. I can get lost in our small town. Yet I was able to organize and document this book, dealing with hundreds of medical references, while conducting a clinical study and writing and contributing to peer-reviewed articles for medical journals. Some of my perpetuating factors I can't eliminate, but I control those I can. I know how to manage the FMS and CMP. You can do it too. You take it one step at a time, armed with the knowledge that you *can* succeed.

What to Do for Fibrofog

You can take some immediate steps to avoid repetitive fog-induced misery. For example, if you are always losing your personal phone book, try using a hole punch and hanging up the book near your phone. If you often forget grocery coupons, salvage the reply envelopes from some of your junk mail. Write your shopping list on the outside of the envelope, and put a pencil and the coupons inside. Keep the envelope closed with a large paper clip until you get to the store. Then you can take out the pencil and use it to cross off items as you put them in your cart. That way, you won't forget what you need. Mostly . . .

If you're in severe fog, don't drive. You may not be able to focus well enough to drive safely. Keep extra food and other necessities on hand, so you don't have to drive to the store frequently. When you know you are going to be overstressing your body, keep well within your limits. Schedule extra mind and bodywork.

Perhaps you've discovered that when you are in fibrofog, you can't trust yourself to write checks. For example, you may forget to enter checks you wrote into your checkbook ledger, or you may enter them in the ledger and then forget to write them, or to send them. I make it a habit to write the information into the checkbook ledger before I write the check. If I am going out to a bodyworker or other place where I know the amount of the check, I write the check and complete the ledger before I leave the house. That makes it easier for me after my appointment, when I may be distracted.

You may need to set up a system of organizing your bills so that you are reminded when they must be paid. If you talk to someone at your bank, you may find that some bills can be paid automatically. Someone at the bank may be able to offer some suggestions for managing your account.

When you are working with numbers, be sure to recheck your calculations several times. Even if you use a calculator, you may sometimes reverse numbers when you're entering them. If you can afford it, consider hiring a bookkeeper to handle your financial record keeping. If your resources are limited, perhaps you can work out a trade with a family member or a friend: a pot of soup, a loaf of bread, or a few hours of childcare in exchange for bookkeeping services.

To avoid spelling problems, make use of the spell checker on your computer. If you are not using a computer, ask a family member or friend to proofread important documents. At times, you may need to decrease sensory input (noise, lights, interruptions) and give your body and mind a chance to catch up with their communications processing. That's one reason we often need to turn off the radio in a car. It's easier to concentrate on driving with less distraction.

Try to minimize chores that can be affected by fibrofog. For example, buy several pairs of identical socks that go with your clothes. They will be easy to match. When one sock wears out, the mate can be matched with another lonely sock.

Singing in the Rain, Laughing in the Fog

Don't ever underestimate the impact of a good sense of humor. It can be one of your best defenses against depression, anger, or other negative moods, and can help you ride out the fog. You can't beat humor for breaking tension. Just make sure that the humor is appropriate. People with FMS often overreact, and other folks may not quite understand our humor.

At times, with fibrofog, it may seem that you can only feel one emotion at a time, because the circuits are jammed with other information. This can lead to mood confusion as well as mental confusion. Every nerve cell requires a specific amount of time for recovery between stimulations, so this confusion is a sign that it's time not only to slow down, it's time to stop. Take a breath, breathe deeply and properly (see chapter 19), and see what you can delete, modify, or delegate.

> I have a self-imposed rule. Anything I buy at a garage sale must be matched by something I take to the garage sale from my own things. This kind of exchange helps to keep the clutter down, and allows life to be more manageable, even during foggy times.

Yeast and Fog

The yeast beast besets many people with FMS. Women and men can be attacked by one candida infection after another. These people often crave sugar and retain water (see chapter 23), which compounds their yeast misery because sugar and water feed the yeast critters.

Taking antibiotics is issuing an invitation to the yeast beast to come for a visit. Use antibiotics only when absolutely necessary. Talk to your doctor about the use of Nystatin when you *must* take antibiotics. Nystatin kills yeast only in the gastrointestinal tract. It won't do anything for an established systemic yeast infection, but it often prevents a yeast infection from invading your vaginal area from your gut. A yeast infection can spread between your genital and anal areas. If you have frequent yeast infections, keep a careful journal. Check for reactive hypoglycemia/insulin resistance.

For more about this nasty beastie, lets turn to Camilla Cracchiolo, R.N., who kindly provided the following information:

> The symptoms that can indicate a yeast problem include water retention, throat irritation, tingling of fingers, irritated bladder and bowel, bloating and gas, body thermostat dysfunction, swollen (crowded) glands, itching and discharge, and muscle pain. Yeast also increases irritable bladder complaints. Yeast most commonly found in the vagina is candida albicans. Yeast overgrowth causes vaginal discharge, itching and burning, although pain can often be the sign of bacterial infection.

> Birth control pills can enhance yeast production. Sexual intercourse can cause mild abrasions, which give the yeast easy access. Your spouse or significant other can be carrying yeast and reinfecting you. It is important to be sure of the diagnosis. There is a painful condition called vulvar vestibulitis syndrome. This causes severe pain in the vulva, the external part of the vaginal opening. This can be mistaken for a yeast infection and anti-fungal treatments may worsen that condition. Corticosteroids cause yeast to spread rapidly.

Here are some steps you can take to avoid being overtaken by yeast infections:

1. Take acidophilus. You can find it at health food stores and some groceries.

2. Shower rather than bathe. If you must bathe, use vinegar in the bath, and dry yourself with a hair dryer rather than a towel.

3. Wear cotton underpants, and iron them after washing. The heat of the iron is sufficient to kill the yeast.

4. You can insert plain yogurt culture or other live lactobacillus into the vagina. Live lactobacillus cultures can be found in many health food stores.

5. You may want to go without underpants at home, at night.

6. Avoid tight clothing, such as panty hose and girdles.

7. Avoid routine douching; it isn't necessary.

8. Use a water-based lubricant during intercourse.

If the yeast is deeply rooted in the vaginal wall, or elsewhere in the body, it may be time for a systemic anti-yeast regimen. Fluconazole (Diflucan) is a prescription drug and it is expensive, but it is safer than other alternatives. You may find that fibrofog clears and water weight drops when you take this medication. Expect a period of extra fog as the yeast dies off and releases toxins into your blood stream This is a message from your body that its time to balance your diet better than you have been doing (see chapter 23).

Trauma

We are just beginning to explore the tip of the iceberg when it comes to post-traumatic *injury*. I'm not talking about posttraumatic stress disorder here. There are changes that come with pain and injury, and these can take a while to develop. A lot of this research has been done on whiplash, but these studies may apply to other injuries as well. Here are some findings from some of these studies and what these findings indicate:

- Whiplash can cause later deficits in attention, concentration, and memory.[17]

- Impairment in brain function is common after head injury, even when the injury has been minor.[18]

- Emotional symptoms as well as brain function may be affected whenever the cervical spine—the spinal cord in the area of the neck—has been injured.[19]

- It doesn't take an auto accident to supply the force required to do damage. Some "psychological" brain-disconnects that are sometimes a part of whiplash aftereffects are a consequence of the whiplash, and not psychological at all.[20]

- Head injuries may add to the risk of later Alzheimer's disease and other dementias later in life.[21]

Seen It All, Done It All, Can't Remember Most of It

You may find that as fibrofog clears, even a little bit, you may notice coexisting myofascial pain and other symptoms even more. Perhaps, as the Flexyx researchers (see chapter 15) have noticed, fibrofog may muddy pain sensations. Fog and mud at the same time! Whew! This does not mean that you should *avoid* your normal stretching or exercise program, or whatever triggers your awareness of painful areas. It does mean that you may need to modify your program for a while.

Stress and Cognitive Deficits: Are You Diagonally Parked in a Parallel Universe?

Stress creates biochemicals called *glucocorticoids*, and they affect memory acquisition and consolidation processes, as well as memory retrieval mechanisms.[22] As your stress level goes up, the fibrofog may rise in tandem. Sensory overload causes stress. Too much of nearly anything causes stress. In many ways, stress is a good defining term of what is "too much." Boosting your mind-work (see chapter 20) and adding other coping mechanisms will help you as you decrease your stressors as much as possible.

Several days of exposure to cortisol at concentrations associated with physical and psychological stress can reversibly affect specific kinds of memory performance in healthy individuals.[23] It is logical to assume that FMS amplifies these effects. It is extremely difficult for us to communicate when we are in some of our dyslexic tongue/brain misconnect *fibromoments*.

For example, I was telling someone about the problem I had been experiencing in my garden. "I think I have a vowel digging in my garden," I told her. "It got a tomato plant and dug up a potato hill last night, and dug up other plants last week." A strange look crossed my friend's face. Hindsight tells me she must have been thinking, did I suspect "a," "e," "i," "o," or "u"? Since it only happened some nights, perhaps "y" was the culprit? "Uh, I wanted to say I think I had a *vole* in the garden," I explained later. Well, I caught that fibroslip, but I know many get by me, and, like the vole, go on to wreak their havoc in our lives. Some slips are not so funny. Lack of restorative sleep, and the side effects of medications, can add to our cognitive impairments.

When you are hurting, you have less tolerance for sensory stimuli, and can't process them as effectively. That may be one of the reasons some of us have a problem with crowds and cities. One study showed that even chronic low back trouble (often due to trigger points) interferes with the functioning of short-term memory, which results in decreased speed of information processing.[24]

The cognitive deficits of FMS may seem overwhelming. What is amazing to me is that, at times, so many of us can function better in some ways than healthy individuals, in spite of our handicaps. The amount of research going on should bring us great hope. We are zeroing in on the reasons for our many symptoms, and that is a big step toward finding ways to relieve or even prevent them.

> When I was in school, we got a speed-reading and memory machine. I spent a lot of time with it. My reading and comprehension were fantastically fast. At least, it seems fantastic now. I belong to Mensa, and even with my FMS-befogged IQ, I qualify in the top two percentile. Yet some days I feel stupid. When I am overworked, especially; my memory is particularly bad for those things on which I am not focused. Every time the phone rings I lose my focus working on the book or research. Sight reading music is no longer efficient for me, because my brain can't comprehend new words and the new notes at the same time. I get dizzy trying to look at both. I know that once the book is done, my pace must slow drastically and my life will come back and, I hope, at least some of my brain will come with it.

Endnotes

1. Lowe, J. 2000. *The Metabolic Treatment of Fibromyalgia.* Boulder, CO: McDowell Publishing Company.

2. Landro, N. I., T. C. Stiles, and H. Sletvold. 1997. Memory functioning in patients with primary fibromyalgia and major depression and healthy controls. *J Psychosomatic Research.* 42(3):297-306.

3. Williams, R. A., B. M. Hagerty, B. Cimprich, B. Therrien, E. Bay, and H. Oe. 2000. Changes in directed attention and short-term memory in depression. *J Psychiatr Res* 34(3):227-238.

4. Mountz, J. M., L. A. Bradley, and G. S. Alarcon. 1998. Abnormal functional activity of the central nervous system in fibromyalgia syndrome. *Am J Med Sci* 315(6):385-396.

5. Heinemann, U., S. Gabriel, R. Jauch, K. Schultze, A. Kivi, A. Eilers, et al. 2000. Alterations of glial cell function in temporal lobe epilepsy. *Epilipsia* 41(Suppl 6):S185-S189.

6. Silver, I. A., J. Deas, and M. Erecinska. 1997. Ion homeostasis in brain cells: differences in intracellular ion responses to energy limitation between cultured neurons and glial cells. *Neuroscience* 78(2):589-601.

7. Grisart, J. M., and L. H. Plaghki. 1999. Impaired selective attention in chronic pain patients. *Eur J Pain* 3(4):325-333.

8. Boucher, T. J., K. Okuse, D. L. Bennett, J. B. Munson, J. N. Wood, and S. B. McMahon. 2000. Potent analgesic effects of GNDF in neuropathic pain states. *Science* 290(5489):124-127.

9. Grigsby, J., N. L. Rosenberg, and D. Busenbark. 1995. Chronic pain is associated with deficits in information processing. *Percept Mot Skills* 81(2):403-410.

10. Kuhajda, M. C., B. E. Thorn, and M. R. Klinger. 1998. The effect of pain on memory for affective words. *Ann Behav Med* 20(1):31-35.

11. Mazer, C., J. Muneyyirci, K. Taheny, N. Raio, A. Borella, and P. Whitaker-Azmitia. 1997. Serotonin depletion during synaptogenesis leads to decreased synaptic density and learning deficits in the adult rat: a possible model of neurodevelopmental disorders with cognitive deficits. *Brain Res* 760(1-2):68-73.

12. Fujioka, M., K. Okuchi, K. I. Hiramatsu, T. Sakaki, S. Sakaguchi, and Y. Ishii. 1997. Specific changes in human brain after hypoglycemic injury. *Stroke* 28(3):584-587.

13. Glass, J. M., and D. C. Park. 2001. Cognitive dysfunction in fibromyalgia. *Curr Rheumatol Rep.* 3(2):123–127.

14. Glass, J. M., D. C. Park, and L. J. Crofford. 1999. Metamemory in fibromyalgia. Poster presented at the *Am Col Rheumatol 63rd Annual Scientific Meeting.* Hynes Convention Center, Boston, MA. Nov 13–17.

15. Cote, K. A., and H. Moldofsky. 1997. Sleep, daytime symptoms, and cognitive performance in patients with fibromyalgia. *J Rheumatol* 24:2014-2023.

16. Gais, S., W. Plihal, U. Wagner, and J. Born. 2000. Early sleep triggers memory for early visual discrimination skills. *Nat Neurosci* 3(12):1335-1339.

17. Kischka, U., T. Ettlin, S. Heim, and G. Schmid. 1991. Cerebral symptoms following whiplash injury. *Eur Neurol* 31(3):136-140.

18 McSherry, J. A. 1989. Cognitive impairment after head injury. *Am Fam Physician* 40(4):186-190.

19. Radanov, B. P., I. Bicik, J. Dvorak, J. Antinnes, G. K. von Schulthess, and A. Buck. 1999. Relation between neuropsychological and neuroimaging findings in patients with late whiplash syndrome. *J Neurol Neurosurg Psychiatry* 66(4):485-489.

20. Radanov, B. P., S. Begre, M. Sturzenegger, and K. F. Augustiny. 1996. Course of psychological variables in whiplash injury—a 2-year follow-up with age, gender and education pair-matched patients. *Pain* 64(3):429-434.

21. Plassman, B. L., R. J. Havlik, D. C. Steffens, M. J. Helms, T. N. Newman, D. Drosdick, et al. 2000. Documented head injury in early adulthood and risk of Alzheimer's disease and other dementias. *Neurology* 55(8):1158-1166.

22. De Quervain, D. J., B. Roozendaal, and J. L. McGaugh. 1998. Stress and glucocorticoids impair retrieval of long-term spatial memory. *Nature* 394(6695):787-790.

23. Newcomer, J. W., G. Selke, A. K. Melson, T. Hershey, S. Craft, K. Richards, et al. 1999. Decreased memory performance in healthy humans induced by stress-level cortisol treatment. *Arch Gen Psychiatry* 56(6):527-533.

24. Luoto, S., S. Taimela, H. Hurri, and H. Alaranta. 1999. Mechanisms explaining the association between low back trouble and deficits in information processing. A controlled study with follow-up. *Spine* 24(3):255-261.

CHAPTER 18

Positive Change

People with fibromyalgia (FMS) and/or chronic myofascial pain (CMP) share many things: we are all in the same boat. But you choose how you to handle this situation. Whether you steer this boat with only a primitive compass or you use a variety of up-to-date navigational aids depends on you. In this chapter, you will explore various options for addressing the key issues in your life so that you may begin the process of creating positive change in your life.

Understanding Depression

If you are living with constant chronic pain that is sometimes so acute as to be unbearable, pain that forces you to give up or to limit many of your former activities (like making love, hiking, working in the garden, or knitting), you have sufficient cause to be depressed. Then, if you are told by your doctors that you are not really sick (as many people with FMS and/or CMP, or "invisible chronic pain," are told), and that you should just put up with the pain, or that it's because you don't exercise enough, insult is added to injury and is further reason to become even more depressed. When neurotransmitter dysfunction, which is understood to be a cause of depression, is added to the scenario just described, you have a prescription for disaster.

Being depressed is like being in the bottom of a deep dark hole; the whole world is bleak and cold. You don't want to do anything, you don't want to be active in any way, you don't even want to move. All the energy seems to have left your body. You ache and you feel ugly and agitated. Despair, pessimism, and hopelessness fill your life. You may hide out, take the phone off the hook, and watch sad stories on television. Perhaps all you do is cry. You may be unable to hold conversations, do chores, pay bills, or keep appointments. You feel that there is no hope and that nothing will ever change. You feel worthless and you may believe that the way you feel is your own fault. You think that your life is over, and you just want to sleep forever and perhaps you want to die.

If this describes how you feel most of the time, you are having more than just a bad day—you are depressed. Depression is dangerous. Suicide is too often the tragic outcome. Get competent professional help immediately, before your symptoms worsen.

The first thing you need to do is to get a complete physical examination. Although having either FMS or CMP is reason enough to be depressed, many other medical conditions can cause or worsen depression. If, after a complete physical exam, other medical causes are ruled out, ask your health care provider to work with you to plan a course of treatment. This may include a strategy that many people find very helpful in preventing and relieving depression—developing and using your own Wellness Recovery Action Plan (see chapter 16). The treatment plan may also include the use of medications and/or counseling, or referral to a psychologist, psychiatrist, or other mental health specialist, and/or other kinds of lifestyle changes.

If you decide to use medications to treat your depression, see chapter 21. If you decide to see a counselor (many people take medications and also see a counselor), make sure the counselor validates your experience of having FMS or CMP, encourages and supports you, and does not criticize you, blame you, or try to control your life.

Positive Changes

There are seven areas in everyone's life amenable to positive changes. The first five have to do with the care and maintenance of your physical body, i.e., what kind of food you eat; how much exposure to bright light you receive; how much exercise you get; how restorative your sleep is; and how comfortable your living quarters are.

Two other areas where positive changes can be accomplished with relative ease have to do with your mind and spirit. Knowing how to change negative thought patterns into positive ones, and how to harness the power of positive affirmations can help you turn your back on depression and allow you to live a richer, happier life in spite of having either FMS or CMP.

Diet

The food you eat definitely affects the way you feel, both physically and emotionally. Poor diet is a key perpetuating factor in FMS, CMP, and many other coexisting conditions. For example, studies have long indicated that excessive carbohydrates are implicated in mood disorders such as SAD.[1] Your diet is an aspect of your perpetuating factors that *you* control. You have to eat. Why eat foods that add to your symptoms, when you can learn to eat responsibly? This requires self-discipline, responsibility, and education. Furthermore, there are numerous support groups available to help you.

The curious thing about diet is that the effects of what is eaten vary widely from person to person. For instance, you may find that dairy foods make you calm and help you to sleep. However, they cause me so much gastrointestinal distress that I become irritable and even depressed. Tomatoes don't affect most people, but some find that eating tomatoes causes them to become agitated. Some people do well when they eat three good meals a day. Others find they do better if they eat five or six small meals throughout the day. Experiment with what works best for you.

It's a good idea to figure out which foods make you feel better or, at least, don't bother you and which foods you may want to avoid because they make you feel worse. Do this by taking the following steps:

1. Observe how you feel right after you eat certain foods and how you feel several hours later.

2. Eliminate from your diet for one week a food that you think might be making you feel badly, then observe how you feel. Then observe how you feel after you begin eating that food again.

3. Study various self-help resources on how foods can affect the way you feel, then make changes accordingly.

4. Address diet issues with a nutritionist or naturopathic physician (many general practitioners have little training in diet or nutrition, and, in the worst cases, may disregard their importance). A nutritionist or naturopathic physician could also advise you on the use of food supplements and herbs.

You will find that work on your diet is accomplished only by trial and error. But as you continue to address this issue, you will customize a diet for yourself that works best for you. Focus on foods that are wholesome, natural, and fresh. Many people complain that these foods are more costly than highly processed and junk foods. They are, however, very high in nutritive value, while processed and junk foods have little or no value and are not worth what they cost. You can stretch your food budget by spending little or nothing on unhealthy foods and purchasing healthy food instead. An added bonus, if extra weight is an issue for you, is that a diet focused on wholesome, natural, and fresh food is a good way to lose weight. Loss of extra weight often correlates with feeling better about yourself and your appearance, and a lessening of symptoms. (See chapter 23 for a more complete discussion of food and nutrition issues.)

Light

If you live in a northern climate, you may have noticed that you have some or all of the following symptoms as winter approaches, the days become shorter, and the amount of daylight decreases:

- a drop in energy level • a decrease in productivity • difficulty getting motivated • difficulty concentrating and focusing • impatience with yourself and others • a hard time getting out of bed in the morning • craving for sweets and junk food • diminished sex drive.

If you experience symptoms like these only in the winter, you may have a form of depression called seasonal affective disorder (SAD) as well as having FMS or CMP. Studies have shown that for most people consistent daily visual exposure to bright light reduces or eliminates symptoms of SAD.[2] It is not clear why bright light works in this way, but it is thought that it has to do with production of the hormone melatonin, which takes place in the pineal gland. Some researchers believe that SAD sufferers are either too sensitive to dim light and manufacture too much melatonin as a response to the dimness, or that they are oversensitive to the normal amount of the hormone that is produced.[3]

Dopamine, a neurotransmitter that transmits information between the nerves in the body and the brain cells, may also play a role in SAD.[4] Also, it is thought that depletion of the neurotransmitter, serotonin, may be responsible for the carbohydrate cravings that often accompany SAD.[5]

A simple program that increases the amount of natural or bright light taken in through the eyes often helps to reduce or completely eliminate SAD symptoms. This includes increasing your exposure to light by putting full-spectrum (grow) lights in your light fixtures, getting outdoors as much as possible even on cloudy days (never look directly at the sun), spending time near windows and in brightly lit rooms when you are indoors, and keeping your work space and home well lit. You can purchase a specially designed light box that many people have found to be helpful. If SAD is a serious issue for you, it may be well worth the expense. You can find light box distributors by searching on the Internet.

Some people spend several hours a day sitting near their light box but not staring at it—they read, write, or engage in some other kind of activity. Others find their SAD is relieved by using full-spectrum lights where they spend most of their time. You may want to turn off these lights late in the day to prevent insomnia. If you become nervous and jittery, turn these lights off. You may be getting too much light.

Some people report an almost immediate relief of symptoms when they begin light therapy. For most people, though, it takes from four to five days to two weeks to work. If it hasn't worked by then, it is probably not your answer. You might consider seeking a physician in your area who has expertise in light therapy before buying either full-spectrum lights or a light box.

Exercise

Exercise is often very difficult for people with either FMS or CMP. Your body may be stiff and achy, and exercise may increase your pain for several days or even longer. Often your pain is so severe that you cannot tolerate any kind of strenuous exercise. But do the best you can. Be gentle with yourself, but move whatever part of your body you can move without causing pain (see chapter 19).

If you can exercise, try to do it every day for at least twenty minutes. In addition to the numerous physiological benefits of exercise, Dr. Edmund Bourne[6] reports the following psychological benefits:

- increased feeling of well-being • reduced dependence on alcohol and drugs • reduced insomnia • improved concentration and memory • alleviation of symptoms of depression • greater control over feelings of anxiety • increased self-esteem

Many people have found that exercising in a heated pool kept at 88 to 94 degrees Fahrenheit works well. When you exercise in water below 88 degrees Fahrenheit, you may find that you experience severe cramping. If a heated pool is available to you, take advantage of it

Remember that with FMS, your sense of time is not always reliable and it is easy to overdo exercise, which could cause you serious problems. Set a timer for specific amounts of time or exercise with a friend who will help you to keep track of the time.

Sleep

A good night's sleep is absolutely essential to avoiding depression, as well as to relieving symptoms related to FMS or CMP. Since sleep problems are almost always a part of FMS and frequently of CMP, getting a good night's sleep can be a real challenge. Do your best to get adequate amounts of sleep. Lack of sleep can make all of your symptoms worse, but too much sleep is not a good idea, either. See "Sleep-Inducing Techniques" in chapter 10.

Living Space

Your living space significantly affects the way you feel. When you have FMS or CMP you need to give special attention to your surroundings. Ask yourself the following questions. Your answers may help you to understand where you need to make some changes in your life that would support your wellness.

1. If you live with others, do you have a space in your home that is your private space to decorate to suit yourself, where you can keep your things and they will not be disturbed, and where you can spend time by yourself involved in your own activities?

2. Is your living space comfortable and easy to clean and keep neat? If cleaning is a problem for you, think about getting a family member or friend to take over your heavy cleaning chores. If possible, hire someone to clean.

3. Do you have too many "things"? Dispose of things you don't need. Lots of "stuff" makes a living space difficult to keep clean and attractive, and a messy living space usually increases stress if only because it makes it harder to find the things you need, such as medications.

4. Do the people you live with support you in your quest for wellness?

Changing Negative Thoughts to Positive Ones

Sometimes you may be your own worst enemy. Almost unconsciously, you may berate yourself again and again. Your moods and emotional states are strongly influenced by what you tell yourself, how you think, and the ways in which you interpret situations. If your personal viewpoints habitually take the form of negative self-talk, self-doubt, and generalized fears and phobias, you can work to change these negative thought patterns and improve your life.

For instance, when you drop things, which may occur often because of trigger points (TrPs), you may call yourself names like "clumsy" or "klutzy." Yet the fact that you function at all with FMS or CMP is often a miracle. Or, when you forget things, you may tell yourself you are stupid. Yet, in spite of neurotransmitter dysfunction and fibrofog, you often are able to navigate through the chaos of life with surprising insight and humor. By changing the negative messages you give yourself into messages that are positive and affirming, you can raise your self-esteem and help yourself to feel better.

How many times do you say to yourself negative phrases such as, "How could I be so dumb?" Are you aware that your subconscious mind believes everything you say to it? If you are constantly putting yourself down, your own habitual reinforcement of negativity can be a considerable obstacle in your journey toward healing. In addition, a strong focus on negativity adds stress to your life. Fortunately, it is in your power to change the destructive habit of reinforcing negative thinking. In many cases, patterns of thinking have become so habitual that you may hardly notice them. Therefore, to begin the process of eliminating thought patterns such as self-doubt, fears, and phobias you must identify them.

Carry a small notebook with you for several days. Every time you notice that you are thinking about yourself or the circumstances of your life in a negative way, write the thought in your notebook. Then, write a positive statement that you want to say to yourself instead of the negative one. At first, this may be hard to do, but after a while, thinking positively can become as much a habit as thinking negatively. Here are some examples:

Negative thought: The holidays are going to be terrible. I will never get my cards sent out on time. That will ruin everything.

Positive response: Even though I probably won't get my cards mailed out in time for the holiday, I can still have a great time.

Negative thought: No one likes me.

Positive response: Many people like me. I am warm and friendly and I treat others well.

Negative thought: It's my fault that my son failed his French test. I should have forced him to study more.

Positive response: My son failed his French test because he didn't study. He needs to learn that his actions have consequences. Perhaps this failure will help him to learn that lesson.

Negative thought: My husband comes home from work at a different time every day of the week. This makes my life more difficult.

Positive response: My husband does the best he can to get home on time. His job requires him to work irregular hours. I am glad about the money he brings home from the job, and he helps me as much as he possibly can.

Negative thought: I don't feel well enough to go to church today. I will probably never feel well enough again to go to church.

Positive response: I will feel better soon. I know I will. Then I will be able to go to church.

Negative thought: I can never lose all this extra weight I've gained.

Positive response: I can and I will lose this extra weight.

Negative thought: I should get the whole house cleaned today.

Positive response: I will do what I can today. The rest will have to wait.

Negative thought: I am stupid.

Positive response: I am smart.

Negative thought: I know I will never be well again.

Positive thought: I know I will be well again.

Negative thinking often becomes so familiar that changing it takes persistence, consistency, and creativity. Spend some time each day working on reinforcing your positive statements. You may want to choose one or two of the ones you use most often, work on them for a while and then work on one or several others. Or you may find that you can work easily on most of them at the same time. Reinforce your positive responses by performing the following actions:

- Repeat them aloud or say them under your breath over and over.

- Writing them down over and over again, ten or twenty times or even more.

- Ask someone you trust to read your positive responses to you.

- Use markers or your computer to make signs which state your positive response, and hang them in obvious places around your home. Be sure to read the signs every time you see them.

- Say "Stop!" to yourself when you say or think a negative thought and then repeat your positive response several times.

After several weeks to several months of daily reinforcement of your positive responses, you will notice that your negative thoughts are no longer an issue for you. If you begin to notice the thought again, return to your daily reinforcement activities for several more days.

There are several excellent resource books that can help you with this process. You can find them in Appendix B: Reading List. You may also want to see a counselor who will support you in the process of changing your negative thought patterns into positive ones.

Affirmations

Affirmations are short, positive statements that describe how you want to feel, and what you would like your life to be like. It's easy to get into the habit of saying affirmations to yourself at all times of the day. For example, they can be repeated while waiting for a street light to change, or washing dishes, upon awakening or at bedtime, and during meditations. Repeating affirmations to yourself stops any negative self-dialogue you might have going. The development and regular repetition of affirmations may seem simplistic, but many people who are challenged by the negativity of chronic pain have used this technique with great success. It is the reverse of negative self-dialogue, and it is noninvasive. It costs nothing and is well worth trying.

Some people carry lists of affirmations in their pockets or purses or tape them to the refrigerator door until they form the positive habit of repeating their affirmations at specific times of the day. It is a good practice to start and end your day with your affirmations. Make them part of your life, and you will fulfill their prophecies.

Examples of Positive Affirmations

Here are some simple sentences that will help you achieve control of yourself and your life. Repeat one or more to yourself whenever you need to assert your rights.

- I am in charge of my life.

- It's okay to make mistakes.

- I can make up my own mind.

- I have a right to ignore the advice of others, even if I asked for that advice.

- My time is valuable, too.

- I deserve the time and space to heal.

- I am a very valuable person.

- I deserve to be treated with compassion, dignity, and respect at all times.

- I am happy.

- Every day in every way I am getting better and better and better.

Creating positive change in your life takes time. You can't do it all at once. Persistence and consistency are your most important assets in this process. Begin by deciding what you want to change in your life. Write down some small steps you can take to begin making these changes. When you have taken these steps, write down and take several more steps. When you have reached your goal or feel comfortable with the work you have done, begin working on creating other change that is important to you. Recognize and reward yourself for your progress.

Endnotes

1. Wurtman, R. J., and J. J. Wurtman. 1989. *Scientific American* 260(1):68-75.

2. Terman, M., and J. S. Terman. 1999. Bright light therapy: side effects and benefits across the symptoms spectrum. *J Clin Psychiatry* 60(11):799-808.

3. Nathan, P. J., G. D. Burrows, and T. R. Norman. 1999. Melatonin sensitivity to dim white light in affective disorders. *Neurophsychopharmacology* 21(3):408-413.

4. Partonen T. 1996. Dopamine and circadian rhythms in seasonal affective disorder. *Med Hypothesis* 47(3):191-192.

5. Arbisi, P.A., A. S. Levin, J. Nerenberg, and J. Wolf. 1996. Seasonal alterations in taste detection and recognition threshold in seasonal affective disorder: the proximate source of carbohydrate craving. *Psychiatry Res* 59(3):171-182.

6. Bourne, E. 1995. *The Anxiety & Phobia Workbook*. Second edition. Oakland, CA: New Harbinger Publications.

CHAPTER 19

Bodywork: Regaining Function

I have tried a lot of different paths to healing. I know a lot of medical care providers, and I have consulted with many of them on my path to better health. This could have resulted in an overload of confusing and/or conflicting instructions. When I went for trigger point (TrP) injections, for example, I was given a set of stretches that take about half an hour to do, and told to do them as the first activity of the morning. I was taught tennis ball acupressure and told to use the ball and take a hot shower as soon as I get up. My nutritionist says I should eat within an hour of getting up. Every bodyworker I have ever met has taught me more exercises that I should do every day, or many times a day—some even *before* I get up. All of these are worthy and helpful. If I listened to them all, I'd never have enough time to eat or sleep, much less get anything done. In addition, I am surrounded by good people, each telling me I should slow down. Each one also wants me to help with her/his project before I do so. But they tell me to stay within my limits, so I can be a good role model. Perhaps that is why I enjoy reading science fiction so much. I'm looking for a planet with a 186-hour day! Each of us has to find stretches and exercise that work best for us, yet allow us some time to live our lives.

You *do* have a high-maintenance body, but there are limits to your ability to attend to its needs. How do you choose? This chapter looks at some options. You will be limited by the expertise available to you, but there are many forms of exercise you can do yourself. Some don't require the expenditure of a lot of time or money. They do take an investment of interest and energy, but you will be repaid with a healthier body and mind. Note that in this chapter I use the term "bodyworker," rather than physical therapist (PT). Many bodyworkers may not have a degree in PT, but may be trained and experienced in just what you need. Some people with PT training may not be familiar with fibromyalgia (FMS) or chronic myofascial pain (CMP), and can do unintentional harm. Inappropriate physical therapy is a major perpetuating factor, and is completely *preventable*. Don't count on a degree to guarantee expertise in these two conditions. Patients, insurance companies, doctors, and physical therapists need to understand this.

> *Carry Tiger, Return to Mountain* is a movement in t'ai chi chuan. T'ai chi is a powerful internal martial art that is healing for body and mind. Each movement has meaning and speaks to the t'ai chi player as she or he develops through practice and intent. The tiger is a symbol of power, energy,

Moving Through Life

Learn to be aware of your body and become aware of repetitious movements. You must learn to move mindfully. Be attentive to and purpose. The mountain is the center of balance and harmony.

To me, Carry Tiger, Return to Mountain represents my mission in life. I believe that God has given me a mission to educate others, both patients and care providers, about fibromyalgia and chronic myofascial pain, and to empower them to identify and control perpetuating factors that are obstacles to the healing process. It is a worthy task. The tiger is hurt, and needs to return to the mountain to heal. Yet at times I feel as if I am personally carrying a very heavy and demanding tiger over broken glass in bare feet, over desert and snow to the mountain. The tiger is frightened and clinging tightly to me with very sharp claws. Even when we get to the mountain, the tiger doesn't want to let go.

This feeling is a signal to me that I need to return to my center. There are often an overwhelming number of people asking me for individual help, and I must be careful to also help them escape the chains of victimhood. This means that I cannot carry each one of them to the mountain. My task is to show them the way and empower them to find the tools they need to reach the mountain, to self-advocate, and to build their own support and medical care teams.

what you are doing. If you use one group of muscles excessively, you will pay. Vary your tasks to give your body variety of motion. The more ways you can find to do a certain task, the less dangerous it will be to do that task repetitively. Your posture is exceedingly important, as are body mechanics. Body mechanics is the study of the physics of the body, and includes how you stand, lift, sit, walk, and so forth. It's about how your body finds its correct balance. If your body is out of balance, strain results. In the management of almost any chronic pain situation, it is vital to restore healthy posture and balance.

Bending. If you are *healthy*, frequent proper bending will strengthen your back muscles. If you have fibromyalgia (FMS) or chronic myofascial pain (CMP), *you must never bend, lift, and twist at the same time*. If you must bend, first turn your feet in the direction you want to bend. Before lifting, look up. This will help your spinal vertebrae to align properly. Check your posture during all of your activities. This means your sleeping posture, your reading position, how you sit at the table when eating, and so forth. You *can* gain a measure of control over your sleeping posture. The use of pillows can help, but the key is the intent to change harmful behaviors. It is very helpful to have a trained trigger point (TrP) myotherapist to help you find your TrP-inciting sleep postures, and to coach you in correcting them. We've all developed bad habits. But, fortunately, there are many techniques for learning posture correction.

Respect Your Limits

Be sure to check with your doctor before starting any exercise program, even walking. At first, any limits your doctor may set may feel very restrictive. Such limits will expand as your health improves. It is important to respect your limits in order to feel your best. There are many ways to do this. One plan is to make a contract with yourself. This can specify when, how much, and how often you will do specific exercises. Don't overdo. Gently, slowly, increase the range of your exercise. Exercise with a friend, or use a timer. Make exercising as pleasant an experience as possible. Most importantly, you must learn to listen to your body.

Do you have a treadmill? Do you even know where it is? Can you plant seeds in the moss growing there? When choosing a form of exercise, pick one you enjoy. Be committed, but not compulsive. Schedule blocks of time for exercise in your daybook. Proceed slowly and gently. There are even exercises you can do while seated. For example, there are a number of seated chi kung exercises. If you have TrPs, remember, *you cannot strengthen a muscle with a TrP*. Your muscles are already contracted. Your bodyworker can teach you exercises to *lengthen* your muscles at first. If you have FMS and TrPs that are affecting your balance and proprioception (the awareness of posture, movement, and changes in equilibrium), you may find balance difficult. Don't despair, but don't sign up for balance beam gymnastics, either.

Immune system effects. Moderate exercise appears to stimulate the immune system, but there is also good evidence that intense exercise can *cause* immune deficiency.[1] Exercise each side of your body equally to maintain balance. Proper exercise can reduce your pain load and even help you sleep better. Be cautious when exercising outdoors in hot, humid, or windy weather, especially if you are taking decongestants and/or pain relievers. These medications can enhance fluid loss. Make sure you replenish your fluid loss with extra water.

Exercise when you feel at your best. Often this is between 10 A.M. and 2 P.M. Any exercise program must be tailored to your needs, and will require modification as you improve. Your schedule may need to be modified during hot weather, to avoid the risk of dehydration. Aerobic exercise, such as walking, swimming, or dancing is great, once your body is ready. Aerobics will help to normalize your sleep cycle and will release your body's internal painkillers, the endorphins.

> I tried water aerobics, thinking that would be easy enough on my body. Wrong. I kept scaling down my idea of "slowly." I couldn't figure out why even the senior citizens' water aerobics did so much damage to my body. Then I found out that being in a swimming pool with a temperature outside of the 88- to 94-degree Fahrenheit range can cause long-range worsening of symptoms in chronic myofascial pain (CMP). Doing the crawl and the breaststroke can also worsen symptoms.

Bodywork You Do Yourself

This first section is about bodywork that you perform yourself, with minimal guidance, as opposed to formal bodywork that you learn from a teacher or in a class. This section starts with some of the most basic bodywork. No matter how basic it is, you still need to do it properly. No matter what bodywork you have done *to* you, it is even more important that you are faithful to the home program that you do for yourself. You can't have a bodyworker with you every minute of every day. You can learn when you need to stretch, when you need to vary your movements, and when you need to do the daily routines that will help not only to maintain your present mobility, but will help extend your limits. Before you begin any exercise program, you must breathe properly. All forms of exercise require coordination with proper breathing techniques.

Breathing: The First Exercise

Proper breathing is the first requirement for optimum health. Because breathing is an automatic function, we tend to take it for granted. You may be breathing well enough to stay alive, but that doesn't mean you are breathing for optimal health. Many people develop bad breathing habits when they are young. Adults often use only a small portion of their lung capacity. Take a moment to consider your breathing. Is it deep, rhythmic, and relaxed? Is it shallow, jerky, and constricted? If any words in the last sentence describe your breathing, you need to relearn how to breathe efficiently.

One of the first things that happen when you are frightened or angry is a change in your breathing rhythm. Your body tenses. If you have FMS, you may live with that particular stress reaction much of the time. Breathing awareness is the key to body relaxation. Unfortunately, in this society, packaging is all-important. There is an emphasis on packaging over substance. So it is with breathing and our bodies. You are told to keep your belly firm and pulled in and to breathe through your chest. This type of breathing, called paradoxical breathing, restricts airflow and worsens TrPs. You can't break the laws of nature without getting caught. If you breathe in this shallow manner, you develop a hunger for air that can cause you to gasp for breath, and to breathe through your mouth. When you breathe through your mouth, your breath becomes even more shallow and rapid. This causes your body to struggle even harder for adequate oxygen. Many people are mouth-breathers and are not even aware of it.

Deep Breathing Exercise

Sometimes it is easier to begin breathing properly when you are lying down. Lie down on your back, in a comfortable position. Place your hand on your belly, right below your navel, so you can feel what is happening. Breathe in. When you breathe in, first fill your belly with air, then fill the middle of your chest, and then your upper chest last.

Now, take a deep breath in through your nose and hold your breath for a few moments. If you are wearing constricting garments, you may have to loosen them to take a really deep breath. This may give you an indication why wearing constricting clothing can be detrimental to your health. You may have developed TrPs in any of your respiratory muscles or their accessories. (If you are not sure, check through the symptoms described in chapter 8.) Your fingers will find the spots, and your body will let you know. You may also run into some TrPs as you do some of the bodywork described in this chapter. They are saying "hello." It's time to learn some techniques to teach them to say "goodbye."

Now, let your breath out slowly through your nose. When you think all of the stale air has been expelled, open your mouth and breathe out the rest of it. Chances are, there will be quite a bit of air that was not expelled the first time. If so, you are probably not using your diaphragm muscle, the main muscle in the body devoted to the breathing process. It forms the base of the chest area and moves up and down with your breath. If you don't use your diaphragm to breathe, you create tension in your body, and you promote shallow breathing. Then your diaphragm develops TrPs, too.

Complete several cycles of breathing in and out, feeling your belly move out as you breathe in, and relax inward as you breathe out. This is a response to the action of the diaphragm muscle. Establish a rhythm. It helps if you keep the front part of your tongue lightly on the roof of your mouth. This helps to prevent mouth breathing. Concentrating on your breath in this way can be a form of meditation. Whenever you catch yourself breathing incorrectly, stop if you can, and breathe properly. Repeating mindful proper breathing for five minutes or so many times a day will help you get into the habit of breathing properly all the time. Think how long you have been breathing incorrectly. Be patient with yourself, but keep at it. You *can* relearn to breathe the way you were born to breathe. Keep practicing this until you are breathing this way all the time.

Oxygen. If your breath is shallow, you don't use your diaphragm fully and you always have some stagnant air in your lungs. Breathing from the belly, using the diaphragm, supplies your body with more oxygen. You need oxygen to create energy. Think of fire. It needs oxygen to burn. So do the energy fires of your body. Deep breathing will help rid your body of waste gases. Breathing correctly massages some of your organs and improves mental clarity and focus. By breathing mindfully and consciously, and slowing and deepening your breath, you can ease anxiety and stress.

The Dangers of Repetitious Exercise

Exercise can be a great help in relieving symptoms, but any type of bodywork you choose should avoid repetitious exercises.[2] Avoid activities that produce repetitive muscular loads, such as shoveling snow, raking leaves, vacuum cleaning, painting walls, or unloading a dishwasher. If you must do such tasks, vary your movements. Use both hands. Alternate sides so that the muscles on each side of your body are used in turn. The number of repetitions of a movement should not exceed six or seven. Rest your muscles between repetitions to allow them to recover. When your muscles are cold or tired, you should not do even gentle *repetitive* activities.

Repatterning movements are not the same as repetitious exercise. An example of repatterning, or modification of bad habits and reflexes through brain programming, is relearning how to breathe correctly. We also have to learn proper posture, and how to move efficiently and in a healthy manner. If TrPs have caused a misalignment, or require some muscles to compensate for others, we may have a lot of relearning to do. This may require a lot of repatterning, but not necessarily one repetition after another. Reprogramming is as much about not using inappropriate muscles as using appropriate muscles. It takes thousands of repetitions to form and reinforce a new body-mind pattern.[3] This is not the same as repetitious exercise. We all must breathe and we all must move, and we must learn to do these correctly.

Stretching

If you have FMS, there is a reduction in body temperature and blood flow to the brain when you exercise. That's the opposite of what most people experience. So, in addition to your normal fibrofog, you may not be able to think clearly enough during your exercise to set sensible limits. And, in fact, FMS patients tend to underestimate the amount of exercise they've experienced. Do not bounce when you stretch. Bouncing can damage your muscles by forcing them to stretch beyond their ability.

Your muscles are supposed to work together in functional units, and they may be out of practice. By itself a single muscle can accomplish nothing. To function, each muscle requires the interactions with the rest of its muscle group. Your muscles need to learn coordination. If one muscle is not functioning as it should, then *all* the muscles in that group are not functioning as they should, because the other muscles modify their actions to take up the role of the dysfunctional muscle. Remember, everything in your body is connected through the myofascia. It will take time to coax your muscles back to healthy function.

Soreness. If TrPs are causing pain even when your muscles are at rest, gentle passive stretches and moist heat may be the only type of bodywork you can endure. It is important that your muscles be slowly stretched to their full range of motion often each day. The stretch should be *within the limits of pain*, and should not produce a lasting ache. When an exercise produces only mild soreness that disappears on the first day, it can be repeated on the second day. Tell your bodyworkers the extent and nature of the aftereffects of your exercise, so that your program can be adjusted accordingly. When the TrPs cause only a mild soreness that disappears quickly, gradual *lengthening* exercises can be added to the daily program.[4]

Muscle strengthening. *You must be out of pain with normal range of motion for two weeks before strengthening exercise is initiated, and then it must be gentle and introduced very gradually.* Janet Travell spoke these words frequently, but I get the impression that they weren't always understood. *The TrPs must be gone before you strengthen the muscle. Not latent, but gone!* When you can perform ten lengthening contractions easily, this daily exercise can be replaced with one muscle shortening contraction. Holding a healthy muscle in maximal contraction for five to ten seconds daily will maintain the strength of the muscle.[5] One additional repetition may be added each day, if the soreness caused by the exercise disappears that day. Exercise must be prescribed carefully and monitored closely. A pause between every repetition to allow the muscle to rest and relax is as important as the exercise itself.

Why Stretch?

Muscles are either lengthened, contracted, or at rest. Leaving a muscle in a contracted condition for any period of time can activate TrPs, especially if illness or some other stressor has weakened your body. Immobility is a fairly common TrP activator, and it's one of your greatest enemies. If you stay in one position for too long a time, your body stiffens because the myofascia forms its own kind of splinting. Stretching the muscle will help to inactivate the central TrPs but may worsen the attachment TrPs by increasing tension on them, so stretch carefully and slowly.

Warming up and cooling down. Warm-up stretching exercises are essential before any exertion. Muscles are designed to work optimally at a warmer temperature, and warm-up stretching prepares them for work. This is true whether you are gardening, hiking, or running the Boston Marathon. When you exercise, as muscles are used, they tighten, that is, they shorten. You need postexercise stretches to get them to lengthen again, or the exercise may do more harm than good. The postexercise stretches will also help you to avoid injuring any muscle the next time you work out. Remember, this is the only body you get in this life—treat it gently.

Referred pain. Any stretch that increases referred pain during or after the stretch should be stopped or modified. Muscles with TrPs start out fatigued and become exhausted more rapidly than healthy muscles.[6] There is a good exercise for just about every TrP, and many bodyworkers who understand TrPs can teach you how to do them properly. Trigger points in the pectoralis and sternalis muscles (see Figs. 8-18 and 8-19), for example, are helped by a doorway stretch that is performed as follows:

Doorway Stretch

1. Stand in a doorway. Place your hands, palms down, on each side of the doorjamb (the upright pieces that form the sides of the door opening) at your shoulder height. Rest your forearms against the doorjamb.

2. Take a step forward and feel the stretch across your chest. Keep your head up.

3. Try this with your hands farther down on the doorjamb, and then with your hands even lower. Do this stretch once or twice a day for each hand height. If you can't do some portions of this stretch, TrPs may be at work. Discuss this with your bodyworker.

Warning: Some people with FMS have hypermobility (see chapter 7). Their joints are loose and pliable. If you have this condition, *don't stretch your muscles*. Everyone must be careful not to *overstretch* muscles, because this may lead to rebound contraction.

Rocking Chair Exercise

Rocking tenses and relaxes the soleus muscle (see Fig. 8-30) in the calf of the leg, which is the secondary pump that helps the heart to circulate blood. Remember John F. Kennedy's rocking chair? In the press, much was made of the fact that he brought his own specially designed rocking chair to the White House. Dr. Travell, one of the founders of myofascial medicine, was John F. Kennedy's White House physician. She designed many pieces of White House furniture to fit the president, including that rocking chair. Rocking is a marvelous activity that prevents immobility and gently stimulates the muscles. It's also low-impact cardiovascular exercise.

Make sure that your rocking chair fits you. It should have arms, and they should be of a height to support your elbows and forearms. The seat should be low enough to allow your feet to touch the ground without cutting off the circulation under your thighs. Footrests don't work well for rocking. Rock gently and slowly, and if you are reading at the same time, make sure that your lighting is adequate and that your book is held in an ergonomic manner. Rocking shouldn't be your only exercise, but it is a good way to start.

Walking

Walking is a great exercise, and it's free. But, like everything else, there is a right and wrong way to do it. Check with your bodyworker. Learn to raise your legs from your hips, not your knees. Trigger points can cause *foot slap* and *foot drop*. These are disturbances of gait that can cause you trip over your own feet, because your body doesn't know how high to lift them to clear the ground (see chapter 8). Trigger points also can cause your knees, ankles, and even hips to buckle. Find someone to walk with, be attentive to how you step, and don't overdo it.

Guidelines for Walking

When you exercise, you increase air intake. If that air is loaded with pollutants, it's damaging to your health. If you live in an area of high air pollution, such as Los Angeles or Houston, you may want to confine your walking to indoor areas with air filters. We *can* control the quality of the air, water, and food we consume. (If you care about your health, become an environmentalist. Help influence corporations and lawmakers to care about the environment. Support companies and lawmakers who are environmentally aware. Don't support the ones who are not.)

Make sure you have well-fitting, supportive shoes with flexible soles. Check your shoes for evidence of wear. Shoes don't last forever. If the heels or soles are unevenly worn, it's time to get rid of them. An imbalance in your footgear will worsen the muscle imbalances in your body. Check to see if you need an insert for your shoes (see chapter 7).

You may be able to manage only a very short walk at first. Relax. If you find yourself breathing through your mouth and gasping, clearly, you are pushing too hard. Remember, people with FMS take much longer to repair damage resulting from overdoing exercise than healthy people do. Start slowly and be gentle with yourself. Anything you do at all is a good start. The most complex, elaborate fitness program begins with a single step.

Guidelines for Longer Walks

- Stretch before you begin your walk. There are many excellent books on stretching. Check your local library and look at several books. Ask your bodyworker to teach you specific stretches that will help your specific problems.

- During the first three minutes of your walk, go at about half the speed you will be walking. This allows your muscles to warm up.

- Tell someone where you are going and about when you expect to return.

- Don't hike by yourself if you're going to walk away from populated areas.

- Wear at least one brightly colored article of clothing, so you can be spotted, if need be.

- Always carry water with you.

- Walk during daylight, and check the weather forecast before you start.

- Carry a police whistle. This can alert others if you fall and need help.

- Breathe as normally as possible when you walk.

- After your walk, stretch again to cool down slowly.

As with any of the therapeutic methods described in this book, it is important to remember that we are providing *guidelines* only. Once you've started walking, you will be able to increase the distance you walk gradually.

Bodywork in General

Bodywork includes any physical therapy techniques that are used to help your body. You can perform some techniques by yourself, once you learn them. There are other forms that you can't do yourself. This doesn't mean that you should view *any* bodywork as a passive process. The little time you spend with your bodyworker must be reinforced with work you do daily on your own. Bodywork includes techniques such as massage, myotherapy, myofascial release, craniosacral release, Spray and Stretch, acupressure, and forms of movement therapy. Start slowly. Add new activities or therapies gradually. Be realistic. The wrong exercise can be as damaging as the wrong medication. Consider all the variables and all your options.

Allow enough time between bodywork sessions to recover before the next one begins. Give your body time to adjust. It will be finding a new balance every day. Even your biochemistry will change. Baby yourself. If you have FMS, all manual techniques described here may need modifying. It is very important that you and your health care team understand this. If you have had TrPs for some time, your tissues may have changed. There may be fibrosis,[7] scarring, and/or calcification. These changes will take a lot of time and work to reverse. The sooner you begin, the sooner you will achieve your optimum range of motion and optimum state of health.

Making Things Easier

You can ease the strain on your body during the course of bodywork by drinking large amounts of good water to dilute and flush out the waste materials. Rest frequently. Avoid strenuous activities (including travel) on the days you have bodywork therapy and for several days thereafter. After your TrPs are broken up, your muscles may be sore for days. If you have many TrPs, you may have to take it easy for a full week after each treatment. Allow time for your body to recover between sessions. Address perpetuating factors, and respect your muscles. Muscles are supposed to relax, contract, and be mobile. Give them a chance to remember how to do this. Your brain must reprogram itself to allow this, so treat yourself gently.

As your muscles improve through bodywork, you will be able to recognize and avoid activities that stress them. Decide which aggravating activities are unnecessary or modifiable. Write down any activity that causes you pain. Then, list ways that you can avoid or modify that activity to reduce or eliminate the pain.

Bodywork and Pain

Electrolytes. Membranes of nerves and muscles constantly exchange biochemicals. They also exchange negative and positive ions, the plus and minus charges that perform the bioelectrical functioning of the body. These ions are in the form of certain minerals, such as sodium, potassium, calcium, and phosphorous, which are called *electrolytes*. When there is a change from a plus to minus charge or a minus to a plus charge, that change releases neurotransmitters and energy. The nerve cells, called neurons, send waves of energy from one place to the next. For communications to be smooth, there must be a continuous flow of circulating materials in and around each cell. If part of a nerve is pinched or constricted, some areas of your body may become numb; others may become hypersensitive. Fibrofog, delayed reactions, and other symptoms may develop under these conditions.

Myelin. There are many levels, or layers, in the nervous system. One layer, called the dorsal column, is coated with insulation, called *myelin*. Myelin gives this tissue a white color. The dorsal column is like an express train. It crosses few nerve junctions and bridges few gaps, and the myelin insulation allows nerve impulses to travel from 40 to 70 meters per second[8] (a meter is 39.37 inches). This is the system that carries sensations of fine pressure, vibrations, and the sensation of body parts in motion.

The gray matter of the spinal cord, which has no myelin insulation, bridges many gaps. This system is called the *spinothalamic system*, and it carries pain, heat and cold, itches, tickles, and sexual sensations. Spinothalamic sensations move at one-fifth the speed of dorsal column sensations. This means that you experience a time lag between the stimulus and the sensation. The lag gives you the chance to flood your consciousness with the more rapidly transmitted touch sensations, and thus to block some of the pain. For example, if you stub your toe, you may rub it. The rubbing sensation travels along a faster track than the pain sensation, so you instinctively try to block the pain sensations with rubbing. (This may be part of why we hug someone when we know they are hurting. I have noticed "fibrohugs," or hugs given to people with FMS by people with FMS, often use rubbing motions on the back, for an extra kind of soothing effect. Some of us with TrP training will hug people on the right and then on the left sides, a kind of CMP hug, to make sure each side is used equally.) This is one reason bodywork is an important part of any therapy program. Be sure to give your bodyworker feedback during therapy.

How Bodywork Helps Control Symptoms

Bodywork is beneficial for more than just pain relief. It can slow and deepen your respiration, so you can take in more oxygen with less effort. Some bodywork will help to break up tightened myofascia. It can help to diminish muscle tension in TrP areas, as well as tension in the entire body. It can improve microcirculation, which also helps the muscles to receive more fuel and oxygen. With most types of bodywork, the resting heart rate will drop. This means that your heart operates with the same degree of functionality, only with less effort.

Here are some guidelines to help you on your way:

- Start only one type of bodywork at a time, self-administered or otherwise.

- Pay close attention to your posture.

- Lie down for at least five minutes a few times a day, if at all possible. If you can, put a cool pack on your neck.

- Use positive imagery and visualization at some time during the day (see chapter 20). Visualize yourself looking healthy, doing exercises effortlessly.

- Play soothing music while you are doing your home program.

- Make every reach a stretch and every movement an exercise.

- Take fifteen-to-twenty-minute warm baths, but be sure the water is not too hot. Try adding a half cup of Epsom salts and two tablespoons of ground ginger in the bath water. It is often remarkably soothing.

Making Progress

As you progress with various physical therapy methods, you will begin to observe changes in your body. Remember, change never comes easily. You might find that as you do bodywork, your pain level increases. This can be discouraging, because, after all, you are doing bodywork to improve the quality of your life. But bodywork often activates latent TrPs. This is one reason why it is vital that perpetuating factors be addressed. If bodywork activates a latent TrP, the next step is for bodywork to get rid of the TrP. Activation of the TrP, in this case, is one step in the process. But if you have something that perpetuates the TrP, all you will feel is worse. Your bodyworker—and your doctor—must understand that the *key* step in the healing process is identifying and addressing the perpetuating factors (see chapter 7).

You may also experience nausea, headaches, and even complete exhaustion after any bodywork has moved a large amount of toxins and wastes from constricted muscles. You may need to nap after a session. Your body is telling you something, so listen. *The bodywork is not what is causing you to feel awful.* Any trauma that you sustain throughout life causes your cells and tissues to accumulate substances in abnormal quantities.[9] Most commonly, such accumulations consist of molecules that are normally present, such as triglycerides, glycogen, calcium, uric acid, melanin, and bilirubin. As you experience bodywork, these substances are released. Be glad that you are getting them out of your system, but remember that your liver and kidneys can handle only so much at one time. Take it easy on yourself. Don't expect an overnight cure. Think of how many years it's taken to get your body into the state it's in today. It will take time and work. The results will be worth it.

Self-Massage

You may find that massaging of your own muscles hurts your hands and arms. Try using a light, soft stroke, just a feathery touch. This can be very effective in releasing tension in your face and head. Sometimes this even results in a light myofascial release of muscle tension. There are ways to support your hands and your fingers to prevent or minimize strain. I have often wished for a book that explained proper self-massage of myofascial TrPs and explained how to find each one. Claire Davies' *Trigger Point Therapy Workbook* fills that need (see Reading List). I believe it will help end a great deal of needless pain and prevent much unnecessary surgery. This book contains clear and simple diagrams and takes you step by step through all the TrPs, explaining how you can work each TrP yourself effectively and efficiently.

Eye Exercises

To check your inner eye muscles for TrPs, stretch them. Put one of your hands on top of your head. Then try to look at that hand. That will stretch your eye muscles upwards. This shouldn't hurt. If it does, remember that muscles with TrPs hurt at the end of their range of motion. These TrPs in the muscles that hold your eyeballs in place are telling you where they are. Trigger points in these muscles can add to eyestrain and headaches.

Next, with your eyes still looking upwards, move your eyes from one side to the other, as far as they will go. Then try moving your eyes in a circular motion, covering as much of your field of vision as you can. Trigger points are more likely to be noticed when you look up, because we don't look upwards often. If you have a lot of TrPs, this exercise can hurt a lot and can even cause a headache or make you dizzy. Your body is telling you to move your eye muscles more often. Be very gentle, but do this exercise once or twice a day. If you concentrate on close objects most of the time, take a little time to gaze at the distance for a short while. Switching your gaze in this manner uses different muscles.

Heat and Cold Therapy

You can use heat or cold to ease muscle tightness and lighten your pain load. These methods of pain relief are based upon the Gate Theory,[10] which states that pain impulses can be prevented from reaching the higher levels of the brain by stimulating the larger nerves, in this case, with heat or cold. Use these types of therapy as you would all others, with caution.

Myofascial muscle pain with nerve entrapment often responds unfavorably to heat. Heat increases circulation, adding more fluids to the area and causing the aggravated nerve to complain even more. If there is no nerve entrapment, heat relaxes the muscles and decreases the pain. It also may increase flexibility. Sometimes deep heat can trigger rebound pain and malaise. Staying too long in a hot bath or hot tub can cause extreme fatigue. If the tub is not too hot, and you limit your time in it to five to fifteen minutes, depending on your tolerance, you may find it relaxing. Find out what works for *you*.

If ice gives you pain relief, this may indicate that there is possible nerve entrapment. You may also be dealing with attachment TrPs, which seem to respond well to cold.[11] Ice massage is often helpful, but you must limit the surface area to be treated, and avoid icing the muscle beneath the myofascia. Go slowly, treating only one area at a time. Cold can be very helpful in easing the pain in the TrP referral zones. You also may find that cool gel packs help.

Warning: Running cold water on the hands can trigger cardiac arrhythmias in people with FMS. There is also the possibility of heat and/or cold intolerance.

Tennis Ball Acupressure

You can do tennis ball acupressure by yourself. You place the tennis ball between one of your TrPs and an immovable object, such as the floor, a wall, or the back of a chair. Then you lean into the ball, compressing the TrP. If, at first, you find tennis balls too hard and painful, try using smaller balls that are used as toys. Some of us have found that harder balls, like lacrosse balls, work better for some areas. It's best to start tennis ball acupressure by leaning against the back of a sofa for back TrPs, or lying down on a sofa for belly, back, leg, and arm TrPs. Compress the points gently, until you meet with resistance. Then hold it until the resistance releases. This may take a few minutes. Be patient.

Walls and floors are, of course, inflexible. A sofa or chair will give a little, so the acupressure will be gentler than if you used a floor or wall. Of course, it won't be as effective either, but it's a good start. The TrPs are painful to compress, but once you have flushed out some of the irritants, you may be able to graduate to a harder surface. Tennis ball acupressure is explained in greater detail in Clair Davies' book (see Reading List).

Tennis Ball Exercise

1. Start by lying on your back with your knees bent and your feet flat on the floor (or sofa). Your knees should be separated by about the width of your hips.

2. Raise your hips slightly and slide a tennis ball under one of them.

3. Come back down and rest on the ball. You can roll it around somewhat, once the pain eases.

Both sides of your body should be treated, and the sides of your hips and front, especially where your legs join your trunk. This means that you will be rolling over on your side or stomach, with the tennis ball between you and the floor or sofa. This treatment on the belly is especially helpful for women who have bloating or pelvic pain. It reduces congestion and frees fluid passages. It is wise to open pelvic constriction with tennis ball acupressure before your period. This helps open fluid passages and decrease bloating. If you lie on a rug with a soft ball or tennis ball under yourself and press gently, rolling up and down over these areas, paying special attention to the area around the pubic arch, you will find that there are TrPs that call out—not gently—for your attention. Go lightly, as they will hurt. Rolling on them will help to break up the myofascial constrictions. Don't neglect your upper abdominals. Try this once a day to help break up these TrPs. *This exercise is not for people who suspect appendicitis, diverticulitis, or other inflammatory abdominal conditions.* It may help relieve irritable bowel syndrome (IBS).

You can even use the tennis ball under your hamstrings when you must sit for a long time, as when traveling or at a meeting. This stretches the hamstrings. It hurts. Keep in mind that you are flushing out the toxins and irritating chemicals in the TrP. Don't leave the ball in one area for longer than longer than two or three minutes to avoid further constriction of blood flow.

Larger Balls

There is a soft ball I learned about from John Barnes' Myofascial Release Center. It is four inches in diameter, and is called the ALL-BALL™. It can be very helpful in applying a different sort of compression to TrPs and can be purchased through your bodyworker, physical therapist, or chiropractor. My chiropractor, Dr. Craig Anderson, introduced me to a large exercise ball and it has been a lifesaver. I used it as one of my chairs for writing this book. I need to be well-balanced to sit on it, so I am aware of my posture. I just wish it had armrests! If you bounce on it, with your legs to either side, you can stretch your pelvic floor muscles. This is the only healthy exception to the "no bouncing" rule that I know.

Formal Exercise Motion Programs

This section begins with exercises you can practice every day at home, but you must first learn them correctly in a formal class. Be careful when you choose an exercise program. It is unlikely that your teacher will be a specialist in chronic pain. Find a teacher willing to be educated about FMS and CMP, who will adapt the standard program to fit your particular needs and limits.

Chi Kung (Qigong)

Chi kung is more than exercise; it is a martial art, a type of bodywork, and a process for integrating the mind and body, with an internal component that must not be neglected. *Chi* translates as the vital life force that flows within and throughout the universe, and it is a difficult concept for Western minds to understand. Chi kung teaches the manipulation of chi and the focus of intention. You may have seen external forms of chi kung. There are many physical postures and movements that are part of chi kung techniques. Internal chi kung can be practiced without external movement. Healthy breathing is part of every process, but the key is always intention, coupled with the movement of the vital force in a steady flow.

Many of us who study both Eastern and Western medicine believe that the chi flows along the myofascia. Remember that myofascia is connected from right under the skin all the way through every part of your body, including the cellular matrix and the structure of the DNA.[12] It is important to keep these energy paths open and not constricted. Improving the flow of the chi reduces pain, removes blockages, enhances microcirculation, and promotes health.

One of the important functions of bodywork is to remove blockages to the flow of chi. Chi kung was developed comparatively recently as a warm up for t'ai chi chuan. It's an excellent exercise to do by and for yourself, but you need a teacher to explain what you are doing, why you are doing it, and how to do it well. Discuss your limitations with your teacher. Some days you may be able to do certain exercises, and other days you may be able to do only crane breathing, arm swinging, or other simple techniques. Some exercises may need to be modified for you. Standing exercises are not recommended for people with CMP because of the immobility required. Even the most physically limited person can practice some types of chi kung.

T'ai Chi Chuan

T'ai chi chuan is a martial art exercise, bodywork, and healing art, but again, it is so much more. In the United States, it is often taught in an incomplete way. T'ai chi, pronounced tie-gee, strengthens muscles and improves endurance, coordination, and balance.[13] It increases flexibility, improves posture, and promotes relaxation and the ability to focus. T'ai chi's physical aspects involve slow, fluid, circular motions in graceful sequences called forms. Some teachers use a more upright posture that I find to be easier on TrPs. Learning the martial arts aspects helps me to understand how I need to move, and what positions I need to find. T'ai chi forms may be frustrating for some people, because there are many movements to memorize, and people with FMS have difficulty with memory sequencing. I allowed this keep me away from t'ai chi instruction for a long time, although I did practice chi kung.

T'ai chi helps me to ward off stress. It develops myofascial suppleness and resiliency, as well as focusing intent. T'ai chi begins as an essay in body mechanics, and then develops into a braiding of mind/body poetry. As you learn t'ai chi chuan, you develop a steady and dependable connection to the flow of universal energy, chi. Master Wang[14] says t'ai chi uses the spine like a spoon, stirring and balancing the chi. Mind and body must move as a single unit, and this movement must originate deep inside, which is why it is so powerful. The movements also help you develop a sense of postural awareness. Once you are adept at awareness, you immediately know when you are in a strained position.

Training of coordination comes about by patterning. You repeat the pattern of performance so often that healthy muscle coordination becomes part of the mind/brain pattern.[15] Training is in the sequence of forms that exercise all the muscles. You repeat the sequences until they are no longer a part of your conscious thought, but occur as a flow. In t'ai chi chuan, a specific movement is often followed by the opposite of that movement. It is important to explain to your teacher that you cannot repeat one movement over and over, but you must learn several so that you can repeat the sequences. You must take care not to stress your muscles, especially if they have TrPs.

Be patient, and find a teacher who is patient. Patience is part of building chi. Explain that you have limited range of motion in many of your muscles. Studies show that long-term regular t'ai chi exercise has favorable effects on balance control, flexibility, and cardiovascular fitness in older adults.[16] There is no reason why it shouldn't do the same for you. I use the t'ai chi forms called *animal frolics* to help me cope in everyday life. These exercises use the motion of animals as a model, which is a common practice in chi kung and t'ai chi chuan. When I need determination and perseverance, my shoulders and my gait become *bear*. If I want to keep it light, I become *crane walking*. If I need agility and cunning, I become the *fox* with quick steps.

Some people become depressed if they can't "do" t'ai chi right away. But t'ai chi is a process that never ends. It is about change, and moving from one posture to another. With FMS and CMP, we don't do that well. At first, your movements may be restricted and choppy, and your balance uneven. You may have trouble shifting your weight from one foot to another. If such is the case, try to use the form as guided imagery. Focus on your intention to flow with the movement. Slowly, you will notice an improvement in your range of motion. As you become more aware of your body, you will feel where any weakness is. You will locate your restrictions. You will learn how to move all parts of your body in unison, as the myofascia lets go, and the chi flows freely and directs your motions. There are no time limits for learning. Patience is at the heart of the art of t'ai chi chuan.

Yoga

There are many forms of yoga. Kripalu yoga combines breath training, meditation, and movement. Prana yoga deals specifically with breath. Hatha yoga and other types of yoga often require sitting in extreme postures for varying lengths of time, or putting pressure and strain on joints and muscles. Before you begin a yoga program, talk to your bodyworker and prospective yoga instructor about which form would be most suitable. I have been to many instructors over time, and all of them assured me that I could do some simple movements and it would be good to stretch my body this way. All of them were wrong. I spent a lot of painful time recovering, with a lot of rebound muscle shortening to show for my efforts. Be cautious.

Bodywork Done by Others

This section starts with some of the traditionally "gentler" methods of bodywork, but this can be misleading. Individual therapists vary. Individual responses to specific therapies vary. Furthermore, there is considerable overlap among some of these methods.

In any bodywork therapy done by others, postural training is one of the first procedures. Your posture must be evaluated while you are walking, sitting, and lying down in addition to your standing posture. A proper evaluation must include your sense of balance, which can be seriously disrupted by TrPs. Your evaluator must understand that TrPs cause pain at the end of the range of motion, and can be responsible for the loss of the normal curves in your neck and low back.

Your bodyworker must also understand that you can tolerate much less mechanical force applied to your body than is customary for patients who do not have FMS. Studies show that for the typical FMS client, posttreatment discomfort can be avoided by maintaining the discomfort level during treatment somewhere between 1 and 5 in a scale of 10.[17] *All forms of bodywork must be limited by what you can tolerate.* If you experience immediate or delayed aftereffects, such as feeling faint, a dramatic increase in pain or other symptoms, weakness, or tremors and sweating, you need to talk with your therapist and doctor *immediately.* If you have a good medical team, they will welcome your feedback.

The length of therapy sessions must be tailored to your tolerance, and sessions need to be carefully spaced to allow for recovery between them. Return home immediately after therapy sessions and take it easy for the rest of the day. If you have severe FMS and CMP, you may need to limit your sessions to once a week or fewer. Only as your tolerance improves and the wastes and toxins are cleared from your system can bodywork increase in length and frequency. Don't allow your bodyworker to talk you into "toughing it out." Some discomfort may be necessary, but abide by the guidelines discussed earlier in this chapter. If your bodyworker doesn't listen, find a new bodyworker.

You may need stronger medication to permit some bodywork while minimizing pain sensations. In my experience, no matter how great the tolerance for pain, and how well you learn to "relax into" the therapy, sufficient pain can produce shock symptoms. If that should occur, it becomes necessary to reduce stimuli *immediately* with lowered lights, quiet, and time allowed for your central nervous system to recover. Don't do anything to aggravate your already hypersensitized nervous system. *Never underestimate the possible effects of FMS allodynia (the condition in which an ordinarily painless stimulus, once perceived, is experienced as being painful) and hypersensitivity on myofascial TrPs and TrP therapies.*

In our experience, some of the most gentle myofascial and craniosacral releases can have profound effects on patients with both of these conditions. These effects may be delayed. You can be remarkably sensitive to what is happening within you, and be a valuable source of insight for the therapist. *Effective and well-tolerated therapy requires the therapist to have both training and experience, coupled with a willingness to learn from and be guided by the patient. Inappropriate bodywork is a totally preventable perpetuating factor.*

Physical Therapy

There are many physical therapists (and doctors) who are not trained to work with TrPs. Many of these care providers make things worse by trying to exercise and strengthen muscles with TrPs. If your muscles are weak, your doctor or bodyworker must determine *why* they are weak, and not immediately start you on a strengthening program.[18] Here is a story about Janet Travell that illustrates this issue. The story was told to me by Tasso Spanos, the founder of the Academy for Myofascial Trigger Point Therapy in Pittsburgh, Pennsylvania.

> I saw her at her last public presentation. There were about 400 people who came, and about 100 of them were physical therapists. I had seen her presentation before, in fact, I had seen it seven times and rarely had I ever seen a physical therapist present. There were always many myotherapists, but rarely physical therapists. But at her last presentation about 100 physical therapists showed up. After three days with Travell they asked her this question: "You've been talking about stretching, stretching, and stretching, and when should we do the work hardening or the strengthening exercise?" She replied, "The patient has to be out of pain for two weeks *and have a normal range of motion or close to a normal range of motion for two weeks.*"
>
> She said that after those two weeks, you can proceed with very light strengthening. Well, five minutes later, a hand came up and someone asked her the same question. Then a couple minutes later someone else asked her the same question. After answering the same question several times, each time phrased differently, Travell stopped it by saying, "Ah, you know, I'm getting old, but I didn't know I was getting deaf!" When she said that, they didn't ask her that question anymore. One of my graduate students turned to me and asked, "Why are all these people asking the same question over and over? Don't they get it?" I told her, "It's not that they don't get it. They just don't like the answer!" When the body is injured, you cannot subject it to a load. In this country, it is against the law to run an injured racehorse. Yet that's what too many physical therapists do. If you can't lift your arm, you practice lifting your arm with weights and repetitions. If you can't turn around, you have to turn around with weights and repetitions. That's wrong. That's what Janet Travell was trying to say. You cannot strengthen a muscle that has a trigger point. You have to get rid of the trigger point first.

Weight Training

Weight training is *not* appropriate if you have active myofascial TrPs. Stretch bands and Nautilus-type equipment also belong on the list of "Things to Avoid," until your TrPs are gone. Softening your muscles without treating your myofascia doesn't work, either. If the myofascia is tight, the muscles have no place to go. They will remain squeezed by tightened myofascia. If your bodyworker is trying to work a TrP, and just focuses on one lump in the muscle, that won't work, either. The bodyworker needs to examine functional muscle groups, and check the fascia for other restrictions. All myofascia is connected.

Don't look to any bodyworker to "fix" you. Make sure your focus is on returning function, i.e., restoring your capability to engage in meaningful interactions with the world. Your therapy is about *you*. You have hired the therapist to help you during this time. If the therapist constantly talks about his or her problems during your therapy, or is frequently distracted from the task at hand by phone calls or unrelated conversation, or even if background music disturbs you, let her/him know that this is inappropriate. Let your therapist know what *you* need. For example, if you can't sleep because of pain, or are unable to sit for long periods and you need to attend meetings. In that way, your most pressing needs can be addressed first. Also, your therapist should always explain what s/he is going to do during a particular session and why.

Reiki

Reiki is one of many types of energy work. The Japanese term *ki* is roughly equivalent to the Chinese *chi*. Reiki is founded on the premise that ki (universal life force) energy is everywhere and can be focused, channeled, and applied to others, promoting harmony, balance, and healing. A reiki master can rebalance the universal life force within a patient by the laying on of hands, but requirements for achieving this stage are not the equivalent to the expertise of a chi kung master. There are many types of energy work. Find the one that works for you.

Movement Therapies

All of the following types of bodywork employ movement as a therapeutic tool. Naturally, the movements vary between the different disciplines, but each discipline is based on a belief in the curative powers of movement.

The Alexander Technique

The Alexander Technique focuses on correcting body mechanics. It improves your posture and movement, thus relieving tensions. During Alexander training, your thought processes and body movements are retrained. You learn to move with greater ease, balance and grace, and to avoid perpetuating factors that can lead to tense muscles and TrPs. It is an exceedingly gentle method. Alexander Technique practitioners have a teacher/student relationship with their clients. Lessons usually run from half an hour to a full hour, once a week, for a minimum of fifteen weeks.

Trager Therapy

Trager is a form of psychophysical integration. Trager bodyworkers use light, gentle motions to release deep-seated physical and mental patterns caused by poor posture, injuries, emotional traumas, poor movement habits, and stress. Trager employs both table work (the patient lies on a massage table), which includes rocking motion and traction, and Mentastics exercises. These dancelike movements are a form of playful mindfulness in motion. These two modes work together for lasting neuromuscular reeducation, integration, and effortlessness.

Feldenkrais

Feldenkrais is an educational movement training technique that enhances the communication between your body and brain. It uses movement and structural training. The movements are slow and gentle, and the focus is on correcting posture alignments. The practitioner verbally guides you through sequences of movement, retraining, or repatterning, your body and brain. This corrects bad posture habits, develops awareness of positioning, and establishes correct patterns by means of one-on-one learning.

Hellerwork

Hellerwork is movement retraining which focuses on the integration of the body, mind, and spirit. Hellerwork restores your natural balance, working from the inside by the systemic release of connective tissue. Movement education is part of the training process.

Proprioceptor Neuromuscular Facilitation (PNF)

Proprioceptors are sensory receptors that inform you about how your body is moving in relation to its environment. They tell the brain which muscles are contracting, and which ones are relaxed. With FMS or CMP, these proprioceptors are often dysfunctional, and neural information often becomes garbled. Proprioceptor neuromuscular facilitation (PNF) retrains proprioceptors. The therapist puts the patient in a comfortable position and then has the patient try to push out of that position. Each time this exercise is repeated, the troublesome muscle stretches a little farther.

An individual muscle is not solely responsible for a single-motion component of a pattern, but it works with related muscles and augments them.[19] The patterns of motion for PNF are large movement patterns, both spiral and diagonal in character, and similar to the movements you use every day. This is another form of repatterning, training several functional muscle groups in coordination rather than individual muscles.

Other Massage and Touch Techniques

There are many forms of massage and related therapies, and books have been written about most of them. Massage can be a relaxing, powerful, healing tool, but it must be respected and carefully managed. The wrong kind of massage, too vigorous a massage, or too short a time between massages can be detrimental to healing. The type and duration of massage must be decided on a person-to-person basis. Remember, *you* must be in control of your own healing path.

After a massage, plan to take it easy for a while. You may be sore the day after, especially if you have a lot of TrPs, but this soreness should disappear by the following day. If it doesn't, tell your massage therapist to take things a little easier the next time. Your body needs time to adjust. Some types of deep muscle massage may be beyond your endurance, and may worsen your symptoms by triggering rebound contraction. Massage and ultrasound therapy might result in degranulation of mast cells, which will release histamine and heparin.[20] This may be part of the reason that patients with both FMS and CMP sometimes bruise easily, and may develop histamine reactions to some forms of fascial bodywork.

Swedish Massage

Swedish massage, which comes in several different styles, is often undervalued. I found it to be gentle but deep enough to be a helpful integrator of other bodywork, but I am fortunate in having a massage therapist who knows TrPs and can help to uncover trouble spots. Her work seemed to soothe my autonomic nervous system. Massage tends to normalize muscle tension.[21] Studies show that with repeated massage, there is a parallel reduction in muscle tension and pain.[22] We must make insurance companies and medical personnel aware of these findings.

Vodder Manual Lymphatic Drainage

This massage technique opens the lymphatic ducts, removing blockages. This reduces tightness and swelling and stimulates lymphatic immune components. It is the optimum treatment for generalized swelling.[23] For more information on this therapy, see chapter 5.

Reflexology

The premise underlying reflexology is that there are areas of the feet and hands that correspond to areas of the body, including the organ systems. These areas of the feet and hands are treated with pressure point therapy to stimulate healing in the corresponding areas of the body.

Craniosacral Release (CSR)

Your craniosacral system is composed of the brain, spinal cord, the dural tube that surrounds the spinal cord, cerebrospinal fluid, a membrane system that separates the brain from the skull, the cranial bones, and the sacrum. The sacrum is a group of five fused vertebrae at the base of the spinal column, right above the tailbone. The fluid in this system moves with a rhythm all its own. The rhythm of patients with chronic pain conditions is often low and fast. CSR can normalize these rhythms.[24]

Crainosacral therapy is based on the premise that the brain expands and contracts with a very gentle pumping that circulates cerebrospinal fluid throughout the brain and spine. This gentle bodywork releases tensions and blocks that have developed in the craniosacral system. Some people with FMS and CMP may be electromagnetically sensitive (see chapter 8). I have observed that when the CSR practitioner is also electromagnetically sensitive, even if the practitioner's hands move the patient's skin only fractions of an inch, it can seem to the patient as though the whole of her or his body is moving. That's because the entire myofascia is adjusting. Often, emotional releases accompany physical releases.

Bowen Therapy

Bowen therapy is a very gentle, noninvasive form of bodywork that doesn't require a long series of treatments. Some therapists who use Bowen therapy treat people only once a week for a month and then once a month for six months. It uses a light, specific touch with a rolling motion on an out-of-alignment muscle. That touch signals the nerves beneath to signal the brain to move the muscle back to where it belongs, like a reset button. In Bowen therapy, some of the areas that are worked on are TrP locations, and some are acupressure meridians. Note that it often takes five to ten days for the muscles to respond after a treatment (see Resources).

Acupressure

Acupressure is the pressing of specific points on the body in order to relieve pain and stress in another part of the body. Although shiatsu often is assumed to be the same as acupressure, it is not. Acupressure uses firm fingers or acupressure implements to exert pressure for a few minutes on an acupoint. These acupoints are found on meridians, invisible channels through which chi flows, that were mapped by Chinese practitioners many hundreds of years ago.

Bonnie Prudden Myotherapy

Bonnie Prudden therapists use the pressure of fingers, knuckles, and elbows on TrPs. They then use passive stretch and special exercises designed for individual patients to enable them to return to function. Every patient must be referred by a physician. Patients are encouraged to bring a helper to help map their TrPs, and learn to work on them (see Resources). Do warn your therapist if you have the hypersensitivity and allodynia of FMS, as well as TrPs. I visited a Prudden-trained therapist in Alaska, and she was very skilled and gentle.

Barrier Release

The second edition of the Travell and Simons' *Trigger Point Manual* advocates for the use of the Barrier Release Method. Treatment focuses on releasing the contractured sarcomeres of contraction knots in the TrP. The *sarcomere* is the basic contraction unit of the muscle. The Barrier Release concept is more "patient-friendly" than old-style "Ischemic compression," and has less chance of sensitizing the nervous system by causing pain, but it requires a high order of skill. The muscle is lengthened to the point of increasing resistance within the comfort zone. Then, the bodyworker gently applies gradually increasing pressure on the TrP until s/he encounters a barrier of increased tissue resistance. This pressure is maintained, but not increased until the barrier releases. The bodyworker then increases pressure enough to encounter the next barrier. This should cause discomfort but not pain. This process must be repeated for each contracted band in a muscle. This therapy may fail if the bodyworker uses too much pressure, if the TrP is too irritable, or if perpetuating factors are present.

Muscle Balance and Function

The Muscle Balance and Function (MBF)® system is a unique method of restoring postural alignment and increased function through a progression of properly sequenced, individualized motions/exercises that retrain the body's neuromuscular system. Most people in chronic pain have postures that are out of normal alignment. These postures lead to excessive muscular imbalance, tension, and fatigue. This can be resolved by retraining your body's neuromuscular system. The MBF system of motions/exercises targets repatterning response levels at the midbrain and spine. This system leads the body to overall restoration, improvement in postural alignment, and reduction of stress/tension in the body. Everyone with FMS and/or CMP can participate. Each person begins from her/his own level of ability and individualized needs and concerns. Eduardo Barrera supplied the MBF™ information for this section (see Resources).

Myofascial Release

John Barnes has developed ways to release tightened and restricted myofascia and return ground substance to its fluid consistency. I have been fortunate enough to visit both his Sedona, Arizona and Paoli, Pennsylvania centers. Both visits were times of learning and recovery. Myofascial restrictions increase pressure on the entire fascial system and on blood vessels that supply the myofascia. As we move through life, the gauzy web of the myofascia turns and twists. Trauma tightens and glues our myofascia in place, and we require unwinding. Scar tissue can create extensive imbalance, affecting the whole craniosacral system. No scar should go unreleased. Even the smallest scar may be just the tip of an iceberg of fascial dysfunction.

John Barnes has found that 90 percent of the people he sees have a twist in their pelvic alignment. The pelvis is the foundation of the body structure, and if it is tipped and/or twisted, the whole body is affected. The fascia becomes torqued around the pelvic floor, creating a twisted crushing tightness around the internal structures, twisting the spinal column in *rotoscoliosis*. Barrier release is an important part of myofascial release therapy. It may take three to five minutes, or even longer, for each barrier to release, and this cannot be rushed.

You may experience a strong emotional release along with a myofascial release. Your body can hold information below the conscious level, as a protective mechanism. Myofascial unwinding allows your memories, associated emotional states, and belief systems to rise to consciousness as your myofascia returns to health. Your body tries to protect you against the pain, keeping you away from positions that are painful or traumatic. Each layer must be released, starting with the most superficial restrictions in the myofascia.

Trigger Point Myotherapy

In the science fiction book I wrote, I created a world where everyone knows what to do for FMS and CMP. That's the way I felt when I spent a few days at the Academy for Myofascial Trigger Point Therapy in Pittsburgh, Pennsylvania. One of the best things you can do for yourself would be to persuade one of the graduates of this school to practice in your locality. That's what I did. The problem is that there aren't enough graduates to go around.

These graduates know how to palpate and treat TrPs. Bodyworkers need extensive, specific training to learn how to palpate a taut band, so that they can locate a TrP. No weekend course can do this. It requires both training and practice to become proficient.[25] This training is available at the academy. Students often have extensive training in physical therapy or massage therapy *before* they begin. I urge bodyworkers to look into this training (see Resources). Classes are small, and the training is intense, emphasizing hands-on training as well as class work. Graduates are entitled to sit for the national certification examination for myofascial trigger point therapy. Many methods of TrP release are taught, including Spray and Stretch.

Spray and Stretch

Spray and Stretch is a form of physical therapy that may be used in conjunction with other therapies, or it can be used alone. In some cases it may provide dramatic and instantaneous relief, avoiding unnecessary expenditures of time and medical costs. In Spray and Stretch therapy, after your myotherapist takes a detailed history and performs an examination to locate your specific TrPs, you are properly positioned for the muscle function group to be treated. The therapist then sprays a vapocoolant in very precise patterns and directions, interspersing the sprays with gentle passive stretching that will increase your range of motion. The cooling of the spray inhibits your muscle-tensing reflexes.

The movement of the spray, the timing of the spray, and the stretching of the muscle are critical to the release of contracted muscle tissue. The spray must be held at the correct angle and distance to achieve the desired effect. The stretching is integrated with the spraying, gradually increasing the stretches, and must be done in a specific manner. The referred pain patterns must be sprayed as well.

After the muscle has been released, it must be rewarmed and taken through three slow, passive, full range of motion stretches. The spray must be done in the proper direction, which changes with the pain referral pattern and the direction of the muscle fibers. The degree of stretch should not be painful. You must reach the full normal range of stretch to inactivate the trigger point. Immediately after treatment, you should return home and stretch gently, and take a hot soak as soon as possible. The change may be accompanied by some soreness, but usually not to the extent of other TrP-release techniques. Note that, like other treatments, Spray and Stretch requires careful training to get effective results.

Too many people have told me, "I've tried Spray and Stretch therapy, and it doesn't work." Too many therapists say the same. But vapocoolant spray has a long and well-proven track record when it comes to dramatic TrP pain relief, even after years of chronic pain.[26] It can even relieve some of the pain from angina and myocardial infarction.[27] *But it must be applied correctly.* For example, for the paraspinals, although the spray is in the direction of the referred pain pattern, you must take a deep breath, hump your back, and then flex and rotate toward the side being treated as the therapist sprays in the designated pattern. You still must pay attention to perpetuating factors.

The complexity of this treatment becomes evident when you consider that there are six Spray and Stretch tapes with Janet Travell, each dealing with small areas of the body, and the lower arms and lower legs are not included in these tapes. If there is a failure with Spray and Stretch treatment, suspect perpetuating factors, inadequate spray coverage, too much tension in your muscles, poor spray technique, incomplete Spray and Stretch, inadequate stretch, incomplete stretch, or poor posttreatment (including the failure to rewarm the muscle).

There are two vapocoolant sprays available in jet spray safety-coated bottles. They are ethyl chloride and Fluori-Methane. Of the two sprays, I prefer the use of ethyl chloride over Fluori-Methane due to environmental concerns, although Gebauer is working on another product that is environmentally friendly. Each spray is available in 3.5 fluid oz. bottles, and should be used with the fine nozzle tip. The sprays are prescription medications. The protocol for this therapy is explained in depth in *Myofascial Pain and Dysfunction: The Trigger Point Manuals*, as well as Janet Travell's "Spray and Stretch" videotape series. Janet Travell used Spray and Stretch as her preferred method of TrP-release, saving TrP injection for those TrPs resistant to other methods of therapy.[28]

Ethyl chloride is flammable, and you must avoid inhaling the vapors. It is possible that with adequate training, responsible patients can learn how to do *some* remedial Spray and Stretch on *some* areas, enough for temporary relief to get them through an acute pain episode until they can see their therapist. This is much healthier, more cost-effective, and patient-friendly symptom relief than a trip to the emergency room, and it has the added bonus of restoring at least some function. Doctors must become aware of this pain-relief option for myofascial TrPs. I have heard of many instances where patients and even myotherapists were denied the use of this spray.

Rolfing

Rolfing used to be too vigorous for FMS-sensitized patients. But I recently learned from my t'ai chi brother, Dameron Midgette, that this is no longer the case. Dameron is a Certified Advanced Rolfer, and he wrote the following for this edition:

Rolfing™ can ease some of the immediate and painful symptoms of FMS, but I believe its strengths lie in a respectful and patient focus on the efficiency of the body as a whole: freeing up reserves of energy, resolving stressful structural problems, and increasing ease and efficiency. Decreasing stress and increasing reserves of energy can have far-reaching benefits. We also explore patterns and habits of physical structure, coping, and relating to stress and the environment, giving the client the information necessary to take an active, empowered role in the process of healing. Spend the time to find a practitioner with whom you are comfortable. Good communication is a very important part of positive outcomes.

For information, contact the Rolf Institute at 1-800-530-8875 or contact Dameron directly at Body Knowledge, Inc., 167 Park Row, Suite 2, Brunswick, ME 04011, 207-373-1236.

Strain-Counterstrain

Strain-counterstrain is a form of physical manipulation to relieve the pain caused by tense muscles. After finding a TrP, the bodyworker moves you into a position where the pain is relieved. You then push against the bodyworker's hand in the direction of the painful position. Then you relax, and are moved slightly closer to the painful position, and the procedure is repeated, until the TrP is released.

Shiatsu

Shiatsu mobilizes your energy systems. It helps circulation, breathing, the nervous system, and the immune system. Shiatsu is not the same as acupressure. If you are fortunate, you will find a certified shiatsu therapist who also knows TrPs. I turned to one of my friends, Andrew Waldie, CST, who is such a therapist, for the following description:

Shiatsu therapy (literally translated as "finger pressure") is a form of manual bodywork originating in Japan early in the twentieth century. During a treatment typically lasting close to an hour, the therapist will apply comfortable pressure with her/his thumbs perpendicular to the soft tissue. At times, the palm, forearm, or elbow can be used as well, depending upon the area of the client's body being addressed. The local response is relaxation of the muscle and an associated increase in range of motion. Should the tissue house a TrP, autonomic nervous system changes may also occur. For instance, in the case of tension headaches in the temple caused by vasoconstriction within the pain reference zone of the upper trapezius, these may be eliminated with effective treatment. Combined with appropriate stretching and attention to perpetuating factors, treatments can help alleviate musculoskeletal conditions related to hypercontracted muscles.

Those readers wishing to contact Andrew for more information can reach him at The Pacific Wellness Institute, 80 Bloor Street W., Suite 1100, Toronto, ON M5S, @V1, Canada or at thewaldies@idirect.com

When you begin any form of bodywork, don't expect an overnight cure. Think of how many years it's taken to get your body into the state it's in today. Be gentle with yourself, and give your body and mind a chance to recover. Choosing the right form of bodywork for youself, and the right type of exercise, is crucial to feeling better. Recent research shows that exercise that is too intense can start a neuroendocrine stress response.[29] This indicates to me that an exercise program that is too intense could trigger FMS in susceptible individuals, or worsen existing FMS. Find one or more forms of therapy that work for you.

Endnotes

1. Boyum, A., P. Wiik, E. Gustavsson, O. P. Veiby, J. Reseland, A. H. Haugen, et al. 1996. The effect of strenuous exercise, calorie deficiency and sleep deprivation on white blood cells, plasma immunoglobulins and cytokines. *Scand J Immunol* 43(2):228-235.

2. Simons, D., J. Travell, and L. S. Simons. 1999. *Travell and Simons' Myofascial Pain and Dysfunction: The Trigger Point Manual.* Second edition. Baltimore: Williams and Wilkins, p. 109.

3. Kottke, F. J. 1980. From reflex to skill: the training of coordination. *Arch Phys Med Rehabil* 61(12):551-561.

4. Simons, Travell, and Simons. 1999. *Op. cit.*, p. 171.

5. *Ibid.*

6. *Ibid.*, p. 22.

7. *Ibid.*, p. 81.

8. Juhan, D. 1987. *Job's Body*. Barrytown, New York: Station Hill Press.

9. Leahy, M., and L. E. Mock III. 1992. Myofascial release technique and mechanical compromise of peripheral nerves of the upper extremity. *Chiro Sports Med* 6(4):139-140.

10. Melzack, R., and P. D. Wall. 1965. Pain Mechanisms: a new theory. *Science* 150:971-979.

11. Simons, Travel, and Simons. 1999. *Op cit.*

12. Finando, D. L., and S. Finando. 1999. *Informed Touch: A Clinician's Guide to the Evaluation and Treatment of Myofascial Disorders*. Rochester, VT: Healing Arts Press.

13. Lan, C. J., S. Lai, S. Y. Chen, and M. K. Wong. 2000. T'ai Chi Chuan to improve muscular strength and endurance in elderly individuals: a pilot study. *Arch Phys Med Rehabil* 81(5):604-607.

14. Yu, G. 2000. Creating power with Yi and Qi. *T'ai Chi* 24(4):10-17. [Translated from interview with Wang, Hao Da.]

15. Kottke, F., J. D. Halpern, J. K. Easton, A. T. Ozel, and C. A. Burrill. 1978. The training of coordination. *Arch Phys Med Rehabil* 59(12):567-572.

16. Hong, Y., J. X. Li, and P. D. Robinson. 2000. Balance control, flexibility, and cardiorespiratory fitness among older T'ai Chi practitioners. *Br J Sports Med* 34(1):29-34.

17. Lowe, J. C., and G. Honeyman-Lowe. 1998. Facilitating the decrease in fibromyalgic pain during metabolic rehabilitation: an essential role for soft tissue therapies. *J Bodywork & Movement Ther* 2(4):208-217.

18. Simons, Travell, and Simons. 1999. *Op cit.*, p. 114.

19. Voss, D. E., M. K. Ionta, and B. J. Myers. 1985. *Proprioceptive Neuromuscular Facilitation*. Third edition. New York: Harper and Row.

20. Awad, E. A. 1973. Interstitial myofibrositis: hypothesis of the mechanism. *Arch Phys Med Rehabil* 54(10):449-453.

21. Danneskiold-Samsoe, B., E. Christiansen, B. Lund, and R. B. Andersen. 1982. Regional muscle tension and pain ("fibrositis"). *Scand J Rehab Med* 15:17-20.

22. Danneskiold-Samsoe, B., E. Christiansen, and R. B. Andersen. 1986. Myofascial pain and the role of myoglobin. *Scand J Rheumatol* 15:174-178.

23. Herpertz, U. 1989. Idiopathic edema in the female. *Z Lymphol* 13(2):65-70. [German]

24. Upledger, J. E. 1983. *CranioSacral Therapy*. Upledger Institute, 11211 Prosperity Farms Road, Palm Beach Gardens, FL 33401-4449.

25. Simons, D. G. 1993. Examining for myofascial trigger points. *Arch Phys Med Rehabil* 74:676.

26. Modell, W., J. Travell, J. Kraus, et al. 1952. Relief of pain by ethyl chloride spray. *NY State Med* 52:1550-1558.

27. Travell, J. G. 1952. Ethyl chloride spray for painful muscle spasm. *Arch Phys Med* May:291-298.

28. Lowe, J. C. 1993. The master of myofascial therapy. *ACA J Chiropractic* (Nov.).

29. Clark, S. R., K. D. Jones, C. S. Burckhardt, and R. Bennett. 2001. Exercise for patients with fibromyalgia: risks versus benefits. *Curr Rheumatol Rep* 3(2):135-140.

CHAPTER 20

Mindwork

The emotional reaction to the diagnosis of chronic illness can be a greater challenge than coping with the physical symptoms.[1] The stresses of chronic illness take you and your loved ones through a grief process. You are forced to assess your support mechanisms, and often find that they need a lot of construction work at a time when you can least afford to don a hard hat. You find out just how resilient you are and how well you adjust to change. If you are a caregiver as well as a patient, coping with your responsibilities in addition to the enormity of adjusting to these changes can leave you feeling like a dry leaf in the wind. Mindwork can supply some of the balance you require. Mind-body intervention and meditation are also a helpful part of fibromyalgia (FMS) symptom relief.[2]

One reader wrote to me that "Finding a sense of wholeness in the midst of a process that leaves you fragmented is mighty hard." This is not something we talk about very much. She asked how I wrestled with that transition. Well, I'm still wrestling. In this chapter, I will talk about that process and I will describe some of the tools I use to build coherence out of chaos.

You've already read about some physical ways to take the edge off your symptoms (see chapter 19). Mindwork can help achieve the same effects. There is an old Chinese proverb that says, "The best way to catch a fish is to have many lines." Some of these techniques may not be for you, and that's okay. Others may be just what you need. There are always options. You may have been taught that the autonomic system's responses of your body are beyond your control. It's time to unlearn that. If you need to slow and deepen your breathing, and to teach your gastrointestinal tract how to behave better, take heart. Many of the body's processes once thought to be completely automatic can be modified by mindwork. Meditation, for example, can give you the capacity to selectively disengage from arousal sensations.[3] You *can* learn to adjust your body's response to stress.

Studies have shown that people with FMS have personalities no different than those with any other chronic pain conditions.[4] Fibromyalgia does tend to amplify sensitivity and, of course, this has ramifications. Many of us were high-energy people before FMS struck. Some of us still are. We need to learn to live with this intensity, and also to take a break from it now and then. Your spirit may still be willing, but your body may need your spirit tempered a little, so that it can catch up. People with FMS can learn to use their hypersensitivity. Use your intuition. I am not advocating that patients with panic disorders and obsessions should listen to their "inner voices," but when you learn to trust healthy intuition, you can often get a lot of help in getting through life. God knows, we need it. It's my personal belief that God will provide it.

Candace Pert, in her book, *Molecules of Emotion*,[5] writes that the strings of a resting violin will resonate when another violin is played nearby. I believe that this may be the case with people who have FMS. We resonate with the emotions of others. It is a form of empathy and is neither good or bad in itself. We simply need to be aware of it, and its effects upon us. Master Paul Gallagher, one of my teachers, says that your resonance is a vital part of your self, connected with chi and electromagnetic force. Everything and everyone is interdependent. We can learn to control and balance our resonance. The primary way to do this, in Chinese terms, is this: Where there is yin create yang, where there is yang create yin. Balance and intention are the keys. This can mean changing a totally structured life to allow time for play and space, or adding self-discipline and order if your life is chaotic. We all need balance. Mindwork helps us to achieve this.

A Different View

In my science fiction novel,[6] planetary explorers are faced with many problems. They approach each one as a puzzle to be solved, rather than as an obstacle they must vanquish. I have observed that people with FMS are often very creative. Use that creativity. As long as you have faith in yourself, your options are open. When a "bad thing" happens, the universe hasn't failed you. Life doesn't always meet your expectations. Can you find logical reasons why the "bad thing" occurred, and prevent it from happening again? Try to do this without judgment. Life is unpredictable. It is made up of changes. If you look at life as a continual learning experience, you may find that obstacles that once loomed large may be smaller, or may even vanish.

Once there was a woman who almost fell into a hole situated directly in her path. She walked carefully around the hole, but she knew it was dangerous. There wasn't much space around the hole, and it was on her daily walk. She tried to fill it, but it was too deep, even when she got help. She and her new helpers tried to build a bridge, but nothing worked. By then, other people who traveled on that path were also looking for alternatives. One person found another path that was safe and pleasant, and it got her to her destination. She went back to the hole with her new friends to rope off the old path, and to put up a sign with the alternative route clearly marked. When you are trying to navigate a hard road, all you may need is a little help to find options.

Attention and Intention

Everyone knows what it feels like to pay attention. Attention focuses the whole of your being. It is an awareness *toward* something. Attention is an important aspect of all mindwork. I have some dear friends who are nuns in a monastery. Some of their prayers start with these words: "Be attentive." That is a profound way to begin any life experience: Be attentive. Life is amazing. We must *want* to know what is happening. We must be curious. Why are we so often not attentive? Why do we go through life on autopilot? What do we learn by being attentive? Perhaps, we learn how to live.

Intention is another quality often missing in our lives. Intention is at the heart of t'ai chi and chi kung. Intention is also at the heart of much mindwork, and the heart of life. Intention means to know what your goals are, and why. Know what you want to get out of what you do. Your goal can be simple and general. Develop a purpose, so every part of your body can get behind your intention and do what needs to be done to make it so. We all have physical restrictions and limitations, but they may become channels to new dimensions in our lives, especially to new spiritual dimensions. I'm not suggesting that we all become mystics, although that wouldn't necessarily be a bad thing. Intention provides the reason to move through life, and it can supply direction as well.

Mindfulness

If you're like most people, you go through much of your life automatically, not consciously aware of how you feel, or what is happening around you. Mindfulness means that with each passing moment you are fully aware of what is happening in the present. Rather than being anxious or worried about the future, or regretting the past, your energy is focused on right now: the sights, sounds, smells, feelings, and thoughts of the present moment. Mindfulness helps you to simplify your life and to enjoy more of it.

Now, stop reading, sit back in your chair, and focus on what is happening at this moment in time. Do this for several minutes. Do you feel relaxed? Are you anxious? What does that tell you about how comfortable you are in the present? Whenever your mind is scattered and you feel overwhelmed, take some time and focus your attention on one thing: a flower, a greeting card picture (you can save your favorites for this purpose), or a piece of art. Study the object intensely for five or ten minutes. When other thoughts intrude, send them on their way and return to studying the object you chose. You can set a timer to let you know when the time is up. For those five or ten minutes, you are practicing being mindful. Mindfulness is a way to enrich your life. It is also a form of meditation that gives you a greater understanding of what life is all about.

Sticks and Stones

Be careful how you use words. Words are powerful tools. Imagine, for a moment, what images these words bring to your mind: wimp, loser, hopeless, helpless, struggle. How do they make you feel? What about these words: joy, power, recovery, freedom, strength, and serenity. Which words do you want as part of your mental environment? Which words will you allow in your "life description"? Become aware of the words that surround you, and don't allow negative ones to creep in and take over.

For example, how often do you say "damn"? Is everything in your life one "damned" thing after another? Do "damned things" surround you? Who do you think has damned them? How often do you say "hell"? How much energy do you put into surrounding yourself with negative imagery? I have found that this form of self-destructive behavior seems to increase proportionally to the amount of pain I am experiencing, which is usually tied to my workload. I have been becoming better at focusing my *attention* on this, with the *intention* to change.

Clutter

Are you carrying unnecessary baggage that is not useful? Clutter, both physical and emotional, can be hazardous to your health. It is amazing how easily and quickly clutter can fill up every corner of your mind and life. Physical clutter can have damaging psychological repercussions, as well as causing you frustration when you try to find things. For example, if you try to hold on to every scrap of paper that comes your way, you may be holding on to a lot of psychological clutter as well. Sometimes mindwork takes some preliminary physical work to get started. Devoting a week or more to scooping up, throwing out, or burning all the unnecessary scraps you have accumulated may give you a great psychological uplift. You don't have to wait until springtime to clean out clutter.

It is the same when it comes to mind clutter. Are you carrying grudges or holding on to bad memories? Are pieces of the past stuck to your mind like rotting food scraps in the back of a refrigerator? When it comes to cleaning out unnecessary "stuff," we are in eternal spring. Give yourself permission to declutter. It may provide you with a feeling of renewal at any time of the year.

The "Little Death" of Chronic Pain

A diagnosis of FMS and/or chronic myofascial pain (CMP) often brings about what is called in hospice work a "little death." You've lost your old self, and you must deal with the same mental states that are common to those with terminal illness while you adjust to your condition and learn to evolve a new self. After diagnosis, you may experience the following stages:

1. Denial/isolation (I don't really have this! Go away, I don't want to talk about it!)

2. Anger (Why me?)

3. Bargaining (Maybe if I do xyz it will go away. . . .)

4. Depression (My life isn't worth much.)

5. Acceptance (Okay, I have this condition. Now let's see what I can do about it.)

When faced with a serious loss in life, it is normal to go through these stages as part of a natural grieving process. It is easy to get stuck in denial. That prevents healing. After the grieving is over, rather than dwelling on what's been lost, it's important to move on. Meditation can help you to move through the stages outlined above to a healthier acceptance.

What Is Meditation?

In the meditative state, breathing slows and deepens, and circulation improves. Meditation and other mindwork can increase blood flow to your muscles.[7] In fact, evidence is rapidly mounting that suggests your state of mind, as well as your diet, your environment, and your occupation can affect the state of your physical health profoundly.

Some people are uncomfortable with meditation, because it's not commonly a part of our Western world's traditions. It isn't difficult to learn, however, and it doesn't require grim training, odd positions, or physical and sensory deprivation. It doesn't even require a lot of time. Meditation offers a way to escape the burden of sensory overload that people with FMS frequently experience, and you need nothing more than an adventurous mind to do it properly.

There are many levels and types of meditation. The time just before falling asleep is a good time to meditate and reflect. At that time you are in a *hypnogogic state*, which is the transitional stage between waking and sleeping. In that stage, your conscious and subconscious minds interact differently than when you are fully awake. If you practice meditating at this time, don't worry if you fall asleep, that's okay.

The process of understanding yourself is a journey, and all journeys, no matter how long, begin with the first small step and then proceed one step at a time. For that reason, it is best to begin meditating with a simple form.

Your First Step

To begin a simple meditation practice, follow these steps:

1. First, find a place where you can be quiet, uninterrupted, and relaxed.

2. Find a comfortable position. It is easiest to start with a sitting meditation. You can sit on a chair if that is more comfortable, or cross-legged on the floor, tailor fashion. The important thing is to find a position that keeps your spine straight, and is stable, comfortable, and easy to maintain for whatever length of time you wish to meditate.

3. Let your body sway slightly from side to side, and then from back to front, until you find your point of balance. That point will feel right to you. This is finding your "root," or center. As you become more adept at meditation and at centering, you will find this point more easily.

4. Breathe in through your nose and out through your mouth. Close your eyes and observe your breathing. Make sure you are breathing from your belly, and that your belly is soft, and not guarded. When you inhale, your belly should swell with the incoming air. When you breathe in through your nose, your tongue should touch the roof of your mouth. Exhale through your mouth, expelling all of the air you took in on the inhalation.

5. Become aware of your body. How does it feel? Mentally scan your body. Don't visualize it, but try to sense it with your mind. Scan your whole body. Start with the top of your head and work your way down to the soles of your feet. Do any sensations cry out to you? If so, don't dwell on them, just observe them, and move on. When you have finished scanning your body, let your body know that things will be getting better. Ask it to let you know what you need. Assure it that you will listen. Treat yourself with gentle respect.

6. Now, let all thoughts leave your mind. At first, you probably will find this impossible. Thoughts will intrude. Just make note of them and let them pass. You are not concerned with them today. If blanking your mind is difficult, think of an affirmation you have chosen, or choose one now. Say it in your mind, not thinking about it, but just letting it rest there in your consciousness. If another thought comes in, note it and then go back to saying your affirmation to yourself.

You might try letting your mind drift for a while, going in and out with your breath, like a fish riding on the waves. Concentrate on your breath. As your thoughts arise, just note them and let them go. Don't follow them. Become a human being instead of a human doing. Practice being for a while. Like anything new, this may seem difficult at first, but it will become easier with time. When you have drifted for a while, bring your mind back to focus on your affirmation again. This type of meditation can be a mini-vacation from the stresses of your day.

Walking Meditation

A walking meditation is a good way to start if you have never meditated before. This walking meditation is an easy one, and not rigidly structured like Zen walking meditations. You make this one up as you do it. When times get tough, go for a walk. As you walk, think of a place that you would rather be. It can be a real place or an imaginary one, perhaps a world you've read about. Make it somewhere you've never been, and some place that would be comfortable. Then, think of what you'd need to bring from your *present* existence that would make that other world perfect.

It's true there are times when life seems bleak and unfriendly, but perhaps that's because you're looking at it through a gray filter of pain and frustration. It's time to clean away the cobwebs and let in the light. Try a walking meditation alone, or try doing one aloud with others.

Meditations on Life

Life is a great teacher. From time to time, you may forget that and become frustrated when your life isn't going the way you think it should. You may find it helpful to think over the event that seems so frustrating and try to figure out what you can learn from it. Use your intent to make it into a lesson. Here is an example of how to do that:

I discovered the walking meditation one day when I was in flare, feeling achy and confused. I was wandering around the woods on our hill, thinking about how miserable life was at the moment and trying to grasp what Heaven must be like, and suddenly I was in the middle of a meditation. That's how meditation works once you've been doing it for a while. It becomes a very positive force in your life and it is there whenever you need it. I was pretty tired of my existence here, and I was comfortable with the idea of Heaven. Then I decided that Heaven must have McCoun apples, though, because they taste so crisp and crunchy and refreshing; it just couldn't be Heaven without them. Just thinking about the way the apple fragrance blossomed when I bit into one brought a smile to my lips. Then I thought about bittersweet chocolate buttercreme truffles (yes, I know many of us shouldn't have chocolate!) and decided Heaven needed those, too. Heaven wouldn't be perfect without soft, purring cats, either. Then, I remembered

Berry picking: When I first began picking wild berries, I was determined to harvest every berry I saw. Yet the ripest, fattest, most luscious berries often fell off the branches before I could pick them. I saw this as a failure on my part. The very best berries seemed to go to waste, and I contributed directly to this by jiggling the branches in my efforts to reach them. Looking back, I see that the best berries became seeds for the future. Mother Nature is wiser than I am. Our berries get bigger, sweeter, and juicier over the years. We do not understand all things. Some things we view as losses or failures may contain the seeds of future joy.

Neal Clark is a resident naturalist at the Harris Center for Conservation Education in our part of the world. He kindly allowed the use of the following (slightly edited) life meditation from one of his newspaper columns.[8]

We have so much to be thankful for, and yet we think about it so infrequently. It's easy to take life's many miracles for granted. If sick, we can still give and receive love, read, write, create, sing and gaze out at the sun. And moon. And think about the hope of another tomorrow.

We should be thankful for clear skies, rainbows, for full moons, allowing us (some of us) to prowl under silver rays; for thunder and lightning that humble and jolt us into the present moment.

In winter, there's snow to ride, ice to glide, and freezing temperatures to keep the bugs down. Late winter offers maple sap running and the chance to enter a misty sugar shack during the boiling-down stage, the sweet aroma enveloping the entire room.

Besides black flies, springtime brings out waves of warblers and other high-flying birds. . . .

We should be thankful for long summer days of toil, sports, berry picking, and watching the Perseid meteor showers.

We can be grateful for autumn and its harvests, for cricket choruses, ripening grapes, brilliant foliage, and wild geese passing overhead.

I'm grateful for environmentalists, sportsmen, teachers, coaches, civil servants, artists, writers, musicians and even politicians. And I can't imagine life without books.

Parks, preserves, sanctuaries, nature centers and museums are all vital in saving what's left of our world and its heritage. Too many people are too far removed from how we got here and what's out there in the real (natural) world.

Let's thank God for this abused, battle-scarred planet that continues to hurtle through our vast yet insignificant solar system. I think there's ample time left to work, learn, and romp before the lights go out. I think there's still hope for our species. I say share the good times while we can. And ponder and vocalize how thankful we are simply to be alive.

Neal takes time to be attentive, and he has intention. Using Neal's meditation as a guide, think over the changes that happen during the months of the year in your part of the world, focusing on the gifts that life has given to you. Take the time to be thankful.

Guided Imagery

Guided imagery is a very effective kind of meditation that has been used successfully to deal with a variety of situations, such as enhancing the healing process, and increasing a general feeling of well-being. You can record this on tape and play it back, have a friend read it to you, or read it over many times until you become familiar with it. When you can't get away but need to, guided imagery provides an option.

> how I enjoy taking a walk in the night after a really cold snow, when snow crystals turn to glitter in the moonlight. By the time I finished my walk that day, I remembered that we all have it within ourselves to create a semblance of Heaven on earth.

A Walk in the Forest

Find a place where you will be undisturbed. Unplug the phone. Turn off the radio or television. Have someone else tend the children. Make yourself as comfortable as you can, either sitting in a comfortable chair or lying down. Loosen any restrictive clothing. Close your eyes. Take five or six deep breaths, releasing the air very slowly. Let your whole body relax completely. Notice any areas of tension and let them relax. You are going on a journey.

Visualize yourself on a glorious, cheerful morning. The sky is soft blue with white, fluffy clouds. You are dressed in comfortable, loose clothes that feel delightful against your skin. You're in a meadow, at the edge of the woods. There is a light backpack at your feet. It holds a tasty, nutritious lunch that has no calories. It also holds something special of yours that no one else knows about. Pick up the pack, and begin your journey.

Visualize and feel yourself ambling down a path bordering the wood. Lush ferns line your way. The forest smells green and inviting. The path takes you into the forest. It's pleasantly cool among the trees. Sunlight filters through the leafy canopy. Birds are singing in the trees. A light breeze blows through your hair. Your path is relatively flat, with only an occasional gentle rise. You walk along, at ease with yourself, breathing in the fragrance of the trees. The forest floor cushions every step. Your walk is steady and your balance, secure.

You come to a clearing and pause, looking over a wide meadow. It is filled with your favorite flowers. A line of trees stands in the meadow, and you can hear the sound of a fast-running brook just beyond them. Multicolored butterflies dance among the flowers, pausing briefly to drink of their nectar. You take the path through the meadow, stopping now and then to appreciate the sounds and smells. You feel light, oh so light.

Soon you approach the trees. You leave the path for a short distance, walking on the soft grasses. The trees are your friends, and they wave their branches gently in welcome. As you reach them, you notice that some of the trees have holes in their trunks, of different sizes. You reach out to touch the closest tree. The ridges of the bark massage your hand as you rub the trunk of the tree, and the tree sighs with pleasure at your touch.

You listen closely and can hear the faint voices of the trees singing softly. The tree voices offer to take your worries and troubles. They instruct you to place your burdens inside the trees' holes. There are large holes for great troubles and small ones for lesser worries. You might find that once you place a burden into a hole, the hole changes size. Maybe a problem bothers you more than you know. Or maybe what you thought was a large burden becomes a much smaller one. No matter. You're just letting the trees hold them for a while. Take some time to think of some of those private, special things you brought along with you. Leave what you wish, and continue on your way to the stream, feeling lighter, and relieved of your burdens.

The brook calls to you, and you sit on the soft grasses beside it, in the shade of a willow. Violets and emerald mosses edge the brook, and there is a little pool created by stones. The water is slower there and warmer, although it is pleasantly cooler than the air. Take off your shoes and dip your feet in the soothing waters of the pool. Feel any remaining tension in your body melt, carried away by the healing waters.

Take a deep breath. Breathe in gently through your nose, letting your belly swell with air. When you can breathe in no more, exhale slowly through your nose. Breathe all the stale air out, and then take in more of the fresh, healthy air. Turn your attention to your body. Mentally scan your body, noticing all the sensations. Observe how the feelings change from place to place, and vary in intensity. If you meet with discomfort, pain, or negative feelings, just observe them. Don't judge them or comment; just note their existence and continue your scanning.

Notice whether your body tries to keep your awareness from focusing on areas of pain and contraction. Is something holding on to the pain or tightness? Be aware of your natural tendency to linger at areas of pleasant sensations, and to skip the areas of pain and contraction. Examine that resistance. What does it feel like? Is there fear? Or anger? Is it dark? What keeps these areas separate? As your awareness encounters areas of discomfort, notice the tight places that are guarding the areas of pain. Gently, allow those tight places to melt like ice on a summer day. Breathe through the tightness, and when you exhale, notice the softening, the letting go. Allow the sensations to float, weightless. Enter the areas of discomfort, exposing the tender sensations inside. Accept them as part of you, and then move on.

When you have finished your scan, imagine all the other beings elsewhere in the universe experiencing these same kinds of discomfort. Don't take on their pain; just link to them and note the connection, and remember that you will never be alone, no matter what your trials. Acknowledge them, and embrace them for all that you share. Then embrace yourself as part of the others. Allow residual pain and discomfort to flow down to your feet, and then out of your feet. Let the pain and discomfort be carried away by the gentle stream. If some of it wants to travel upward, let it go. Float it on the breeze to the trees, and let the trees carry it away.

Hold on to your connection to others, but watch the pain drift away on the breeze. You are part of a vast family of beings, struggling to make the best of life, in spite of difficulties. Let your thoughts flow through the universe, brimming with compassion. You feel light, nearly weightless. Breathe deeply, and know that whenever you feel alone, you can come back to this healing brook.

Now, if you wish, you may savor the delicious food from your pack and drink from the pure, refreshing stream. Linger as long as you like. This is a safe place for you. If you wish, you may return to the trees and resume your burdens. Or you may decide to let the trees hold on to them. That's your choice. Just note the size of the holes containing each burden. What does that tell you? Perhaps you will decide to pick up a few of the burdens, or only one, and let the trees keep the others until you are ready to deal with them. You are in control.

When you are ready to come back from your trip, take another deep breath, and let it out slowly. Move your fingers and toes, and, if you wish, stretch. When you are ready, return to the room and open your eyes.

Focusing

Focusing is a simple, safe, free, noninvasive, yet powerful self-help technique. Using a series of well-defined questions or steps, it helps you focus on the *real* issue of most importance at any given time, not what may seem to be the real issue. The question sequence then connects you with the feelings generated by that issue. When you make the connection, you can achieve positive change.

Have a person you trust and with whom you feel safe slowly read the following instructions to you, giving you time between each step to follow the instructions in your mind and body. If no one is available, tape-record the instructions yourself, allowing time to perform the actions.

1. Do whatever is necessary to make yourself comfortable. Lie down or sit on a comfortable chair. Loosen any clothing that is tight or restrictive. Take several deep breaths and relax fully.

2. How are you feeling? What's between you and feeling fine? Don't answer in your mind: Allow what comes up in your body to do the answering. Several issues may arise. Greet each concern that comes to your mind. Put each aside in your memory, acknowledging but not addressing it. Except for these things, are you fine?

3. Review the list of concerns that stand between you and feeling fine. Which has the most effect on how you are feeling? Focus on that problem. What do you sense in your body when you think about all aspects of that problem? Where do you feel it in your body? What does it feel like?

4. What one word, phrase, or image describes and fits that feeling best? Take several minutes to find the one that feels right.

5. Go back and forth between the word or image and the feeling. Do they match? If they don't quite fit together, explore further until you arrive at the right word or image.

6. Ask yourself, what it is about the problem that is causing this feeling. If an answer doesn't come easily, ask yourself, what is the worst part of this feeling? What's so bad about this? What does it need? What should happen? Don't answer immediately; wait for the feeling to give you an answer. What would it feel like if it were all okay? What is in the way of feeling that it is all okay?

7. Feel the change that comes from having this new information. Welcome and feel the feelings and information that come. Be glad your body spoke. This is only one step in solving this problem. Now that you know where it is, leave it, and come back later. Don't analyze it or criticize it.

8. Ask your body if it wants more focusing, or is this a good stopping place?

> Focusing therapy was brought to my attention by friends in England. Based on their strong recommendation, I attended a focusing workshop. It was led by Dr. Neil Friedman, a student of Eugene Gendlin, the founder of this method, who teaches and writes on focusing.
>
> Once I had basic instruction in this technique, I began my own regular practice of focusing. Whenever things feel too busy, confused, or hectic, I find myself a comfortable space and go through the steps of a focusing exercise. It helps! Instead of feeling "so scattered," I get a sense of what is really bothering me.
>
> M.E.C.

Prayer

How can you cultivate an "attitude of gratitude" when you "hurt like hell"? When you can't sleep at night, where does your thankfulness lie? How can you turn around the negativity that may surround you? I frequently pray to know the way God wants me to live my life. I also remind God to be very clear and elaborate in the instruction, due to my FMS fibrofog. Sometimes, though, I still feel as if I'm getting mixed messages.

I am a very New Age Judeo-Christian mystic. I believe that all mainstream churches should have at least one mystic to keep them honest. I manage to fill this role while being an Episcopal lay minister. Matthew Fox, the great present-day religious teacher, says a mystic is doing a good job if she/he is always in trouble. By all accounts, I'm doing really well.

There is a significant correlation between health, spirituality, and the ability to cope.[9] There seems to be less of a chance for depression to set in if you have *Someone* to lean on, who is there all the time and will never let you down. A conference on Spiritual Dimensions in Clinical Research was held at Georgetown University School of Medicine. One conclusion they reached is that spirituality is important and should be considered whenever developing a therapeutic program.[10] If some degree of a religious practice is used to cope with chronic pain, you are less likely to become depressed. You might not understand how it works, but there is healing in prayer. Medical science can't explain why this is so, but it is.

Fortunately, prayer requires faith, not understanding. How often have you worried about how electricity works? You take it on faith that whenever you plug in a toaster or the television set, it will work. No matter who you are and what you do in life, you learn to use things you don't understand. There is some comfort in accepting that there are some things you don't know, and that's okay. That's what faith is all about. Search for and find your own form of a spiritual discipline, and discover what works for you. Then "plug in" to your cosmic source regularly.

I do believe in the value of unconditional love and unconditional forgiveness. But I am aware that I have negative people and events in my life. Sometimes they get to me. This is unavoidable when you travel apart from the crowd, especially if you are leading others on a path that is new. One humorous prayer that helps me is, "Lord, I'm not asking you to smite my enemies, but please get them out of my way!" This prayer is useful for things like computer malfunctions or negative personalities. Dealing with these kinds of issues can distract you from your intent and your life work. It can be hard to keep your balance in the face of an unreasonable world. Negativity surrounds us at times, but if we have a positive force within, nothing can prevail against us.

One difficulty you may face in your prayer life is the temptation to fill every moment with conscious thought or talk. Take time to listen for answers. You will get them, if you allow the space for them. Prayer and meditation can be times of listening to the universe, or to God, or to your inner self. Understand that your inner self, the universe, or God, won't use a fax, UPS, or Special Delivery to get back to you. The answer will come, but you have to be ready and open to receiving it in whatever form it arrives. Make sure you haven't put up any blocks to understanding that answer.

Check out your past. Are you carrying a grudge or ill feelings toward anyone? Let it go. Your load is heavy enough without carrying needless baggage. Tie up loose ends and mend fences when you can. Accept that there are some people who want to hang on to negativity. That is their problem. Let it go, and let them go as well.

Think about your connection to all that is positive, and to God, whatever you believe God to be. There is power in the presence of the Cosmic Force. You can touch that power. The peace that is beyond all your understanding is there for you, but it's not a passive gift. Any gift must be taken before you can make it your own. Accept the gift and give thanks, for you are very special and you are loved. Return that love. Think of prayer as a form of communication with that cosmic love. Pray not only for yourself, but also for all who are united with you, afflicted with illness and in pain.

Using Your Imagination

One woman told me that she felt she was at the end of her rope. Let's take that image and see what we can do with it. Visualize *your* rope in your mind. What's it made of? Is it sturdy? Does it end in space with no support? Look carefully. It's your rope, so you can change it. Make it strong, but don't let it wrap around you. Turn it into a swing, with a nice comfy seat. You are riding it—not the other way around. Don't let it bind or chafe. What color is it? Would you like it to be braided with many colors? Make it so. Is it bare, or are there flowers and decorations woven into it?

Are you secure? Are you swinging a little too fast? Perhaps you want to pump with your legs a little less. Relax. Breathe deeply. Life can be quite a ride, if we don't pump too hard, and don't allow others to push us where we don't want to go. Play with the swing awhile, and realize that it isn't too bad to be on the end of it.

We all have our ropes, each with its own unique texture and identity. Each of us also has a sturdy seat, if we care to use it, and don't try to "go it alone." But sometimes we have to help craft that seat ourselves, or ask someone else to help us make it. I also believe that when it's time to slip off that rope, we have a Heavenly Parent waiting with open arms to cradle us and carry us home.

Visualization and Imagery

As you saw with the image of the rope above, visualization can be a powerful tool for powerful mindwork. You need to stretch your imagination's muscles and enter a world that is real to your inner senses. Get comfortable, and let's take a trip inside to visit your informational substances. Close your eyes and look within to see neurotransmitters, peptides, and hormones. What do they look like? Remember that they are always busy and that the receptors are never still. There is also constant movement through the cellular membranes, and the informational substances are in constant communication with each other, and with your body and brain. Can you see the vast, complex web that flows through your body? Can you feel the electromagnetic sparks that hum through the wires of your consciousness?

Do you sense any rush? Any confusion? Are things moving too fast? Are there any bottlenecks? Take a tour through your body. At first you will be on a fact-finding, reconnaissance mission; so don't try to fix anything just yet. Can you sense any resonance in your body? Any pulsing and swaying of the movements and flows? As you travel around your body and mind at the submicroscopic level, are you aware of the network of conversations going on between the informational substances? How does it sound? Is it like the roar of ocean waves reaching the shore, or is it a whispering?

Once you feel comfortable in this interior environment, find an area that seems congested or stagnant. See if you can visually change the flow, and open it up. Work gently, changing a little at a time. You can come out whenever you wish, but trust your intuition on this. You may want to stay within until at least one area is cleared. Don't try to change too many things in one trip. You can always come back later.

Humor

Laughter does a lot more than make noise. A sense of humor is a survival tool. Cultivate it as you would a fine flowering plant. Don't let illness stop you from living and trying new things. So what if you drop something, or stumble? So what if you make a mistake? The world will continue. Learn from it and move on. One comic strip I especially like is *Garfield*. In one episode, Jon says to Garfield, "Everything I did today went wrong." Garfield looks smug. "Not me!" he replies. "You didn't do *anything* today, did you?" Jon accuses. "A minor detail," the cat replies. We must guard against Garfielding. Life is a gift, but we must accept that gift, and not waste it. Comedy movies, television, and books are also excellent resources for distraction. Humor helps us cope.

Dream Weaver

When you dream, different parts of your body/mind exchange information, clearing the decks for the next day. If you have a dream that you remember, try to interpret it. Is your body/mind trying to tell you something? You can learn to interpret your dreams, and you can also learn to influence them. If you have a bad dream that keeps recurring, it is within your power to change it. Review the dream just before you fall asleep, and rewrite the script, changing the troublesome or frightening parts. If you deal with the issues *before* you sleep, you may not have the dream again. It may take some time to accomplish this, but give it time. It will be well worth the effort.

You can use your dreams to travel. Is there a special place you always wanted to see? Get a library book, and read all about it. Many libraries lend travel videos. Immerse yourself in foreign lands. Just before you go to sleep, visualize your destination. Think about what it looks like. What it smells like. How it sounds. You might discover that you can program your dreams and visit faraway places.

Having Fun!

It has been said that it is pleasure that binds one to existence. To make life more worthwhile, spend more of your time having fun. This may seem like a formidable task when you have to deal with chronic pain. Start simply. Engaging in an activity that makes you happy and keeps you totally focused is an excellent distraction from chronic pain. What do you really enjoy doing? Maybe it's something you haven't done since you were a youngster, like reading comic books or arranging the furniture in a doll house. Make a list of the things you enjoy doing *now*. It is terribly difficult to think of amusing or interesting things to do when you are in the midst of crisis, such as when you are in flare. But if you had such a list to refer to at crises times, it might be easier to distract yourself, when you most need to be distracted.

Plan to have distractions available for those times when you must cope with extra pain or negativity. Buy the paints. Set up the workshop. Start a (small) garden. Be sure that your activity is one that will not present you with an insurmountable challenge. If you aren't able to do what you want, find a way to modify it to fit in with your current limitations. Take a few minutes every day to do something you enjoy. You will feel better if you make a special time for yourself *every day*. Even a few minutes a day spent in pursuit of that which brings you pleasure can change your life.

Become a kid for a day. Play. You may find out that you have forgotten how to play. Observe children at play. They are intent on their own world. They are focused. Find something you enjoy and focus on it. Forget your responsibilities for a while. Give yourself permission to be silly. Make a sand castle. Make a snow angel. Play with finger paints. Use a coloring book. Explore your world.

Biofeedback

Studies have shown that those patients who can identify their own physiological responses, such as changes in skin temperature, blood pressure, and brain-wave activity, also can learn to control those responses by mental effort.[11] During biofeedback training, a machine is attached to your body to monitor your blood pressure, brain waves, skin temperature, and/or neuromuscular activity. You don't feel anything while you are hooked up, but you learn how to influence the biological parameters that are being monitored by making changes in your mental and emotional states.

In one study, patients were able to raise their skin temperature and increase muscle relaxation at trigger point sites, and decrease their pressure-pain sensitivity.[12] Electromyographic (EMG) biofeedback is the most common type of biofeedback used in medical settings. Studies show that this type of biofeedback is helpful for FMS patients, and may reduce pain and muscle tension, leading to an improvement of quality of life.[13]

Self-Hypnosis

Self-hypnosis can be a safe and effective way to control or diminish chronic pain,[14] as well as the negativity that often comes with it.[15] Hypnosis and self-hypnosis are not about the loss of conscious control, as some may fear. You have complete control at all times. In a way, all hypnosis is self-hypnosis.

The hypnotized brain is different from the normal brain, both waking and sleeping.[16] Brain scans show increased activity during hypnosis, especially in areas connected to mental imagery. Every time you daydream, you are in a self-hypnotic state. Sometimes you hypnotize yourself when reading or watching a movie; you experience accelerated heart rate and breathing just as though you were participating in the real events. Hypnosis is a tool you can readily access to assist in your healing process. You simply need to learn how to channel something you may have been doing all along.

Self-hypnosis can enable you to channel your ability to put your whole brain to work for you when you need it. The goal of hypnosis is for you to gain control—over behavior, emotions, or physiological processes. Before you decide to use hypnotherapy in any form as part of your healing process, learn about it. There are excellent books you can borrow from your library, either on site or from interlibrary loans. If you choose to work with a therapist, choose one who is certified (see Resources).

Subliminal Tapes

If you have FMS and use subliminal tapes, your hypersensitive neurotransmitters and nerve endings may work to your advantage. They come in both audio and visual modes, and some audiotapes can be played while you are doing chores. I have found the ones that aim at banishing negativity or frustration very useful. Some audiotapes have the subliminal messages on one side and the same messages with the audible words on the other side. If you tend to be extremely analytical, or to "second guess" yourself, subliminal tapes can be a way to open your mind to the power of subconscious healing.

Pacing and Boundaries

It can be quite difficult to build healthy boundaries. Many of us take in abandoned animals, and our hearts go out to anyone in need. We understand what it is like to need help. Empathy

> In our house we post strategic signs, such as the one in our bathroom: "We have many cat water bowls but only one toilet. Please close the lid." I have found out that I can get away with nearly anything if I do it with a sense of humor.

can be a great gift but we need to have a firm knowledge of what our responsibilities are in life, and which responsibilities belong to others.

Many people with FMS and CMP are needy and have boundary issues. It's hard to be compassionate and understanding and still maintain healthy boundaries. It can be especially difficult if you are a support group facilitator or other caregiver, as well as a patient. In the world of chronic pain there is a constant struggle to find answers. Your impulse is often to give and give and give. This can drain you, because, if you don't empower others to serve themselves, the demands on you will be endless. It is important to remember that the first patient in line must be you. Take care of yourself so you can take care of others. Keep your goals and your intention in mind, and search for a workable, sustainable balance. Ask for help. You can't do it all alone.

As you learn to set boundaries for yourself and not allow others to encroach on them, at times you are going to feel guilty. You are also going to upset others. This may be hard to accept, but it is true. This is part of the price of growing up, and part of the price of our own growth.

Fibromyalgia and CMP are time-consuming illnesses. These past years I haven't taken enough time for myself. My "self" time has been diminished, or even eliminated. I need time to meditate, do t'ai chi, read, and declutter. I must be very careful to set boundaries, so that others don't intrude upon the time I need to restore and replenish myself. I need alone time to restore my own sense of balance. One book, *Boundary Power*,[17] has been particularly useful in this quest.

Time and Space Enough?

It may seem as though you need to work twenty-four hours a day just to take care of yourself. It takes longer to accomplish tasks because of FMS and CMP. It pays to do tasks mindfully, or you will be spending even more time cleaning up spills and undoing that which you did not mean to do. Mindwork, bodywork, attention to meal planning, building and maintaining a support structure—when will you have some time just to live and enjoy life?

Sometimes you must slow down and focus on doing one thing at a time. This is a hard lesson. You may want to do too much, and now you have limitations that make you pay huge fines if you exceed them. At times, you may have to "stop the world" and get off, to find your center. But by taking the time to restore your own internal balance and harmony, you may find that once you decide to "get back on" the world, life will be more meaningful and much happier.

To stop the world, take some time to just *be*. Notice the world around you. What do you smell? What sensations do you feel on your skin? Stretch your mental ears and concentrate. How many sounds can you hear: Then *listen*. Is there a difference in quality if you are listening, rather than just hearing? Do the same with your sense of sight. What can you see close by? Far away? At a moderate distance? Look at some objects you tend to take for granted, and really *observe* them. What is the air like around you? What are you feeling emotionally right now? Don't judge, just notice it. Does it help you to feel that way? If you can't answer any of these questions, that's an answer in itself.

> Working on this book has been a challenge. I've pushed my limits and have been enlightened as to how ill I am. I have had to institute the "Law of Rectangles": While I'm focused on the book, parts of the house will be a wreck and other parts will be tangles.

Sacred Space

A sacred space is a space where you can be alone to explore your thoughts and dreams. You need a place to go where you can be alone and safe. This can be a real place, in your backyard, or in a park or by a brook. If you don't have this kind of place handy, you may find it useful to make a sacred space indoors. It could even be a shelf for special pictures and objects that have meaning to you. I have a "sacred shelf" in my office, and pictures of some of my healers on the wall. You can even put special objects in a basket and hang it from the ceiling, if you don't have a shelf. Take the time to create a sacred space in your mind. This is the place that is safe and special that you can visit with no preparation. Help your supporters to cope by allowing them to have their own space, and by making your needs specific and clear. Understand that your supporters have needs too.

Explore different ways to "go somewhere else," where you can take a vacation from FMS and CMP. Where can you go to escape? Some of us lose ourselves in novels, nature shows, other books or movies, gardening, or grooming our pets. Listening to music may help you escape. Making music can even more so. You don't need to take formal lessons. When was the last time you picked up a harmonica? Most people can pick out simple folk tunes on a harmonica and get real pleasure from it. Did you ever try playing with a bamboo flute? It can provide a lot of pleasure. Collect music, books, and videos that you find inspirational, uplifting, and empowering. Go to them to restore your sense of self and your need for balance.

Remember, too, that those who have FMS are hypersensitive. Listen to your inner self. Do certain types of movies, books, conversations, and even certain people make you feel edgy or ill? Think about it. Your inner self is telling you something. Don't subject yourself to more negativity than you need to handle.

You can learn to use mindwork to help quiet your mind, lessen the effects of hyperstimulation, and deal more effectively with your symptoms. In addition, mindwork can bring you a measure of focus and control, help you restore emotional balance, and enhance the quality of your life. You may find that these and other forms of mindwork are not enough to restore your sense of balance. There is help available. Assess your needs. You may require peer counseling, psychiatric help, cognitive behavioral therapy, pastoral counseling, marriage counseling, or another form of guidance. It is available and can help you change your attitudes and focus.

> When I first started my support group, I invited people to my home for free counseling sessions, to help them cope. I thought there would be a limited number of people. Before long, I found that this activity was not only perpetuating my TrPs and FMS, it was making things dramatically worse. Now I know that there is no way I can see everybody who wants to come. That is part of what this book is about. I found that I must schedule time for my first patient, me, or I will have nothing left for others.

Endnotes

1. Lewis, K. S. 1998. Emotional adjustment to a chronic illness. *Lippincotts Prim Care Pract* 2(1):38-51.

2. Singh, B. B., B. M. Berman, V. A. Hadhazy, and P. Creamer. 1998. A pilot study of cognitive behavioral therapy in fibromyalgia. *Altern Ther Health Med* 4(2):67-70.

3. Austin, J. H. 1999. *Zen and the Brain*. Cambridge, MA: MIT Press.

4. Amir M., L. Neumann, O. Bohr, Y. Shir, and D. Buskila. 2000. Coping styles, anger, social support, and suicide risk of women with fibromyalgia syndrome. *J Musculoskel Pain* 8(3):7-20.

5. Pert, C. B. 1997. *Molecules of Emotion*. New York: Scribner's.

6. Starlanyl, D. J. 1999. *Worlds of Power, Lines of Light*. West Chesterfield, NH: Devstar.

7. Davis, M., E. R. Eshelman, and M. McKay. 2000. *The Relaxation & Stress Reduction Workbook*. Fifth edition. Oakland, CA: New Harbinger Publications.

8. Clark, N. 1999. Adapted with permission from the *Keene New Hampshire Sunday Sentinel*, November 14, p. D-5.

9. McBride, J. L., G. Arthur, R. Brooks, and L. Pilkington. 1998. The relationship between a patient's spirituality and health experiences. *Fam Med* 30(2):122-126.

10. Marwick, C. 1995. Should physicians prescribe prayer for health? Spiritual aspects of well-being considered. *JAMA* 273(20)1561-1562.

11. Sarnoch, H., F. Adler, and O. B. Scholz. 1997. Relevance of muscular sensitivity, muscular activity, and cognitive variables for pain reduction associated with EMG biofeedback in fibromyalgia. *Percept Motor Skills* 84(3 pt 1):1043-1050.

12. Albright, G. L., and A. A. Fischer. 1990. Effects of warming imagery aimed at trigger-point sites on tissue compliance, skin temperature, and pain sensitivity in biofeedback-trained patients with chronic pain: a preliminary study. *Percept Mot Skills* 71(3 pt 2):1163-1170.

13. Mur, E., A. J. Drexler, F. Gruber, V. Hartig, and V. Gunther. 1999. [Eletromyography biofeedback therapy in fibromyalgia]. *Wien Med Wochenschr* 149(19-20):561-563. [German]

14. Nickelson, C., J. O. Brende, and J. Gonzalez. 1999. What if your patient prefers an alternative pain control method? Self-hypnosis in the control of pain. *South Med J* 92(5):52152-3.

15. Faymonville, M. E., S. Laureys, C. Degueldre, G. DelFiore, A. Luxen, G. Franck, et al. 2000. Neural mechanisms of antinociceptive effects of hypnosis. *Anesthesiology* 92(5):1257-1267.

16. Carter, R. 1998. *Mapping the Mind*. Berkeley: University of California Press.

17. O'Neil, M. S., and C. E. Newbold. 1994. *Boundary Power*. Antioch, TN: Sonlight Publishing.

CHAPTER 21

Medications

Medications are one form of therapy with which you can gain some measure of control over your symptoms. They may enable you to handle a greater amount of bodywork and exercise, and can be used to restore greater levels of function. Until recently, much of the medical world regarded complaints caused by fibromyalgia (FMS) and chronic myofascial pain (CMP) as psychological. Today, one result of that attitude is that very few drugs have been established as effective for these conditions. Medications that have been developed for other conditions, however, often prove helpful. Antidepressants have pain-relieving effects independent of changes of mood, for example, and are prescribed for pain in lower doses than are used to treat depression.[1] They may be effective in reducing pain associated with FMS.[2] Medication should never be considered as the only form of pain control for FMS and CMP. It must be part of a holistic strategy, with sound nutrition, bodywork, mindwork, healthy lifestyle adjustments, and other nonmedicinal options for pain control.

Before adding any new medication, review your current medications with your doctor. Discuss your options. It is crucial to address all of your perpetuating factors, and consider whether there may be one that has not been identified. For example, you may have been put on a medication such as Tagamet, Zantac, or Prilosec for heartburn and esophageal reflux (see chapter 7). These drugs may be good short-term symptom relievers, but they can decrease your ability to digest foods and add to your symptoms in the long run. If you have reflux, look into the possibility that you may have insulin resistance/reactive hypoglycemia. If you crave carbohydrates and have other symptoms of these conditions, try diet modification. Eliminate excess carbohydrates. Check for possible trigger points (TrPs) in the area around the base of your breastbone. With a change of diet and some myotherapy, you may be able to avoid having to use these expensive medications.

Medications that affect the central nervous system are appropriate for FMS. These medications target the symptoms of insomnia, pain, and fatigue. Also, if you have FMS, pain sensations are greatly amplified, so if you have TrPs or other instigators, your total pain level may be severe. Fibromyalgia patients may react in an unusual manner to medications. Discuss your reactions with your doctor and pharmacist.

Side Effects

If you develop side effects from any medication you're taking, it's important to know the difference between minor and major side effects. The following medical side effects could be serious or dangerous, and must be reported to your physician or to another qualified medical professional immediately:

- blurred vision • rapid or irregular heartbeat • rash or hives • sore throat or fever
- constant intense fatigue and/or sleepiness • restlessness • lack of coordination
- confusion • giddiness • fainting or seizures • hallucinations • numbness or swelling in your hands or feet • nausea and/or vomiting • slurred speech • stomach pain • stumbling • jerking of the arms and legs • ringing in the ears • large increase/decrease in urination • infection • change in your sex drive/impotence
- change in your menstrual cycle

Managing Side Effects

You can take steps to reduce or eliminate side effects that are not serious, but that may be uncomfortable or difficult to endure. Call your pharmacist if you aren't sure. In many cases, a healthy lifestyle can reduce the incidence and severity of many medications' side effects. When life begins to get out of control, side effects tend to worsen. Many side effects are most severe when you first start taking the medication and your body is still adjusting to it. After a week or two, the side effects may diminish or disappear. Ask your pharmacist or physician if this is to be expected with the medication(s) you are taking. Keep records of your medicines that note the following:

1. Generic name

2. Product name

3. What are the risks associated with taking this medication?

4. Why are you taking this medication?

5. What short-term side effects does this medication have?

6. What long-term side effects does this medication have?

7. What symptoms indicate that the dosage should be changed or the medication stopped?

8. Is there a way to minimize the chances of experiencing side effects? What are they?

9. What dietary and/or lifestyle restrictions will you have on this medication?

10. What medications might interact with this one?

11. If blood tests or other tests are required, how often will you need them?

12. What tests do you need prior to taking the medication?

13. What information is available about the medication?

14. What options do you have?

As your health improves, you may have to readjust the amounts and types of your medicines. During flares, you need to reduce your stress load and probably will need to increase your medications *temporarily*. Such variations are typical, and should not alarm anyone. As soon as the flare lifts or the unusual stressor is removed, you should reduce your medication dosage again.

Sensitivities and Interactions

Epinephrine and ephedra. Many people with FMS have contacted me about sensitivity to epinephrine. If you see an increase in your symptoms after undergoing local dental anesthesia, ask your dentist to try using a local without epinephrine. The related herb, ephredra, also triggers an adrenaline surge. Ephedra is not safe. Ma huang is a form of ephedra. It can cause insomnia, motor disturbances, and impaired cerebral circulation. Results of ephedra use include high blood pressure, seizures, stroke, irregular heart rhythms, seizures, permanent disability, and death.[3] If you have insulin resistance, be aware that ephedra, related herbs, and epinephrine can cause adrenaline surges and worsen your symptoms.

It is important that you don't mix nonprescription medications, like herbal remedies, with your prescription medications without discussing it with your health team first. There is no cookbook recipe for prescribing medications for FMS and CMP. A medication that works well for one person can be completely ineffective for another. A medication that puts one person to sleep may keep another awake.

To find a combination of medications that works for you, you need both a doctor and a pharmacist who are willing to work with you until an acceptable level of symptom control is reached. Patients with FMS may have difficulty metabolizing drugs. Your doctor may wish to mix the metabolic routes. For example, it would be easier on your liver if your kidneys metabolize some of your medications. You may have insufficiencies of certain biochemicals along the metabolic path that are needed to break down the medications.

Smoking. Tobacco smoke can have a profound impact on absorption, metabolism, and the actions of some medications. For example, smokers who take acetaminophen or tricyclic antidepressants have lower levels of these medications in their plasma than nonsmokers who take the same dose. Smokers also eliminate ascorbic acid and benzodiazepines and their derivatives like Valium more rapidly than nonsmokers.[4] This varies a great deal in different individuals. Drug absorption can be influenced by what you have eaten, or by antacids or minerals that you have taken at the same time. Anything that affects the rate that your body metabolizes any given medication may influence how well it works for you, and for how long.

Medications and Foods. Everyday foods and vitamins sometimes can interact dangerously with prescription drugs. For example, never drink grapefruit juice less than two hours before or five hours after taking the drugs called calcium channel blockers (see "Prescription Medications" below). Grapefruit and grapefruit juice can interact with several medications.[5] Grapefruit juice should never be taken with antihistamines because the combination can cause serious heart problems.[6] High doses of vitamin E or garlic can inhibit platelet function and increase serum insulin, which may be dangerous if you already have insulin resistance as a perpetuating factor. Antidepressants called MAO inhibitors can cause a potentially fatal rise in blood pressure when taken with foods high in the chemical, tyramine, such as is found in cheese and sausage. Certain antibiotics like Cipro or the ulcer drugs Tagamet, Zantac, and Pepcid can increase caffeine levels, causing the jitters and stomach irritation. Too much caffeine can amplify theophylline, a bronchodilator, causing nausea, palpitations, or seizures. Soy proteins may affect thyroid function at the thyroid gland, without creating differences in TSH.[7]

Doctors often decide if patients need thyroid supplementation by measuring their TSH (thyroid stimulating hormone) levels. Most doctors believe that if their patient has serum TSH lab test results above a certain level, s/he does not need thyroid supplementation. Often the use of thyroid supplementation is monitored by measuring TSH, and doctors try to keep that level in the middle of the "normal" range. In cases of FMS, this is not valid.[8]

In most cases of FMS, the hypothalamus-pituitary-thyroid axis is not functioning normally (see "FMS and the Thyroid Connection" in chapter 15). If your thyroid gland is producing adequate amounts of hormones, but you require large doses of thyroid supplement due to your cells' inability to metabolize them efficiently, the results of the TSH test can be dangerously misleading. The low TSH is typical of hyperthyroidism, but this does not mean that you are overstimulated. Doctors need to understand that hyperthyroidism and thyrotoxicosis are different conditions. John Lowe writes, "In all of diagnostic practice, probably no other confusion of concepts likely results in more mistaken diagnoses and improper treatment of patients."[9]

Calcium and other minerals can also interfere with oral thyroid supplementation. You may have to time the intervals that you take these medications and supplements. Discuss possible food interactions with your pharmacist when you pick up any medication.

Herbal Remedies

As indicated above, herbal medications must be treated with respect, just like prescription drugs. Be very cautious, as some herbal remedies can vary greatly in bioavailability, stability, and other qualities that may be unknown. Each herb you buy, if sold in a commercial over-the-counter preparation, may be labeled with the milligram amount of the main active ingredient. But such herbs can contain many components that act in different ways. Some of these ways may be helpful. Some may not. Some of the components may even interact with other medications that you take. For example, licorice is a natural diuretic, and if you are taking a prescription diuretic, it can cause low potassium and muscle cramping. It could even cause a stroke.

Herbal remedies are not regulated under federal drug laws. There is no guarantee that the product is safe and effective. The time the herbs are harvested, the processing, and the location of their growth may be important. For example, St. John's wort should not be harvested close to a major road because it can absorb diesel and other vapors. Even the packaging can affect an herb's potency. Regulated drugs undergo stability testing, which tests the medication in its packaging. For unregulated herbs there may be no check on adulteration of the product, which includes contamination with foreign materials.

If an herbal product is standardized, the specified level, or potency, of the herb is usually on the label. This does not mean that amount specified is *bioavailable*. Bioavailability refers to the amount of the medication in a readily absorbable form. The number of milligrams on the package may simply indicate the amount of herb instead of its potency. The active ingredient can vary enormously from lot to lot. Some of this confusion can be avoided by finding a reputable herbal company that is very careful with its standards. Still, you are often in the position of accepting the word of the company.

Herbs can be very effective. For example, St John's wort has been shown to be effective for depression (but there are many kinds of St. John's wort). Hypericum, the active ingredient in St. John's wort, can be an effective treatment for seasonal affective disorder (SAD).[10] but it may interact with birth control pills, seizure medication, and other drugs. Valerian may sometimes be useful for the relief of insomnia.[11] Ginko biloba may be helpful to increase the blood supply to the brain, but it may also cause excess bleeding. Feverfew may be helpful to prevent migraines, but it is also a serotonin antagonist. It must be used with caution if you take anticoagulants. Doctors need to become more familiar with the use and potential interactions of common herbals.[12] Many herbs still need to be studied thoroughly before we understand their mechanisms, although some have been in use for thousands of years.

Capsaicin is an active ingredient that heats up hot peppers. It seems to deplete substance P, which is involved with neurological information transfers and pain. Capsaicin ointment may be too fierce for people with FMS, although the burning may ease up after first few days of use. You don't need to further sensitize your nervous system. I know one woman who puts a spoon of cayenne pepper in her coffee every morning; she says it helps to lower her pain level.

Chai is tea with an (East) Indian spice mix, which can include ginger and cayenne. Mine does. Every chai mix is different, so you may want to experiment. Find out whether any help you.

Ginger may aid digestion. It may also provide nausea relief, and help with sensitivity to cold. I find that putting a few tablespoonfuls of ground ginger into bath water and soaking in it eases muscle soreness.

Herbals can vary tremendously in their processing and their origins. For example, Dong quai (Angelica sinensis) sold in the United States, for example, may be heavily sulfited, and must be properly washed before use. "Ugly dong quai" is not preserved with sulfites, and is shipped with its "skin" on.[13] Dong quai is often used for sore muscles, sciatica, and pinched nerves. But, like other herbals, dong quai has side effects and can be dangerous for some people.

Devils claw root (Harpagophytum procumbens) is another herb that may have significant pain-relieving properties.[14] Some people with FMS report that it helps them. I read about a medical abstract that indicated edible chrysanthemum might be effective for insulin resistance.[15] The article was written in Kanji. I was fortunate that my friend and teacher, Paul Gallagher, was able to read this. He told me that the herb is not the edible yellow Japanese chrysanthemum. "Jiangtangkang" is a white chrysanthemum, and the flower is the active part. I am now looking for a reliable seed source.

I do not want to discourage the use of herbal medications. There are doctors who specialize in herbal treatments, and I strongly urge you find one to help you. If you are going to try herbals on your own, please proceed very cautiously. There are some excellent reference materials available (see Appendix B: Reading List).

Over-the-Counter Medications and Supplements

There is a misconception that a drug purchased over-the-counter (OTC) cannot cause harm. This isn't true. If you have FMS, your body and mind are already out of balance. You must be careful not to add to these imbalances. Too many doctors tell patients to take OTC remedies for pain. This could be due to habit, lack of training in pain management, lack of training in FMS and CMP, or fear of prescribing stronger medications.

If you take OTCs, you may need less prescription medication. This does not mean that you will endure fewer side effects, or that the OTC medications are as efficient. Often, the bioequivalency and side effects of OTC medications and health food nutrients have not been studied as extensively as FDA-approved medications. Many of the considerations for herbal medications may apply. Be sure to check with your doctor or pharmacist before you use them along with prescription medications.

Currently, researchers are examining some supplements carefully. For example, early evidence indicates that folate, tryptophan, and phenylalanine enhance the effectiveness of prescription antidepressants. S-adenosylmethionine (SAM-e) seems to have antidepressant effects, and omega-3 polyunsaturated fatty acids, particularly docosahexaenoic acid, may have mood-stabilizing effects.[16]

Some doctors have found that omega-3 fatty acids can considerably reduce total cholesterol levels and even pain levels in FMS patients.[17] Only a few common OTC remedies are discussed here, but there are some excellent references available (see the Reading List). Vitamins and minerals are discussed at greater length in chapter 23.

Benadryl (diphenhydramine). This is a helpful sleep aid/antihistamine that is safe to take during pregnancy. The starting dose is 50 mg, taken one hour before bed. About 20 percent of patients are stimulated rather than sedated by Benadryl. Patients have reported urinary hesitancy while taking this medication, which was relieved when they stopped taking it.

Calms Forte. This is a mix of herbs, calcium, and magnesium phosphates. It may be effective as an alternative medicine to take to promote sleep before going to bed.

Chromium Picolinate. This mineral supplement may be effective in decreasing the "carbocraving" that some of us experience. It seems to improve the efficiency of insulin in the body.[18] Glucose intolerance, related to insufficient dietary chromium, appears to be widespread.[19]

Coenzyme Q10. This is a vitaminlike substance. Some people have found it helps to reduce fibrofog. It's an important part of the mitochrondrial membrane, but we don't understand all of its functions yet.

DHEA (dehydroepiandrosterone). This turns into estrogen and testosterone in your body. High doses (25-50 mg/daily) of DHEA can trigger heart palpitations and irregular heartbeat, or even a heart attack.[20] Some FMS patients report that it gives them increased energy, better sleep, and a sense of well-being.

Digestive Enzymes. If you have problems digesting food, try taking papain or a natural enzyme combination to help your gastrointestinal system break down foods. Some preparations contain hydrochloric acid, and you may want to find one that does not. Read your labels. There is no logic to taking a prescription or OTC medication for reflux to inhibit your stomach acid and then taking an OTC pill containing more acid.

Glandular Extracts. These extracts for boosting immunity may carry a danger of prion transfer between species. Prions are extremely small particles that carry infectious diseases. Discuss this issue with your doctor before you consider taking any of these preparations.

Glucosamine and Chondroitin. These two biochemical supplements are often packaged together. They may be beneficial in cases of inflammation, bone or cartilage degradation, or problems with ground substance. Glucosamine may cause worsening of symptoms for FMS patients who have high levels of hyaluronic acid (see chapter 15).

5-Hydroxytryptophan (5-HTP). Your body converts this to serotonin. It easily crosses the blood-brain barrier and effectively increases synthesis of serotonin.[21]

Human Growth Hormone (HGH, somatotropin). This is an endocrine hormone that declines with age. It is produced by the pituitary gland, released during early deep sleep, and converted into insulinlike-growth-factor-1 (IGF-1). There are dangerous implications with OTC use.[22] The use of OTC growth hormones is not to be confused with the legitimate FMS research that has uncovered a subset of FMS patients who have low insulinlike growth hormone. IGF-1 deficiency occurs in about 30 percent of FMS patients.[23] *Replacement* treatment for these patients improves some FMS parameters, including the number of tender points. Defective growth hormone secretion in these patients appears to be due to a dysfunction in the hypothalamus. Studies show that most FMS patients do not have severe growth hormone deficiency as a significant contributor to their illness.[24]

Malic acid and magnesium hydroxide. These are used in energy production and energy use. Malic acid plays a key part in the metabolism of carbohydrates, as well as in the formation of adenosine triphosphate (ATP). Magnesium and vitamin B6 must be present for malate to help the transfer of electrons across the mitochondrial membrane.[25] One study showed that this combination is safe and may be beneficial in the treatment of FMS.[26]

Melatonin. Melatonin is a neurotransmitter secreted by the pineal gland, located in the center of the brain. The body changes it to serotonin. It is nontoxic and may make the antidepressant Elavil more active or effective. It may help reduce tender point count and severity of pain as well as improve sleep significantly in FMS patients.[27] Patients with FMS may have low melatonin secretion during the hours of darkness. This may contribute to impaired sleep, daytime fatigue, and changed pain perception.[28]

Melatonin in sufficient dosage may inhibit ovulation. Up to one-third of those who try melatonin become depressed. If depression occurs, *stop taking it immediately* and alert your doctor. Melatonin stimulates the immune system and should not be taken by people with autoimmune conditions.[29] It may, however, help to reduce seizurelike symptoms.

NSAIDS. Nonsteroidal anti-inflammatory agents (NSAIDS) have their uses, and they can be very effective in some cases for *inflammatory* pain, but there are problems with chronic use on a daily basis. Neither FMS nor CMP are inflammatory conditions. NSAIDs include medications such as ibuprofen and naproxen. NSAIDS have some very serious side effects including: asthma, direct cell toxicity, chromosome abnormalities, and phototoxicity.[30]

A large majority of the patients who develop serious gastrointestinal complications on NSAIDS never had previous mild side effects. *Prophylactic treatment with antacids and H2 receptor antagonists such as Zantac™ (ranitidine HCl), Pepcid™ (famotidine), and Tagamet™ (cimetidine HCl) may increase the risk for subsequent serious GI complications.*[31] In animals, treatment with NSAIDs delayed fracture healing.[32]

SAM-e (S-adenosylmethionine). One study found that SAM-e had no effect in patients with FMS, but it was a short-term study.[33] SAM-e may need to be taken long term. This is a sulfur-rich metabolite of an amino acid that is involved in the regulation of some hormones and neurotransmitters, and with DNA. We don't know all that it does. Be careful. Some people say it helps with arthritis pain. If arthritis is a perpetuating factor of your FMS and/or CMP, it may be worth considering.

Simethicone. When gas and bloating are a problem, Phazyme™ and other brands of simethicone may be useful. Try it before eating foods that normally cause bloating. Make sure that you are chewing your food carefully, eating a healthy diet, and taking enough time to eat. Bloating and other digestive symptoms are ways that your gastrointestinal system lets you know that something isn't right.

Guidelines for Taking Medications

Before you start any medication, be sure your doctor has the following information:

- The names of all your medications, including all over-the-counter medications and supplements, and a list of bodywork, electrotherapies, and other forms of healing that you use.

- If you are pregnant, could become pregnant, or are planning a pregnancy in the near future. Also, are you or will you be breast-feeding?

- Any allergies or sensitivities you have.

- Any other illness or medical condition you have.

- Whether you need any change in normal medication routines, such as the addition of an antiyeast medication whenever you take antibiotics.

If you need to discontinue or change medication, make sure you discuss the following with your doctor and pharmacist:

- Whether your medications require periodic blood tests. If so, ask about testing frequency.

- Any physical or emotional side effect that may occur.

- Any possible food or drug interaction.

If you plan to add another medication to your regimen, ask about the following:

- Should you fill only part of a new prescription until you know whether you can tolerate it?

- Should you inform your other doctors, dentists, therapists, etc., of your new medication?

Also ask about the following:

- Any planned vacations, and any extra medications or medical needs you might have to ensure your traveling and vacationing comfort.

- Any vacations your doctor has planned. Be sure you know who will be covering for him/her.

Safety Rules for Medications

- Store your medications in a dry place, at room temperature.

- Store medications up high to avoid having to use childproof caps. (The road to hell is paved with pain medications in childproof caps.)

- Don't share your medications. Don't take medications prescribed for others.

- The first time you take a medication, alert someone nearby that you are taking it. If possible, have someone else in the house. Side effects happen.

- Always keep a medication in its original container.

- If a medication is outdated, throw it away.

- Don't mix medications in one container.

- Don't take medications in the dark.

- Check the medication's label each time you take it to make sure you have the correct one you need.

Be sure to take sufficient water with medications. An 8 oz. glass of water will help ensure the usefulness of the medication. Use room-temperature water. Studies on the availability of medication, as it breaks down in the stomach, are done with room-temperature water to dilute the medication. If a tablet dissolves in your throat, you might get a cough reaction that could send burning powder to your lungs, throat, and esophagus. You may get unusual reactions if you take your medications with hot or cold liquid. Some medications are rendered ineffective if taken with milk, and taking timed-release medications with hot liquid may affect the timed-release mechanism.

Prescription Medications

People with FMS and CMP often take many medications to control their symptoms. Each of these medications may have side effects. For example, SSRIs (selective serotonin reuptake inhibitors) appear to be beneficial for chronic pain, but they can lower the seizure threshold.[34] If you already have seizurelike symptoms, you may want to consider your options carefully before you take an SSRI.

You may have to try many medications in different combinations before you find the right balance. Your doctor may become frustrated trying to find the right combination of medications that works for you. Remind your doctor that it's frustrating for you, too, and ask for patience and support. I have observed that people with FMS may take less time before they know whether a medication is effective or not (or if it has an unacceptable side effect) than the amount of time needed by people with other illnesses. When your doctor prescribes a new drug for you, you may want to ask for a small amount to try at first. Try nonmedicinal symptom relievers as well. If your health improves, you may need to adjust your medications, and perhaps be able to drop some of them. During flares, you may need to reduce your stimuli and temporarily increase your medications.

If you've been on a medication for a while, it may seem as though its effects don't last as long as they once did. This may mean that your metabolic system has become more adept at breaking it down. Discuss this with your doctor and pharmacist. Ask for advice. Let them know if you forgot to take your medication several times, or didn't renew your prescription on time. Let them know if you couldn't afford to renew it. This will help to ensure accurate assessment of the medication's effects. If you tend to lose track of what you have and haven't taken, your pharmacist has options to help prevent this.

Pharmacies and Pharmacists

Have all your prescriptions filled at one pharmacy so your pharmacist can warn you of any possible drug interactions, no matter how many doctors you have. Your pharmacist can be a great ally and teacher. Learn all you can about your medications. It's important for you to know, for example, that amitriptyline, ibuprofen, and other medications, as well as FMS itself, can cause water retention. Many medications should not be taken together, and even vitamins and minerals can affect prescription medications. Check with your pharmacist, and develop a working relationship based on mutual respect and trust.

Educate your pharmacist about FMS and CMP as well. If you have a copy of *The Fibromyalgia Advocate*,[35] the handout, "What Your Pharmacist Should Know," may be helpful. Set good boundaries. If your pharmacist treats you like a drug addict or malingerer, let him/her know that this is inappropriate, and that you do not allow inappropriate behavior from your health care providers. If the behavior continues in spite of educational efforts on your part, talk to the pharmacy manager or change pharmacies.

Compounding Pharmacists

Compounding pharmacists are different than standard pharmacists. They are like the ancient apothecaries, only with all the present-day knowledge and technology available. All pharmacists learn something about compounding prescriptions, but compounding pharmacists are specialists in the formulation of pharmaceutical compounds from basic ingredients, in the exact dosage form, strength, and combination you may require. For example, you may need a dye-free, sugar-free, alcohol-free or preservative-free formulation.

When you take a medication orally, you dose the whole body. Often this is not necessary for localized symptoms. Oral medications often go from the stomach through the liver before they are used. The liver metabolizes many medications, and the *metabolites* that are created may not be as potent as the initial form. This may mean that you have to take a higher oral dosage to get the amount of the medication you need. The transdermal (through the skin or topical) form of medications allows you to bypass the liver the first time around, which means you may need a much lower dose to achieve the same effect. A transdermal medicine also gives your liver and stomach a rest.

It isn't sufficient for a pharmacist to put a drug into a topical form. The drug must be bioavailable in this form, and a true compounding pharmacist knows how to do this. Standard topical preparations compounded include NMDA inhibitors and calcium channel blockers, medications like Neurontin, NSAIDs, and opioids. The International Academy of Compounding Pharmacists can help you find the name of a local compounding pharmacist in your area (see Resources). Your doctor may not be utilizing this option, and you may be able to provide him/her with an important contact.

Generic Medicines

Generic and brand-name drugs are not always exact equivalents. Some FMS and CMP patients are sensitive to the differences. It is important that your doctor and pharmacist be on the alert for this. It is also important that your doctor believes you if you require the brand name, so your pharmacist can be advised. In recent years, because of attempts to lower drug prices, doctors have been under a lot of pressure to substitute generics for brand-name drugs.

If a company wants to market a generic as being exactly the same as a brand-name drug (this is legal after the drug patent expires), it must pass the Food and Drug Administration (FDA) bioequivalency program. This means that it isn't sufficient for the generic to be made of the same chemical components in the exactly the same strengths as the brand-name product. The company that manufactures the generic must prove that when someone takes the drug, the amount of the active substance released by the generic is the same as would be obtained with the brand-name drug. Doctors and patients have been led to believe that the generics are the same as the brand names, except perhaps for packaging. *This is not always true.* The FDA considers two formulations as bioequivalent when the rate of adsorption varies no more than -20 percent or +25 percent.[36] This means that there can be 20 percent less usable medication in a dose, or 25 percent more! In this study, based on a questionnaire sent to 3,639 physicians nationwide, only 17 percent of the physicians responding knew this. Physicians need to understand the issues surrounding generic substitution and remain empowered to influence decisions to substitute generics. You may find that most generics are fine, but one or two of your medications may work better if they are the original brand. Listen to your body.

Specific Prescription Medications

The list presented here is only a partial listing of medications used to treat FMS and CMP. It would take a whole book to describe them all. You may not have heard about some of these medications. For details on the use of common pharmaceutical and nonpharmaceutical medications for chronic pain, see *The Chronic Pain Control Workbook*[37] and *Pain: Clinical Manual.*[38]

Ambien (zolpidem). This is a hypnotic for insomnia. It can be a tremendously effective sleep aid, but you may have to get into bed right after you take it. A hypnotic can cause you to lose all memory of what you do from the time it takes effect until it wears off. You may eat food you don't need, shouldn't have eaten, and won't remember eating. You may not have conscious control over what you do or say. Some people have had wonderful sexual experiences, or so their partners say, but they can't remember them because they had taken a hypnotic beforehand. One study showed that short-term treatment with Ambien (5 to 15 mg) doesn't affect FMS pain, but is useful for sleep and subsequent daytime energy.[39] William Dement, a leading researcher in the field of sleep medicine, writes that Ambien is the safest and most useful sleep medication for long-term use.[40] Studies show that Ambien has a low abuse potential compared to other hypnotics.[41] There have been some reports of serious depression from taking Ambien. Some patients have reported difficulty discontinuing it; they had to decrease it by a quarter pill a night. Others have had no problems.

Atarax (hydroxyzine HCl). This suppresses activity in some areas of the central nervous system to produce an antianxiety effect. This antihistamine and anxiety-reliever may be useful when itching, rashes, or hives cause problems.

BuSpar (buspirone HCl). This drug may improve memory, reduce anxiety, and help regulate body temperature. It is not as sedating as many other antianxiety drugs.

Calcium Channel Blockers. Short-term use of topical calcium channel blockers may be a safe and effective method to treat myofascial TrPs. When resistant TrPs are broken up, if the perpetuating factors are controlled, it may require only temporary or periodic use of the calcium channel blocker on the TrP itself. *This use is new and experimental.* Use caution until clinical studies have been done. Some doctors may wish to try it as an office procedure on resistant TrPs. Its use may be limited by muscle cramps, especially in the lower legs. We hope to see research on this.

Catapres (clonidine). This may be effective treatment for restless leg syndrome (RLS) patients who experience sleep-disrupting periodic limb movements and sensations.[42]

Celexa (citalopram). One study found this medication gave FMS patients significant relief from pain after two months of treatment, but after four months the effect diminished.[43] Also, there have been reports of hallucinations.

COX-2 medications. Ariva, Vioxx, and Celebrex are supposed to be easier on the gastrointestinal tract than earlier NSAIDS (nonsteroidal anti-inflammatory drugs). There have been some indications that their use carries a greater risk of heart attack, stroke, or other cardiovascular problem.[44]

Desyrel (trazodone). This antidepressant may help with sleep problems. It must be taken with food. It should not be used by women who are or may become pregnant.

Diflucan (fluconazole). This antifungal medication penetrates all body tissues, including the central nervous system. Short-term use can be helpful if systemic yeast is suspected, especially if reactive hypoglycemia and/or insulin resistance is present, but diet modification is important for lasting yeast eradication.

Effexor (venlafaxine HCl). This is an antidepressant and serotonin and norepinephrine reuptake inhibitor. Food has no effect on its absorption. When discontinuing this medication, taper off slowly.

Elavil (amitriptyline). This is an inexpensive antidepressant. It can cause photosensitivity, morning grogginess, weight gain, and dry mouth, and may slow normal intestinal movements. It may cause restless leg syndrome.

Ethyl Chloride. This vapocoolant spray is useful for Spray and Stretch treatment (see chapter 19), to inhibit pain impulses, and to aid passive stretching (see Gebauer in "Products" section of Appendix A: Resources).

Flexeril (cyclobenzaprine). This may ease spasms, twitches, and muscle tightness. It generates stage-four sleep, but it may cause gastric upset and feelings of detachment.

Guaifenesin. This is the active ingredient in many expectorants, and is being used experimentally to treat FMS (see chapter 15). Unfortunately, most of the OTC guaifenesin preparations contain sugar and alcohol, and may also contain pseudoephredine. These should be avoided. The pure form is available by prescription, and OTC from Hyrex (see Resources).

Inderal (propranolol HCl). This medication can help reduce pain, although it may also lower blood pressure. Antacids block its effect.

Klonopin (klonazepam).). This is an antianxiety, anticonvulsive, and antispasmodic medication. It may ease muscle twitching, restless leg syndrome, and teeth grinding.

Lidocaine, intravenous. Studies have shown that, in animals, intravenous lidocaine can provide prolonged relief of some types of allodynia (where an ordinarily painless stimulus is experienced as painful).[45]

Neurontin (gabapentin). This anticonvulsant is effective for hyperalgesia (excessive sensitivity to pain) and allodynia (experiencing pain from an ordinarily nonpainful stimulus).[46] You may be able to lessen any side effects by drinking extra water. As dosage increases, bioavailability *decreases*. A 400 mg dose is about 25 percent less bioavailable than a 100 mg dose. This medication should not be discontinued abruptly.

NMDA (N-methyl-D-aspartate) inhibitors. Chronic pain due to nerve or soft tissue injury may result in the sensitization of the central nervous system, caused partly by excitatory amino acids glutamate and aspartate. NMDA antagonists can moderate or eliminate effects like secondary hyperalgesia,[47] and may be effective in the treatment of some types of chronic pain.[48] NMDA inhibitors include ketamine, dextromethorphan, memantine, amantadine, methadone, dextropropoxyphene, and ketobemidone. Ketamine reduces pain in a subgroup of FMS patients.[49] Dextromethorphan, an ingredient in some cough medicines, can inhibit skin hyperalgesia which can develop after trauma.[50] There have been reports of sexual dysfunction from dextromethorphan,[51] and it can temporarily stop bowel motility and add to mental fogginess.

Opioids. Because of the fact that some doctors still consider the use of opioids to be controversial for treating FMS and CMP, these medications are covered in a separate section later in this chapter.

Pamelor (nortriptyline HCl). This tricyclic antidepressant is used to help patients with insomnia. Some people find it stimulating, however, and must take it in the morning to allow restorative sleep that night. There have been some reports of it causing depression.

Paxil (paroxetine HCl). This serotonin reuptake inhibitor may also reduce pain, and has been found helpful for menopausal hot flashes (see chapter 11). Some people find it stimulating, and they must take it in the morning to allow for sleep that night.

Piracetam. This is an extract of ginko biloba. It may step up the flow of messages between the two halves of the brain. It may stimulate the cerebral cortex and increase the rate of metabolism and energy level of brain cells.

Procaine injection for TrPs. Trigger point injection protocols can be found in Travell and Simons' *Trigger Point Manual*s. Trigger point injections *must* be given in the proper manner, with the patient properly positioned for *each specific muscle*, and performed *with* bodywork (see chapter 22). Perpetuating factors must be addressed for lasting effects. Trigger point injections are *not* to be done with steroids.

Relafen (nabumetone). This NSAID (nonsteroidal anti-inflammatory drug) may be better tolerated than others because it is absorbed by the intestine, thus sparing the stomach.

Remeron (mirtazapine). This antidepressant is unrelated to SSRIs, tricyclics, or MAO inhibitors. It seems to cause fewer occurrences of common side effects.

Restoril (temazepam). This hypnotic may be useful for improving sleep. There have been few reports of "hangover" effect.

Serzone (nefazodone HCl). This antidepressant is unrelated to SSRIs, tricyclics, or MAO inhibitors, and is prescribed for FMS symptoms. *Caution: It has a low bioavailability, which may vary considerably. It may cause a drug reaction with other medications.*

Sinequan (doxepin HCl). This tricyclic antidepressant and antihistamine combination can produce marked sedation effects. It may enhance the effects of Klonopin, and can reduce muscle twitching by itself.

Soma (carisoprodol). This helps patients to detach themselves from their pain, and can moderate the sensory overload of FMS. This central nervous system muffler works rapidly, but it should not be used as the only pain control. Except for the rare patient with sensitivity to it, it is well tolerated. There have been some reports of dependency. Soma may cause drowsiness and raises the seizure threshold. It is not recommended for children under twelve years old. It can cause respiratory depression given in conjunction with propoxyphene. Studies show the treatment of FMS with the combination of carisoprodol, acetaminophen, and caffeine is effective.[52]

Sonata (zaleplon). This is a short-term-acting hypnotic. You can take it at bedtime or even later on those nights you have difficulty sleeping. You do need four hours to sleep it off. It doesn't cause rebound insomnia or withdrawal symptoms when discontinued.[53]

Ultram (tramadol HCl). This medication for moderate to severe pain acts on the central nervous system. Side effects may be constipation, nausea, dizziness, headaches, weariness, tightening of jaw and neck muscles, and vomiting. Some doctors have reported psychological addiction to Ultram that is even harder to break than a narcotic addiction. This medication can lower the seizure threshold.

Wellbutrin (bupropion HCl). This antidepressant is sometimes used in FMS, but it can promote seizures.

Xanax (alprazolam). This benzodiazepine is used for anxiety, panic disorder, muscle tension, and autonomic nervous system hyperactivity. It raises the seizure threshold. It must not be used during pregnancy. If you stop taking it, taper off gradually.

Zanaflex (tizantidine hydrochloride). This muscle relaxant may help with restless leg syndrome. It may help to reduce muscle tightness, and may have sedative effects. This is another medication you may have to take just before bed, as there have been reports of loss of muscle control. Some patients also have mentioned hallucinatory effects.

Zofran (ondansetron). This medication appears to be effective in about 50 percent of primary FMS patients, according to one clinical study.[54] The response was not the same with posttraumatic FMS.

Zoloft (sertraline HCl). This medication is commonly used to help with sleep problems. There have been several reports of night sweats with strong ammonia odor. It may be useful to relieve symptoms of PMS.[55]

Note: Most people who find Benedryl stimulating rather than sedating seem to have the same response to Pamelor, Paxil, and Ultram. I don't know why, but I suspect it may be a clue to one subset of FMS.

Medications and Pain

It is the rule rather than the exception that patients with FMS and CMP save strong pain medications prescribed for use after surgery or injury for those times when they *really* need painkillers. This is one indication of an inadequate medication program (see chapter 9). Too often readers write, "My doctor would not prescribe this medication because he said it is too hard to get someone off it." It has been my experience that it's very hard to stop taking a medication that will relieve your pain. It's nearly as hard as trying to figure out why any doctor in his/her right mind would want to do so.

Some doctors believe that opioids are inappropriate for treatment of FMS and CMP. I have never heard a logical argument to support that belief. Some of these doctors have come down hard on the fact that I have information on opioids in my books. They say that opioids are not approved for chronic noncancer pain. They claim there is no basis in the literature for the use of opioids in treating FMS and CMP. These same doctors will probably go ballistic, but I include this information and these references because my readers tell me that their doctors are denying them access to these medications.

In the best of all possible worlds, early FMS and single TrPs would be promptly diagnosed and treated. In our present reality, central nervous system sensitization and the hypersensitivity to pain of FMS coupled with the pain generated by TrPs can make this world a living hell for patients who have not been promptly diagnosed and treated.

Slowly but surely health care providers are becoming better educated in the early diagnosis and treatment of FMS and CMP. With the aid of central nervous system modifiers currently being developed, topical T3 (see chapter 15), topical calcium channel blockers, guaifenesin, bodywork, lifestyle modifications, mindwork, and attention to perpetuating factors including diet, in the future opioids might not be needed to treat FMS and CMP. However, we must deal with reality as it is today. *Pain control is imperative to reduce any further sensitization of the central nervous system, as well as to allow some of these auxiliary therapies to be provided without adding additional shock to the pain-sensing system.* It hurts when your body is undergoing massive readjustment and alignment, even when this realignment is a positive change.

I am not advocating the use of opioids as a first line method of pain control, or as the singular method of pain control. *When other options have failed, medical literature documents that opioids, in conjunction with a thorough pain control program including bodywork, mindwork, and lifestyle adjustment, are a logical and humane option in the treatment of severe FMS and CMP.* If some doctors don't agree with these references, they can argue with them, or refuse to read them, but they can't say that they don't exist.

Opioids

The word "narcotics" is often confused with the term "illegal substances." The term "opioids" is preferred, as it does not, and should not, carry negative connotations. Who makes the judgment as to how much pain relief is enough? Is it adequate pain control if all you can do is whimper in the corner? When does ability to function come into play? There is no way any doctor can give a numerical objective value to someone else's pain level, as can be done with cholesterol level or blood pressure. Numerical scales are comparative and there is no way of judging what your base line of pain is.

Sometimes, narcotic analgesics are more easily tolerated than NSAIDs. Prolonged use of narcotics can result in physiological changes of tolerance or physical dependence, but these are not the same as psychological dependence. Presently the world of chronic noncancer pain management is ruled by outmoded ideas and myths. The word "addictive" seems to be imbedded in some heads, and the word "effective" doesn't seem to be an issue. I am not asking anyone to take my word on this. The rest of this section is culled from my readings in medical journals. There are many more statements I would have liked to include, but there is only so much space. For more information on this subject, see *The Fibromyalgia Advocate*.[56]

- Opioids taken to relieve chronic noncancer pain can enhance mood without impairing mental function.[57]

- There are times when opioids are the only logical option for relief of chronic noncancer pain, but these must be used appropriately.[58]

- Studies show that instead of fogging the mind, the appropriate dosage of opioids, even morphine, may help clear the mind by removing the distraction of pain.[59]

- High levels of opioid use are not linked with greater incidence of disability or depression.[60]

- Patients with chronic pain may suffer needlessly because of lack of doctor training, prejudice, and politics concerning the use of opioids.[61]

- Of the effective medications now available, appropriate opioids may cause the least danger from side effects.[62]

- When a patient is in chronic pain, the focus must be to restore patient function with minimal pain, not to eliminate opioids. Opioids are of use to chronic pain patients to restore function, not impair it.[63]

- Addiction behaviors are not common in chronic pain patients.[64]

- State laws often impede appropriate use of opioids by regulations on prescriptions such as multiple-copy requirements.[65]

- The combination of morphine and the NMDA inhibitor dextromethorphan (MS:DM) provides twice the pain relief of the morphine dose in a longer-lasting and faster-acting form, and appears safe for chronic pain conditions.[66]

There are possible side effects with opioids, and some people do have a tendency toward becoming addicted, but, according to these and many other references, this is fairly uncommon in chronic pain patients. Opioids often slow intestinal motility. Measures should be taken to prevent constipation. Temporary sleepiness and confusion is common during the first forty-eight hours or so after initial opioid therapy, and after an increase in dose. Nausea may occur for the first three or four days of therapy.

Some opioids are available in suppository form if nausea and vomiting occur. Transdermal patches are also available. The liquid form may be very useful because of the ease with which you can vary the dose. For example, hydromorphone hydrochloride 5 mg per ml is available. It also has 100 mg guaifenesin per dose with it, because this formulation was designed as a cough syrup. Hydromorphone, the opioid component, is a cough suppressant. My doctor suggests this dosage for moderate chronic pain control in appropriate cases, because it isn't combined with NSAIDS, and she wants to avoid the potential side effects of NSAIDS. On days when pain is severe you may need to use a full dose, but on good days you can take a lesser amount. Codeine and codeine-like substances such as hydrocodone require an enzyme, CYP2D6, to break them down into their working metabolite. Some drugs, such as Prozac, Darvon, Lamasil, Haldol, and Paxil suppress this enzyme. Care providers should be aware of this interaction, and discuss options with the pharmacist. Higher dosages may be required. This interaction may be partly responsible for the mistaken belief that opioids don't work in FMS.[67]

Marijuana and Other Cannabinoids

Marijuana is illegal. I believe that one objection to marijuana is that it is uncontrollable. Anyone can grow it. Nobody makes a profit. It is tremendously variable in strength. People need to learn to use it wisely. It needs to be studied honestly, without prejudice. Little of that has been done. I offer the following:

- There is a sizable quantity of medical literature supporting the use of marijuana pharmaceuticals for chronic and acute pain. They offer selective suppression of pain neurotransmission.[68]

- Studies show that over the long term, there are no significant differences in loss of permanent cognitive function between users and nonusers of marijuana.[69]

- One study proposes a six-month trial program of prescription-controlled marijuana use for chronic pain and other indications. This would help gather evidence for possible FDA approval.[70]

FMS and Antibiotics

I, like many others in the health care community, am concerned about the increasing inappropriate use of antibiotics. There are many symptoms of FMS and CMP that might appear to be due to infection if the treating doctor is untrained in the scope of these conditions. The neuroendocrine nature of FMS means that the hypothalamus is often dysregulated, and fevers or low body temperature may occur in cycles. Many neurotransmitters such as histamine may be dysregulated, as well as many hormones, and some of these may cause symptoms that appear to be similar to infectious agents.

The answer for the situation described above may be to check for lack of restorative sleep, and to find a lifestyle change and/or medications that will enable the return of delta sleep, *not* to dose the patient with repeated antibiotics. The effects of CMP on the autonomic nervous system may also mimic infectious symptoms, and some of the direct TrP effects may also. One person I know was in the hospital being treated with intravenously administered antibiotics for meningitis, when what she had were TrPs in the levator scapulae and facial muscles.

Fibromyalgia or CMP may be initiated, perpetuated, or aggravated by infections. If an infection is the precipitating or perpetuating stressor, a course of the specific antibiotic, antiviral, or antifungal systemic to which the organism is sensitive is appropriate. *This does not mean that the infectious organism per se causes either FMS or CMP*; it simply means that the effect of any stressor *may* start the neuroendocrine cascade of FMS or the TrP cascade of CMP. It is important to make this distinction.

Recently, researchers have uncovered other reasons how antibiotics may work in other ways to help someone feel better, without an infection being present. The antibiotic minocycline can significantly slow the progression of Huntington's disease, an illness that we know is caused by autosomal dominant genetics. Minocycline indirectly inhibits caspase regulation. Caspases are enzymes encoded by genes, and the genes are affected by the minocycline.[71] Without the benefit of this research and the knowledge of the mechanics of Huntington's, it would seem that there was some organism causing Huntington's, because it responds to the antibiotic. It is very easy to break a leg leaping to conclusions.

I have seen many cases where the overuse or inappropriate use of antibiotics and the results (yeast or other fungi/bacterial infection) were responsible for initiating either the neuroendocrine cascade of FMS or the TrP cascade of CMP. I want to be absolutely clear about this. *Neither antibiotics nor steroids are to be given routinely for FMS or CMP.* They are to be used the same way as in patients with other nonautoimmune chronic pain conditions: carefully, and with respect, and only with due cause. I have seen many people who had their lives ruined by overuse or improper use of antibiotics. There is a clear and present danger in the emergence of resistant strains of pathogenic organisms due to the overuse of antibiotics.

Maintenance Costs of FMS and CMP

Most health insurance policies do not cover all health care costs, especially supplements and some medications. The cost of medications keeps rising. As our daily newspapers keep reminding us, we are in a health care crisis. We have not focused on preventive medicine and healthy lifestyles, concentrating instead on treating disease. I believe that is one reason that FMS and CMP are so widespread today. Our medical care providers have been trying to "stamp out fires," but if they look up they will see that the roof is ablaze and ready to collapse on us all.

According to Congressman Bernard Sanders of Vermont, the average elderly person pays 81 percent more than Canadian consumers for prescription drugs (quoted in the *Brattleboro Reformer,* July 29, 1999). Something has to give, and chronic pain patients just can't give any more. The most common reason patients don't take their prescribed medication (or don't take it as often as prescribed) is financial. There may be some resources available, however, if you are willing and able to jump through the paperwork hoops.

The Directory of Prescription Drug Patient Assistance Program is available free. Call 202-835-3400 to obtain a copy. Or look it up on the Internet. This directory will give you the name of pharmaceutical companies that will supply free medication for those in need. Talk to your doctor about this program. If you or a companion can do the bulk of the paperwork, and you can prove your financial need, you may be able to get at least some of your medications free. Most doctors' offices can't deal with the paperwork that pharmaceutical companies require, although your doctor must send in the initial request. The newest and most expensive medications may not be offered, but your doctor and/or pharmacist may be able to find an alternative. If it works, go for it. It may take a while for you to get the financial aid you need.

Many states have prescription-assistance programs for low-income residents. Ask for help from your local research librarian to research this possibility. If you are over fifty years of age, check with the AARP (see Resources). They are a great resource and are concerned about their members' needs. Veterans may be eligible for low-cost medication even if their illness isn't service-related. Contact the Department of Veterans' Affairs, toll-free, 800-222-8387, or contact the nearest VA facility in the phone book. The price of medications can be staggering, and we have enough balance problems. One of the best ways to cut down on medication expenses is to identify your perpetuating factors and get them under control.

Because physicians' understanding of FMS and CMP has been so slow and is still so incomplete, information about effective medications is also incomplete. It is essential to find a physician and pharmacist who understand that your pain is real and should be addressed with appropriate medications. Your medications must be tailored to your specific symptoms and must also be monitored to meet your changing needs.

Endnotes

1. Fasmer, B. 1990. [Do antidepressive agents have analgesic effects?] *Tidsskr Nor Laegeforen* 110(18:2370-2. [Norwegian]

2. Fishbain, D. 2000. Evidence-based data on pain relief with antidepressants. *Ann Med* 32(5):305-316.

3. Haller, C. A., and N. L. Benowitz. 2000. Adverse cardiovascular and central nervous system events associated with dietary supplements containing ephedra alkaloids. *N Engl J Med* 343(25):1833-1838.

4. Lipman, A. G. 1987. Effects of smoking on drug therapy. *Mod Med* 55:185-186.

5. Ameer, B., and R. A. Weintraub. 1997. Drug interaction with grapefruit juice. *Clin Pharmacokinet* 33(2):103-121.

6. Cardona Pera, D. 1999. [Drug-food interactions.] *Nutr Hosp* 14(Suppl 2):129S-140S. [Spanish]

7. Barth, C. A., K. E. Scholz-Ahrens, M. de Vrese, and A. Hotze. 1990. Differences of plasma amino acids following casein or soy protein intake; significance for differences of serum lipid concentrations. *J Nutri Sci Vitaminol (Tokyo)* Oct. 26(Suppl 2):S111-117.

8. Lowe, J. 2000. *The Metabolic Treatment of Fibromyalgia*. Boulder CO: McDowell Publishing Company, pp. 981-986.

9. *Ibid.*, p. 809.

10. Wheatley, D. 1999. Hypericum in seasonal affective disorder (SAD). *Curr Med Res Opin* 15(1):33-37.

11. Fugh-Berman, A., and J. M. Cott. 1999. Dietary supplements and natural products as psychotherapeutic agents. *Psychosom Med* 61(5):712-728.

12. Zink, T., and J. Chaffin. 1998. Herbal "health" products: what family physicians need to know. *Am Fam Physician* 58(5):1133-1140.

13. *Ibid.*

14. Lanhers, M. C., J. Fleurentin, F. Mortier, A. Vinche, and C. Younos. 1992. Anti-inflammatory and analgesic effects of an aqueous extract of Harpagophytum procumbens. *Planta Med* 58(2):117-123.

15. Chen, S., Y. Sun, X. Chen, et al. 1997. [Effects of Jiangtangkang on blood glucose, sensitivity of insulin and blood viscosity in non-insulin dependent diabetes mellitus.] *Chung Kuo Chung Hsi Chieh Ho Tsa Chih* 17(11):666-668. [Chinese]

16. Fugh-Berman, A., and J. M. Cott. 1999. *Op cit.*

17. Ozgocmen, S., S. A. Catal, O. Ardicoglu, and A. Kamanli. 2000. Effect of omega-3 fatty acids in the management of fibromyalgia syndrome. *Int. J Clin Pharm Ther* 38(7):362-363.

18. Striffler, J. S., J. S. Law, M. M. Polansky, S. J. Bhathena, and R. A. Anderson. 1995. Chromium improves insulin response to glucose in rats. *Metabolism* 44(10):1314-1320.

19. Anderson, R. A. 1992. Chromium, glucose tolerance, and diabetes. *Biol Trace Elem Res* 32:19-24.

20. Sahelian, R., and S. Borken. 1998. Dehydroepiandrosterone and cardiac arrhythmia. *Ann Intern Med* 129(7):588.

21. Birdsall, T. C. 1998. 5-Hydroxytryptophan: a clinically-effective serotonin precursor. *Altern Med Rev* 3(4):271-280.

22. Ng, E. H., C. Y. Ji, P. H. Tan, V. Lin, K. C. Soo, and K. O. Lee. 1998. Altered serum levels of insulin-like growth-factor binding proteins in breast cancer patients. *Ann Surg Oncol* 5(2):194-201.

23. Bennett, R. 1998. Disordered growth hormone secretion and fibromyalgia: a review of recent findings and a hypothesized etiology. *Z Rheumatol* 57(Suppl 2):72-76

24. Dinser, R., T. Halama, and A. Hoffman. 2000. Stringent endocrinological testing reveals subnormal growth hormone secretion in some patients with fibromyalgia syndrome but rarely severe growth hormone deficiency. *J Rheumatol* 27(10):2482-2488.

25. Lowe. 2000. *Op. cit.*

26. Russell, I. J., J. E. Michalek, J. D. Fletchas, and G. E. Abraham. 1995. Treatment of fibromyalgia syndrome with Super Malic; a randomized, double-blind, placebo-controlled, crossover pilot study. *J Rheumatol* 22(5):953-958.

27. Citera, G., M. A. Arias, J. A. Maldonado-Cocco, M. A. Lazaro, M. G. Rosemffet, L. I. Brusco, et al. 2000. The effect of melatonin in patients with fibromyalgia: a pilot study. *Clin Rheumatol* 19(1):9-13.

28. Wikner, J., U. Hirsch, L. Wetterberg, and S. Rojdmark. 1998. Fibromyalgia: a syndrome associated with decreased nocturnal melatonin secretion. *Clin Endocrinol (Oxf)* 49(2):179-183.

29. Lapin, I. P., S. M. Mirzaev, I. V. Ryzov, and G. F. Oxenkrug. 1998. Anticonvulsant activity of melatonin against seizures induced by quinolinate, kainate, glutamate, NMDA, and pentylenetetrazole in mice. *J Pineal Res* 24(4):215-218.

30. Leach, M. W., D. W. Frank, M. R. Berardi, E. W. Evans, R. C. Johnson, D. G. Schuessler, et al. 1999. Renal changes associated with naproxen sodium administration in cynomolgus monkey. *Toxicol Pathol* 27(3):295-306.

31. Singh, G., D. R. Ramey, D. Morfeld, H. Shi, H. T. Hatoum, and J. F. Fries. 1996. Gastrointestinal tract complications of nonsteroidal anti-inflammatory drug treatment in rheumatoid arthritis. A prospective observational cohort study. *Arch Intern Med* 156(14):1530-1536.

32. Banovac, K., K. Renfree, A. L. Makowski, L. L. Latta, and R. D. Altman. 1995. Fracture healing and mast cells. *J Orthop Trauma* 9(6):482-490.

33. McAdam, B. F., H. Volkmann, J. Norregaard, S. Jacobsen, B. Danneskiold-Samsoe, G. Knoke, et al. 1997. Double-blind, placebo-controlled cross-over study of intravenous A-adenosyl-L-methionine in patients with fibromyalgia. *Scand J Rheumatol* 26(3):206-211.

34. Jung, A. C., T. Staiger, and M. Sullivan. 1997. The efficacy of selective serotonin reuptake inhibitors for the management of chronic pain. *J Gen Intern Med* 12(6):384-389.

35. Starlanyl, D. *The Fibromyalgia Advocate*. 1998. Oakland, CA: New Harbinger Publications.

36. Banahan, B. F., III, and E. M. Kolassa. 1997. A physician survey on generic drugs and substitution of critical dose medications. *Arch Intern Med* 157(18):2080-2088.

37. Catalano, E., and K. Hardin. 1996. *The Chronic Pain Control Workbook*. Oakland, CA: New Harbinger.

38. McCaffery, M., and C. Paseo. 1999. *Pain: Clinical Manual*. St. Louis: Mosby.

39. Moldofsky, H., F. A. Lue, C. Mously, B. Roth-Schechter, and W. J. Reynolds. 1996. The effect of zolpidem [Ambien] in patients with fibromyalgia: a dose-ranging, double-blind, placebo-controlled, modified cross-over study. *J Rheumatol* 23(3):529-533.

40. Dement, W. C., and C. Vaughan. 1999. *The Promise of Sleep*. New York: Delacorte Press.

41. Soyka, M., R. Bottlender, and H. J. Moller. 2000. Epidemiological evidence for a low abuse potential of zolpidem. *Pharmacopsychiatry* 33(4):138-141.

42. Wagner, M. L., A. S. Walters, R. G. Coleman, W. A. Hening, K. Grasing, and S. Choroverty. 1996. Randomized, double-blind, placebo-controlled study of clonidine in restless legs syndrome. *Sleep* 19(1):52-58.

43. Anderberg, U. M., I. Marteinsdottir, and L. von Knorring. 2000. Citalopram [Celexa] in patients with fibromyalgia—a randomized, double-blind, placebo-controlled study. *Eur J Pain* 4(1):27-35.

44. McAcadam, B. F., F. Catella-Lawson, I. A. Mardini, S. Kapoor, J. A. Lawson, and G. A. FitzGerald. 1999. Systemic biosynthesis of prostacyclin by cyclooxygenase (COX)-2: the human pharmacology of a selective inhibitor of COX-2. *PNAS* 96(1):272-277.

45. Chaplan, S. R., F. W. Bach, S. L. Shafer, and T. L. Yaksh. 1995. Prolonged alleviation of tactile allodynia by intravenous lidocaine in neuropathic rats. *Anesthesiology* 83(4):775-785.

46. Attal, N., L. Brasseur, F. Parker, M. Chauvin, and D. Bouhassira. 1998. Effects of gabapentin on the different components of peripheral and central neuropathic pain syndromes: a pilot study. *Eur Neurol* 40(4):191-200.

47. Oestreicher, M. K., J. Desmeules, V. Piguet, A. F. Allaz, and P. Dayer. 1998. [Genetic and environmental effects of neuromodulation and the antinociceptive effect of dextromethorphan.] *Schweiz Med Wochenschr* 128(6):212-215. [German]

48. Sang, C. N. 2000. NMDA-receptor antagonists in neuropathic pain: experimental methods to clinical trials. *J Pain Symptom Manage* 19(1 Suppl)S:21-25.

49. Graven-Nielsen, T., K. S. Aspegren, K. G. Henriksson, M. Bengtsson, J. Sorensen, A. Johnson, et al. 2000. Ketamine reduces muscle pain, temporal summation, and referred pain in fibromyalgia patients. *Pain* 85(3):483-491.

50. McConaghy, P. M., P. McSorley, W. McCaughey, and W. I. Campbell. 1998. Dextromethorphan and pain after total abdominal hysterectomy. *Br J Anaesth* 81(5):731-736.

51. Rafols, A., J. A. Garcia Vicente, M. Farre, and M. Mas. 1999. [Dextromethorphan-induced sexual dysfunction]. *Aten Primaria* 24(8):495-497. [Spanish]

52. Vaeroy, H., A. Abrahamsen, O. Forre, and E. Kass. 1989. Treatment of fibromyalgia (fibrositis syndrome): a parallel double-blind trial with carisoprodol, paracetamol and caffeine (Somadril comp) versus placebo. *Clin Rheumatol* 8(2):245-250.

53. Elie, R., E. Ruther, I. Farr, G. Emilien, and E. Salinas. 1999. Sleep latency is shortened during 4 weeks of treatment with zaleplon, a novel nonbenzodiazepine hypnotic. Zaleplon Clinical Study Group. *J Clin Psychiatry* 60(8):536-544.

54. Hrycaj, P., T. Stratz, P. Mennet, and W. Muller. 1996. Pathogenic aspects of responsiveness to ondansetron [Zofran] (5-hydroxytryptamine type 3 receptor antagonist) in patients with primary fibromyalgia syndrome—a preliminary study. *J Rheumatol* 23(8):1418-1423.

55. Yonkers, K. A., U. Halbreich, E. Freeman, C. Brown, J. Endicott, E. Frank, et al. 1997. Symtomatic improvement of premenstrual dysphoric disorder with sertraline treatment. A randomized controlled trial. Sertraline Premenstrual Dysphoric Collaborative Study Group. *JAMA* 278(12):98393-8.

56. Starlanyl. 1998. *Op. cit.*

57. Haythornthwaite, J. A., L. A. Menefee, A. L. Quatrano-Piacentini, and M. Pappagallo. 1998. Outcome of chronic opioid therapy for non-cancer pain. *J Pain Symptom Manage* 15(3):185-194.

58. Shannon, C. N., and A. P. Baranowski. 1997. Use of opioids in non-cancer pain. *Br J Hosp Med* 58(9):459-463.

59. Lorenz, J., H. Beck, and B. Bromm. 1997. Cognitive performance, mood and experimental pain before and during morphine-induced analgesia in patients with chronic non-malignant pain. *Pain* 73(3):369-375.

60. Ciccone, D. S., N. Just, E. B. Bandilla, E. Reimer, M. S. Ilbeigi, and W. Wu. 2000. Psychological correlates of opioid use in patients with chronic nonmalignant pain: a preliminary test of the downhill spiral hypothesis. *J Pain Symptom Manage* 20(3):180-192.

61. McQuay, H. 1999. Opioids in pain management. *Lancet* 353(9171):2229-2232.

62. Horning, M. R. 1997. Chronic opioids: a reassessment. *Alaska Med* 39(4):103-110.

63. Seas, K. L., and H. W. Clark. 1993. Opioid use in the treatment of chronic pain: assessment of addiction. *J Pain Symptom Manage* 8(5):257-264.

64. Fishbain, D. A., R. Cutler, H. L. Rosomoff, and R. S. Rosomoff. 1999. Chronic pain disability exaggeration/malingering and submaximal effort research. *Clin J Pain* 15(4):244-274.

65. Shapiro, R. S. 1994. Legal bases for the control of analgesic drugs. *J Pain Symptom Manage* 9(3):153-159.

66. Dickenson, A. H. 1997. NMDA receptor antagonists: interactions with opioids. *Acta Anaesthesiol Scan* 41(1 pt 2):112-115.

67. Walker, J. M., A. G. Hohmann, W. J. Martin, N. M. Strangman, S. M. Huang, and K. Tsou. 1999. The neurobiology of cannabinoid analgesia. *Life Sci* 65(6-7):665-673.

68. Supernaw, R. 2000. CYP2D6 and the efficiency of codeine and codeine-like drugs. *J Am Acad Pain Manage* 11(1):30–31.

69. Lyketsos, C. G., E. Garrett, K. Y. Liang, and J. C. Anthony. 1999. Cannabis use and cognitive decline in persons under 65 years of age. *Am J Epidemiol* 149(9):794-800.

70. Hollister, L. E. 2000. An approach to the medical marijuana controversy. *Drug Alcohol Depend* 58(1-2):3-7.

71. Chen, M. V., O. Ona, M. Li, R. J. Ferrante, K. B. Fink, S. Zhu, et al. 2000. Minocycline inhibits caspase-1 and caspase-3 expression and delays mortality in a transgenic model of Huntington's disease. *Nat Med* 6(7): 797-801.

CHAPTER 22

Complementary Medicine

Basic Western allopathic medicine doesn't know everything about the healing process. No discipline does. Admitting that there are some things you don't know is the first step to greater knowledge. Why waste time reinventing the wheel if someone else has already perfected the radial tire? Some alternative/complementary forms of treatment are presented here, but there are now so many that, clearly, we can't cover them all. See the Reading List and the Resource section for more sources.

Complimentary Disciplines

Medical care is changing. Now, there is often a focus on preventive medicine, as well as on curing disease. The arts of observation and taking a medical history, almost lost in the world of hi-tech medical practice, are once again gaining respect. To find the best complementary medical program for yourself, you may wish to look into several ways you can support your own healing. When choosing different disciplines to explore, try to keep an open mind. You never know when something will work for you, so a flexible and open approach can be very helpful You may need to educate your primary care physician and your insurance company, so there are some references included in this chapter to help you in your self-advocacy. Studies show that it is appropriate and sound practice to allow patients access to multiple pain therapies.[1] If health care providers offer guidance, patients are responsible health care consumers.[2]

Acupuncture

There are many types and varieties of acupuncture. Classical acupuncture teaches that wherever there is pain, the chi (life force and energy) is not flowing freely. For the free flow of informational substances, e.g., neurotransmitters, to take place between muscles and connective tissue, the free flow of chi is essential. Acupuncture may be effective for treating both osteoarthritis and fibromyalgia (FMS).[3] For some FMS patients, ten to fourteen acupuncture sessions seem to provide benefits.[4]

Electroacupuncture is effective in relieving symptoms of FMS.[5] Relevant acupuncture combined with heat contributes to modest pain reduction in myofascial neck pain.[6] Functional MRI (magnetic resonance imaging), which maps the brain at work, shows that there is a correlation between specific acupuncture points and the area of the brain connected to functions associated with those specific acupuncture points.[7]

I enjoyed reading *A New American Acupuncture: Acupuncture Osteopathy*, by Mark Seem.[8] It was delightful to read an acupuncture book for patients written by someone trained by Janet Travell in trigger points (TrPs). This author practices meridian acupuncture from a myofascial perspective. During an acupuncture session, as in myofascial TrP injection therapy, when the needle hits a TrP, the myofascia actually "grabs" the needle. In acupuncture, this is called *de chi* or "arrival of chi." Dr. Seem believes that his method of acupuncture accomplishes the same results as myofascial release, and will free myofascial blood vessel, lymph, and nerve entrapments. He has observed that when laboratory tests rule out visceral causes of abdominal symptoms, many physicians erroneously assume that the symptoms are psychosomatic, whereas they are often caused by soft tissue problems. Dr. Seem generally treats chronic pain patients only once a week, as the tissue needs time to heal between treatments. Before beginning any acupuncture treatment, first check to ensure that the National Certification Commission for Acupuncture and Oriental Medicine certifies your practitioner.

Ayurveda

Ayurvedic medicine originated in ancient India. It is based on balancing spiritual and physical activities. Ayurvedic belief holds that illness may be an expression of your life and how you react to what life gives you. Some of the exercises are similar to the asanas (postures) of hatha yoga. Ayurvedic practitioners also use herbal medicine, massage, meditation, and aromatherapy. Using a mix of lifestyle changes, diet modifications, purification practices (including the use of herbal laxatives, enemas, therapeutic vomiting, and bloodletting), and harmonic balancing of the five elements—earth, air, fire, water, and ether—Ayurveda practices are aimed at harmonizing the balance between your body and mind, so that your body can heal itself.

You might want to try the use of a "netti-pot," an Ayurvedic long-spouted pot that is used to irrigate the nasopharangeal and sinus areas with salt water (see chapter 8). For more information on Ayurveda, contact www.ayurvedic-association.org.

> I know exactly where I'd be without chiropractic medicine—in a lot more pain. If I'm going on a trip or planning something that will place unusual stress on my body, I visit my chiropractor before I leave for the trip. I do everything to ensure that I am in the best possible condition *before* I tackle something difficult—chiropractic can be great preventive medicine. I also schedule an appointment following a stressful activity. My body needs that alignment help before it can begin to heal itself.

Chiropractic

Chiropractic medicine is based on the fundamental idea that if the bones (especially the spinal column) and muscles of the body are in proper alignment, the recuperative powers inherent in the body will take over, and the body will heal itself. Chiropractors are *doctors* who are also bodyworkers. They often refer patients to an M.D. or to another health care specialist, but unfortunately, this process is rarely reversed.

This is sad, considering the mounting evidence that many patients are greatly helped by chiropractic care. Such care is seldom covered by insurance, although some policies do offer a chiropractic rider. Chiropractic practice is well integrated with other therapies. For example, chiropractors often can straighten extremely tight areas so that other bodyworkers can then loosen extremely tight myofascia. My chiropractor helps me to maintain a high level of function.

Studies have shown that chiropractic management of FMS can improved patients' range of motion and reported pain levels,[9] although I believe some of this study pertains to chronic myofascial pain (CMP) rather than to FMS. Another study suggests a role for chiropractic care in the management of FMS.[10]

One study found that spinal manipulation has a significant positive effect in cases of headache caused by tight neck muscles.[11] Chiropractic treatment as the primary therapy achieved the same results with about the same costs after six months as physiotherapy.[12] Manipulation for relieving symptoms and enhancing spinal flexibility can be a valuable tool for low back pain.[13] Also, for women with chronic pelvic pain, chiropractic treatment can be very effective.[14]

Your first visit to a chiropractor should include a careful, detailed medical history, a thorough physical examination, and sometimes X-rays. Only then can a treatment plan be formed. Chiropractors use many methods to coax the bones back into their proper position and to ease muscle tightening, including heat, cold, vibration, and other types of bodywork discussed elsewhere in this book (see chapter 19). Electrical stimulation (see below) can be especially effective in eliminating or minimizing TrPs, and this is often part of a therapeutic chiropractic regimen. Many chiropractors can also help with exercises and nutritional advice, and many specialize in areas such as kinesiology (the study of muscles and body movement).

One gentle method used in chiropractic treatment is called blocking. Blocking can help realign your bones. In this treatment, wedges are placed under your hips, and your muscles are gently coaxed to allow the bones to slide back into place. Blocking is especially good for those of us with chronic myofascial pain (CMP). Traction usually does not provide permanent relief for CMP, since the muscles revert to the same tightness and misalignment after traction is released.

At first, chiropractic treatment may seem frustrating. For example, if you have pain in your right hip, your chiropractor may find that one leg is short due to torsion of your pelvis, so s/he will use adjustments to equalize leg length. If your left hip has been overworking and compensating for the right hip, as soon as your right hip is relieved, your left hip may start to hurt. This pain can travel back and forth, as the muscles slowly adjust to a healthier balance. Also, liberated metabolic toxins and wastes can cause you to feel ill and exhausted after a treatment, as do most successful treatments of other kinds of physical therapy. You may ache a little after the treatment and for part of the next day. Bones follow muscles, so when your bones are coaxed into alignment, tight and contracting muscles can pull them out again rather quickly. If this happens after repeated treatments, you may have a perpetuating factor that must be addressed.

Manual adjustment is the familiar "cracking" of body manipulation to align bones properly. If there is nerve entrapment, cracking can cause great (and lasting) pain. But not all chiropractors use manual manipulation for all patients. One of the kindest innovations in chiropractic medicine is the Activator.

The Activator is a small (pen-sized), handheld instrument that delivers a low-force tap where directed. It's the most widely used low-force chiropractic technique. Some people say it looks like a mini-pogo stick. (Others say it looks like a metal hypodermic without a needle.) When used expertly by a Doctor of Chiropractic Medicine, it can realign your skeleton almost instantly. The Activator works faster than the body's ability to tense and resist. Most people can tolerate Activator adjustment. If I am going to travel or do something else that usually results in activating a TrP, I make sure I get a "tune up" at my chiropractor beforehand. This often helps to prevent a great deal of distress later.

Electromagnetic Sensitivity

I have never been shy about going out on a limb. Now, I am about to levitate out from that limb. That's okay, though. From what many of you have told me, I will not be alone. If chemistry is the language of the body, electromagnetism supplies the vocabulary used. We are electromagnetic (EM) beings. Fibromyalgia is a sensory amplifier, and myofascial TrPs are points of high conductance (low resistance).[15] We are all different, in demonstrable ways. It is wise to look at the effect EM may have on us—for good or ill. We don't know what lies beyond what we can presently measure, but even what little we know gives us plenty of food for thought.

There is a phenomenon that, although not restricted to FMS and CMP, I have observed consistently in people with these conditions. For want of a better term, I call it EM sensitivity. Many of us have difficulty with electronic devices. Some of us stop watches. Some of us can't sleep if the moon is full. We are energized by electrical storms, and the noise of fluorescent lights can drive us to distraction. Some of us can feel EM fields, and we have an edge when it comes to manipulating chi energy. Animals sense this and seem to be drawn to us. Many readers have written to me about paranormal experiences, wondering if we are more in tune with other vibrations. Readers recognize "EM sensitivity." Pigeons kept in iron cages don't "home" properly. Their sense of direction becomes skewed. What happens to us in airplanes and cars?

I don't know why these things are so. I only know I have EM sensitivity to a great degree, and I can feel its presence in others. This is a mixed blessing. I seem to react to the northern lights, even when due to inclement weather I can't see them. I get a pain pattern and buzzing in my brain that is fairly specific. My myotherapist has noticed that my temporalis regions swell.

New theories give us possible clues to some of the mechanisms of EM sensitivity. Electromagnetic energy can activate a type of connective tissue cells called mast cells, causing the release of a number of biochemicals including hyaluronic acid, vasoactive intestinal polypeptide (implicated in keeping our HPA-axis in the "fight or flight" stress mode), and histamine (adds to swelling, itching, pain, allergic manifestations, and hypersensitivity). Electromagnetic energy causes other cells to release somatostatin, which can enhance sensations of inflammation and light sensitivity.[16] We know that EM fields can affect the way cell membranes interact with hormones, antibodies, and neurotransmitters.[17]

There was a study done on EM activity and the serotonin irritation syndrome.[18] The researchers (all M.D.s) who did this study found that weather-sensitive people reacted to certain types of winds that were high in EM activity. These included the fohn in Central Europe, the sharav in Israel, the sirocco in Italy, the mistral in France, the Chinook in the Rockies, and the Santa Ana in California. Signs and symptoms of these sensitivities were caused by an increase of serotonin brought about by positively charged winds. The researchers found that high-voltage lines also cause this phenomenon.

We are living in a universe of changing EM fields. Solar flares dump quantities of charged particles onto Earth. Flashes of lightning release energy bursts. The surface of Earth and the ionosphere act like the charged plates of a condenser, producing another electromagnetic field. We live inside that field. Potential interactions are staggering. If one nervous system could sense the nervous system of another, would that explain the realm of ESP? This may be why many of us with FMS and CMP seem to have an empathic sense.

Trees cast tremendous low frequency electrical fields. Some patients with FMS have reported that touching trees and living near trees help them to cope better. Bioelectromagnetics may be the future of medicine. Minute electrical fields and ionic exchange play key roles in our structural and cellular integrity and function. Earth pulses with a strong EM beat, and some animals can sense changes in the earth before earthquakes happen. Just as in my science fiction, who's to say sensitive people can't develop this hypersensitivity for good purposes?

What of chi, the vital energy called by so many names but recognized in nearly every non-Western culture? Chi energizes and organizes. We can't measure it yet, although researchers are working on it. Perhaps it exists outside the parameters we presently recognize as EM energy. These comments from recent studies may be relevant:

- Trigger point pain can be relieved successfully and promptly by local application static magnetic fields of 300 to 500 Gauss.[19]

- Exposure to electric and magnetic fields caused changes in the cerebrospinal fluid of dairy cows consistent with a weakening of the blood-brain barrier.[20]

- Humans do react to changes in the direction of Earth's magnetic field. This may be related to the sensitivity of some animals to magnetic orientation.[21]

- Microwaves can affect cognitive functions such as attention, learning, memory, and time perception.[22]

- Chronic exposure to 60-hertz electric and magnetic fields can significantly affect neurotransmitters and the biochemicals that influence their function.[23]

The magnetic Earth grid system resonates at 7.8 Hz. Do we resonate with that pulse? Evidence-based medicine is an important thing. It is also important to realize that there is more about science we don't understand than we do. Simply because we cannot measure something does not mean it does not exist. Stretching is as good for your mind as it is for your body.

Electronically Speaking

We've known that electromagnetics can be involved with the tightness of muscle ever since Dr. Willard Travell (Janet Travell's father) discovered that, if directed properly, an interrupted rhythmic electrical discharge produces a vigorous exercise of the muscle. Alternating muscular contractions and relaxations increase blood flow through the muscles. Sustained contraction, which occurs with TrPs, decreases blood flow. There are many kinds of electrical therapy, but there is no way to predict which type will work best on any specific patient. Only skilled practitioners and those they have trained should use electronic devices. Note that some gels used with electrical bodywork devices contain salicylate and/or aloe. Do not use these if you are taking guaifenesin (see chapter 21).

Electrical stimulation has positive effects on myofascial TrPs.[24] Electrotherapy for myofascial TrPs in patients with mild to moderate pain may be very effective for pain as well as muscle tightness.[25] I have observed that TENS (transcutaneous electrical nerve stimulation), does not work well for either FMS or CMP. Electrotherapy units are small (about the size of a pager) and relatively cheap, and are often used for other pain conditions. Physicians are familiar with TENS units, so they often order them for FMS and CMP patients, and then mistakenly assume that electrical stimulation of all kinds will not work on these patients. Many doctors and patients have told me that various forms of electrotherapy can worsen symptoms of FMS. Some of this may be the result of liberation of metabolic toxins and wastes. We need more research on this.

In chapter 15 of *Myofascial Pain and Fibromyalgia Trigger Point Management*,[26] Dr. Joseph Kahn writes that continuous electrical stimulation is effective for relief of myofascial TrPs, as long as the frequency is greater than 50 Hz. This produces relaxation of tense myofascial tissues and enhances production of endorphins for relief of pain. You can feel the targeted muscles contracting when you have this therapy. Microampere stimulation (Microstim) enhances the healing of damaged tissues.[27]

> When I'm in flare, I can turn on the computer from across the room. The phone beeps when I pass it. I affect electronic equipment, not always well, although I was able to get into the hospital earlier this week when the electricity was off and other people were standing around waiting for the emergency generator. Animals are attracted to me—even wild ones. Unfortunately, this includes mosquitoes and black flies. Naturally, I am interested in discovering why this is so.

Neuromuscular electronic stimulation (NMES) is also called Microstim. It delivers a very low electrical pulse through electrodes applied to the skin. It is beneficial for relaxing muscle spasms and muscle tightness, increasing circulation, and increasing the range of motion. NEMS requires a prescription and should be used only under a doctor's guidance. There are small, patient-use electrical stimulators available. When it is applied to TrPs, the stimulator assists the muscle to contract fully, and helps to relax the tightness of the myofascia. This allows for the return to a fuller range of motion (see "Products" section of Appendix A: Resources).

Interferential therapy uses two medium frequency currents of slightly different frequency, mixed in such a way to produce a single frequency equal to the difference between the two frequencies. The interference field that develops from this mix covers a fairly wide area, and can be used to enhance delivery of medications to the tissues.

There are two new treatment techniques, automated twitch-obtaining intramuscular stimulation (ATOIMS) and electrical twitch-obtaining intramuscular stimulation (ETOIMS), that can help control spinal nerve entrapment in both FMS and CMP.[28] These methods work by reducing muscle tension.

The use of ultrasound[29] and high voltage pulsed galvanic stimulation[30] to break up TrPs has been suggested. Travell and Simons theorized that rhythmical contractions may increase local blood flow and help to equalize sarcomere length, and that the galvanic stimulation may be used effectively to interrupt the pain/contraction cycle.

In cases of TrPs in localized muscle groups, the treatment regimen is relatively straightforward. Muscle stimulation should be set to patient tolerance. If FMS symptom amplification is present, patient tolerance may be quite low, so obtaining patient input is vital. The clinician must raise the setting slowly, with the gelled probe-face kept in motion over the suspected TrP area to avoid overheating the tissue in any one site. (If the probe is kept stationary, heat will build up and may burn the tissues beneath the probe.)

Craig Anderson, my chiropractic physician, has found that TrPs are often responsive to a setting of 1 to 1.5 watts/cm^2. Galvanic muscle stimulation (GMS) or ultrasound with low-volt muscle stimulation can also be used in a diagnostic "search and destroy" mode. Deep TrPs and latent TrPs will respond to this method, and can be located and broken up in this way.

With more superficial TrPs, the patient will feel either a pins and needles sensation or feel as if there were a raw sore deep inside the tissue at the site of the TrP when the probe travels over it. When the TrPs start breaking up, the muscles will need toning; they've been in the "TrP straitjacket" too long.

During the course of treatment, the pain may shift from side to side as more TrPs are revealed under the softening musculature. As the TrPs break up, they release chemical toxins. If too much therapy is done at one time, nausea and/or low-grade fever and flulike symptoms may appear. Even a five-minute treatment may leave an especially toxic patient fatigued. The patient should take it easy for the rest of the day.

Dr. Saul Liss has done work that shows neurotransmitters and neurohormonal release can be affected by electronic impulses, resulting in reduced pain levels.[31] For patients with chronic neck and shoulder pain who were not helped by conventional TENS, high frequency high energy pulses resulted in a 62 percent rapid reduction in their pain level.[32] The Liss Bipolar Body Stimulator is small and patients can be trained in its safe use (see Resources).

Warning: Electronic devices should not be used on patients with cancer, heart trouble, or seizure disorders. Also, they should not be used near patients who are wearing pacemakers. Electronic equipment should not be used in the lower trunk area of a pregnant woman, nor around the cardiac or carotid artery areas. All manufacturer contraindications and precautions should be followed.

Healing and the Arts

Never underestimate the power of creative expression. Inspiration is all around us. In one episode of *Touched by an Angel*, Della Reese's character, Tess, tells Roma Downey's character, Monica, that God never said we had to make a perfect noise unto the Lord, just a *joyful* one. So it is with all artistic expression. It is a health-giving and life-enhancing experience, and one in which we should all feel free to take part. Other cultures use the arts for healing, too. Chanting, "singing" bowls, gongs, hymns, dance, carving, and painting are all used for spiritual and healing purposes. Writing is another way to be creative and to heal.

I don't know that we'll ever be able to quantify scientifically all that the arts can do for us, but studies do show that music which evokes specific emotions can cause physiological changes that may aid relaxation and behavior therapies.[33] Sounds can profoundly influence your mood and your health. Think of the negative energy generated when someone yells at you, or if your personal space is invaded by blasting music.

Music can be a powerful motivator. If your life is "out of key," either sharp or flat, or you are out of harmony with your environment, find the right kind of music to bring you "back in tune." Dance can also promote wellness by strengthening the immune system. It helps to moderate, eliminate, or avoid tension. Dance can help the healing process as it aids in gaining a sense of control.[34]

The best book I have read on healing and the arts is *Illness and the Art of Creative Expression*,[35] by Dr. Graham-Pole. He can help you to unleash the artistic forces trapped within yourself. If you have forgotten how to have fun, this book will help you to remember. You can catch the flavor of the author's teacher, Patch Adams (he wrote the foreword), and remember how being silly can be very healing. Take this book, add laughter and creativity, mix in equal portions of adventure and delight, and enjoy!

Homeopathy

Julian Jonas, homeopathic physician, was kind enough to supply the following information:

There are several kinds of homeopathy. Constitutional homeopaths believe that the body will generate its own best possible response to a challenge, and that remedies must enhance this. In homeopathy, chronic illness symptoms are not treated per se. Homeopaths believe that drives illness deeper, and a new illness would replace the old one. They look for something unique to the patient to find the best remedy. Remedies are not substance-based. They are extreme dilutions that are said to contain the essences of the substances, that is, their vibrations, or some other quality that we cannot yet measure.

Homeopathy is based on the Law of Similars. If a healthy person experiences a certain symptom after taking a particular substance, a sick person with similar symptoms will be cured by that same substance. Homeopaths perceive an intelligence, variously called "the dynamic principle," "the dynamis," or "vital force," which is responsible for the coordination and activities of life. The greater the dilution, the stronger the remedy. To the homeopath, symptoms are an expression of the vital force of a person. They surface as an attempt by the vital force to stabilize or cleanse the entire system when it becomes disordered, but they are not the disorder itself. Ideally, when the system is adequately stabilized or cleansed, the symptoms disappear.

Sometimes in chronic or inherited conditions, the best the vital force can do is to maintain a semblance of balance by manifesting symptoms as chronic disease. It does not resolve on its own without some assistance from the vital force.

Symptoms are not the only way in which a homeopath becomes familiar with the vital force of a patient. The nature of the vital force also manifests itself in a myriad of traits, habits, or signs in every individual. These might include the types of food that a person likes or dislikes, the nature and position of sleep, temperament, and a host of other details that seem otherwise insignificant to the problem at hand. The homeopath seeks out the characteristics of a person that are unique, that are individual to that person, in order to understand the nature of his/her vital force.

Constitutional homeopathy requires giving a single medication at a time. Ten patients with asthma could be given ten different remedies. One may have attacks in the middle of the night, and another in the morning. One may have developed it after birth, and another after the death of a loved one. Once the nature of the vital force is perceived, a suitable remedy is chosen which will invigorate it. The end result will be that not only are the symptoms thrown off, but that the person feels generally healthier and more energetic.

There are practitioners who only prescribe according to the remedy that best fits the chief complaint. A variation of this method is to prescribe remedies to strengthen a particular organ or system of the body. These practitioners employ homeopathic remedies, but their model is more akin to the traditional medical approach.

Julian J. Jonas, CCH, CA, is a practicing constitutional homeopath. He can be reached at jjjonas@sover.net, or at Saxons River Natural Health Care, POB 515, Saxons River, VT 05154.

Magnets

I admit to skepticism when it comes to magnet therapy. Some people say it works, others that it doesn't. I have tried different kinds myself, including magnetic blankets, magnets on TrPs, and magnets in my shoes, and have felt no effects. Logic tells me that it should work, however, but that we don't yet know how to use it. Electromagnetic effects work on the ion channels in the body, including actin filaments in the muscles.[36] Researchers have been able to enhance DNA repair using magnetic fields.[37]

There are many different types of magnets, with different polarities. All uses are experimental. One study was done on the use of magnets in low back pain, but they had no effect.[38] In the first controlled study of magnetic therapy for chronic pelvic pain, the results suggest that magnets can provide pain relief related to the duration of magnet exposure.[39] Keep an open mind.

Native American Healing Traditions

Each Native American tribe has different, specific healing traditions, so it is impossible to generalize about their healing traditions. However, in many Native American tribes, illness is not considered a state of being but a process of transformation. You must surrender to the path you are on: there is no way out but through. Accommodate and optimize life within your limitations. Use your downtime wisely. Eventually, you will be restored to harmony. Your passage through the illness will give you a greater understanding of life, and bring wisdom. Concentrate on the discomfort instead of ignoring it; learn what it has to teach you. It will keep trying until you learn the lessons you need.

Some Native American peoples treat those individuals who are sensitive to changes to Mother Earth with respect. They are considered as having a special link to the spirit world, and may be consulted on matters of importance. Attributes of this hypersensitivity are similar to what I call "electromagnetic sensitivity," discussed earlier in this chapter. Many tribes have terms for this vital energy, similar to what the Chinese call chi. For example, the Athabascan name for this concept is *coen*.

Local heat, massage, and pressure were used therapeutically in many ancient cultures. American Indians often used such techniques as a first-line approach in many of their treatments. The medicinal manuscripts of the Cherokee give a new understanding of this tribe's healing traditions. Persimmon wood "stampers" were used as massage tools to treat rheumatism, possibly in a form of acupressure on TrPs. Hand pressure on pulsating body sites was also used to break up disease.[40]

The "Swimmer" manuscript of the Cherokee details these modalities of treatment. Typical instructions include pressing a warm palm on a colicky abdomen or using repeated thumb pressure over the site of toothache. The healer would place warmed hands on an affected abdominal area to feel the pulsations of the disease and cause it to break up under the touch.[41]

Many modern Native American shamans emphasize creative dreaming and visualization as forms of healing. Herbs, smudging with smoke, singing, and drumming are often parts of healing rituals. I know many Native Americans with FMS and CMP, and many of these people have reactive hypoglycemia as a perpetuating factor.

Naturopathic Medicine

Naturopathic doctors (NDs) have four years of medical training, which follow three years of standard pre-med studies. Naturopathic physicians use the same diagnostic techniques as allopathic physicians do, such as X-ray and laboratory testing. Naturopathy is a prevention-based style of medicine, and often uses botanicals, nutrition, homeopathy, and lifestyle counseling to help patients heal. Some NDs specialize in Ayurvedic medicine, traditional Chinese medicine, manipulation, acupuncture, or other forms of healing. Naturopaths are not licensed in many of the United States, but this is changing. There are certifying examinations given by the Council on Naturopathic Medical Education. Some insurance companies in the United States and Canada provide ND coverage.

Kathleen Janel, ND, told me that all patients with chronic invisible illnesses must be approached as individuals, even though their illnesses may have similar core features. It is important to identify the individual stressors that affect the patients, and to address them. She has observed that patients with FMS and CMP often have glands that are stressed by the constant demands of a hyperstimulated system.

She uses a twenty-four-hour periodic saliva test to determine a specific patient's cortisol fluctuations. If the adrenals are fatigued, this must be remedied before other factors can be treated. This is important, because the symptoms of excess cortisol and depleted cortisol can appear to be similar, and some patients fluctuate between the two stages. She found that blood testing isn't as accurate as saliva testing, because the stress of the blood test itself can provoke an adrenal reaction and give a misleading reading.

She finds *Siberian* ginseng helpful as a balancing agent in cases of both adrenal excess and deficiency. Vitamin B5 (pantothenic acid) is also helpful, as is buffered vitamin C. Both of these vitamins are found in high concentrations in the adrenals. Supplementation helps to replenish what has been used. She has found that the wisdom of the body will tell you how much vitamin C is needed by what the bowel will tolerate.

To find healing, a patient often must commit to significant lifestyle changes. Dietary changes are often crucial. This naturopath also has found that insulin resistance is a pervasive coexisting condition. To uncover this problem, she orders insulin levels when she does a glucose tolerance test.

Check with the American Association of Naturopathic Physicians (AANP) to find a licensed naturopath in your vicinity (see Resources).

Occupational Therapy

The phrase "occupational therapy" (OT) can be misleading. The work of OTs is not confined to the workplace, but is also for people who need help in their daily home and community life. Occupational therapy includes the restoration of disturbed muscle function and psychosocial aspects, as well as advice and training with technical aids and adapting the home and workplace according to a specific disability. The use of occupational therapy is indicated for soft tissue rheumatism.[42]

If you have CMP, it is important that your OT understands myofascial TrPs, as this will have a direct affect on your therapy. For example, you need to avoid immobility and repetition.[43] Note that there are even OTs who specialize in proprioceptor dysfunction.

Osteopathic Medicine

Doctors of Osteopathy (DOs), hold a degree equivalent to an M.D. They often share the same hospital privileges and do everything an M.D. does, including diagnosis, prescribing medications, and performing surgery. Osteopaths complete a one-year residency and then pass state licensure. Training emphasis is on palpation diagnostic skills and manual medicine, such as myofascial release, muscle energy techniques, and lymphatic drainage. Classical osteopaths avoid standard allopathic medications if possible. They rely on natural medicinals and manual medicine to help the body heal itself. Most DOs work as primary care physicians, although there are pediatricians, obstetricians, and neurologists who are also DOs.

Some DOs specialize in cranial osteopathy. Cranial osteopathy focuses on sensing and influencing the cranial rhythmic impulse. The living skull is made up of separate bones that fit together in areas called *sutures*. Layers of connective tissue surround these bones, and these layers allow tiny motion between the bones. The movement in the sutures affects the rhythmic movement of spinal fluid through the brain, central nervous system, and body tissues, as well as the ability of the sacrum and pelvic bones to move in sync with everything else.[44] Osteopathic care focuses on restricted movement in these and other musculoskeletal connections in the body. For more information, contact the American Osteopathic Association (see Resources).

Pet Therapy

Many people with FMS and CMP report amazingly positive effects from having a pet. There can be something incredibly satisfying about being owned by a pet. (Let's not kid ourselves here.) Pets seem to sense when you are ill and offer moral support. With an animal there is always something to smile about. Dogs can help you stick to your exercise routine by needing (and demanding) to be taken for walks and, when you are outside, you may feel safer with a dog. The soft purr of a warm kitty can be just what you need to cheer you up on a gloomy day. Pets are always there for you, even when you are in a bad mood and it feels as though the rest of the world is against you.

Here are some of the advantages you can expect to reap by inviting a pet to share your home:

- Petting an animal is relaxing. • Pets are not critical, threatening, or judgmental.
- Pets help to reduce your tension and stress levels. • Pets can improve your state of mind and help you see your problems in perspective. • Pets love to be loved, touched, and held. • Pets remind you that you are lovable. • Pets can give life new purpose

and meaning. • Pets encourage play and laughter. • Pets may even help boost your healing process.

Cats and dogs are the most popular pets. However, guinea pigs, rabbits, and birds are also popular. Also, many people find that watching fish is relaxing. Animal shelters are an inexpensive source of pets, especially for dogs and cats. When you get a pet from such a shelter, the animal is usually in good condition, has been checked for medical problems, and may have received the necessary shots. The shelter will provide information on pet care.

Unfortunately, tenants are often not allowed to keep pets in many rental housing units, even though a well-managed and maintained pet is no dirtier or more offensive than your average run-of-the-mill human being. Sometimes, a landlord will make an exception to the rule if you have been a good tenant, or will allow a smaller pet such as a guinea pig or a bird.

Not everyone likes animals or enjoys pets. Don't force yourself or anyone else to get a pet. Make sure you can properly take care of a pet before you consider acquiring one. Pets are a lot of extra work, and extra money, and a great deal of responsibility. Be sure you understand what it involves. Once you adopt a pet, it's a twenty-four-hour-a-day, seven-days-a-week contract, even when you don't feel well. Lives are not disposable, even little furry, feathered, or scaled ones, and the pet you contract to care for will depend on you to keep your part of the contract.

Traditional Chinese Medicine

China is a large country, and there is no *one* "traditional Chinese medicine" (TCM) approach. There are many different ways of healing. Lao-tzu laid the foundation for TCM in the sixth century B.C., and the complexities of TCM have grown with the passage of time.

Many Chinese healers view FMS or CMP as a disturbance of chi energy. Chinese disease categories comprising FMS are: *bi zheng*, muscle-joint pain; *bu mian*, insomnia; *xu lao*, chronic, severe fatigue; and *yu zheng*, depression.[45]

Restoring harmony is the essence of Chinese medicine. The balance of yin and yang is the foundation, but yin is only yin in relation to yang, and yang is only yang in relation to yin. When balance and harmony are disrupted, and the flow of chi, the universal energy, is blocked, dysfunction and dis-ease results.

In FMS and CMP, the chi becomes blocked and discolored by pain and by toxic, stagnant wastes in the chi flow. The chi kung master teaches the student ways to clear and balance the chi, and to encourage chi flow with specific movements and body positions, so that the interior channels re-open. These channels must be properly open and insulated so that the chi may flow unimpeded.

Many forms of massage are used in TCM. Two of the oldest are *an-mo* and *tuina*. An-mo massage features pressing and rubbing massage. *Tuina* involves more joint thrusting and rolling massage. Traditional Chinese medicine also uses herbs, acupuncture, acupressure, diet, and equalization and balance of energies to unblock the flow of chi. Herbal preparations must be gathered and processed at special times and in precise ways. There is no *one* Chinese FMS herb, or even a single FMS formula. Chinese medicinals are individually prescribed, based on a person's pattern discrimination, not on a disease diagnosis like FMS.[46] One of my t'ai chi brothers, Rob Zilin, explained that many Chinese herbs are given in mixtures and packets that are often tailored to the individual. Herbs may even be prescribed as a sequence of mixtures to be taken at specified times.

Chi kung and t'ai chi and other forms of chi work can help to regain and maintain good health. Nei gong is the exercise of moving the chi with the mind rather than with breath. It opens all the hundreds of chi channels at the same time, and seeks the integration of mind, body, and spirit. Traditional Chinese practitioners are licensed on a state-by-state basis throughout the United States.

Trigger Point Injections

There are many doctors who "do" trigger point (TrP) injections. There are not many who can do them properly. For example, one reader told me, "My doctor gives the trigger point injections while I sit upright on the exam table without an assistant stretching me. When I asked him about the stretches you mentioned, he said 'That's right. I inject. Then you go home and stretch.'"

There is no way to explain the frustration I feel when I hear or read about this sort of practice. This is *not* the way to give TrP injections. Doctors must *study* the *Trigger Point Manuals*, *not just look at the pictures*! Each muscle must be properly positioned before injection, and the TrP must be carefully palpated. This may necessitate pillows and props, and you may need to have a limb or two hanging over the treatment table, or placed in another unusual position, depending on the TrP. Often, many of the TrP loci (see chapter 3) can be treated with one needle insertion.

The doctor uses *very* small amounts of local anesthetic (*not steroid*) in each TrP. The TrP injection is immediately followed by compression to prevent bleeding, then the muscle is massaged and put through three passive range of motion stretches (often accompanied by Spray and Stretch and ubsequent rewarming). After a TrP injection, individual muscles from the functional muscle unit must *always* be stretched to their full passive range of motion. Otherwise, the TrPs can recur due to residual dysfunction. This is all in the *Trigger Point Manuals*.

The *Trigger Point Manuals* explain each TrP carefully, why each TrP occurs, what perpetuates it, and *how to treat it*. Trigger point injections are used only when other methods have failed. In cases of acute TrPs, *manual methods* are to be used first. The International Association for the Study of Pain has published recommended standards for TrP training (see Resources). To minimize bleeding, Vitamin C is given for at least three days *before* injection therapy. All TrPs in a functional muscle unit should be addressed by a combination of manual techniques and, if necessary, injection. Stretching is an *essential part of the TrP injection*. Applying moist heat will reduce postinjection soreness.[47]

Trigger point injections are no fun. Procaine is the anesthetic of choice, because it is metabolizes locally and doesn't numb the area for long. Local anesthetics should be free of epinephrine. Doctors can use 1 percent lidocaine instead of procaine, but the numbness lasts much longer. One study showed that commercially available lidocaine at 1 percent is even more effective and less painful in TrP injections if it is diluted to 0.25 percent with sterile distilled water.[48] "[T]he injection of steroid into central TrPs rarely appears to prove more beneficial clinically than nonsteroid needle techniques. . . ."[49] "The use of long-acting (Deposit) steroids is not recommended for the injection of TrPs. Such a preparation may, by itself, be destructive to muscle fibers."[50] "Epinephrine severely increases myotoxicity without adding anything."[51] TrP injections should not be done with Marcaine (bupivicaine). It is toxic to muscles.[52] Adding steroid to the bipuvicaine increases the initial muscle tissue damage, and will lengthen the time needed to heal.[53] This information was in The Fibromyalgia Advocate. Ask your doctor what is in that syringe. Care must be taken to avoid needless pain. "*Even brief exposure to considerable pain can cause long lasting neuroplastic changes in the spinal cord that tend to enhance pain.*"[54]

Consider getting a preinjection block to relieve pain, or premedication. Patients must be warned that when the needle hits the TrP, a flash of pain and often a muscle twitch will result.

I have found that if I inject a tiny amount of anesthetic into the area immediately around the TrP, it doesn't hurt so much when I inject the TrP itself. I have never read about anyone else doing this, and the only experience I have giving TrP injections is on myself.

Because I have severe FMS, I have a personal interest in trying to find the least traumatic method of TrP injection. I would like to know if any others have tried this method and found that it reduces the amount of pain of the TrP injections, especially for patients who have FMS as well as TrPs. Some doctors use pre-injection nerve blocks for the same effect. Then, the TrP injections are far less painful, and they don't rattle the central nervous system as much. There are dry-needle techniques, and some doctors are masters at them, but I don't think that they are the logical choice for patients with coexisting FMS.

There are contraindications for TrP injections. People who smoke tobacco, for example, should never be given TrP injections, nor should people who have recently taken aspirin.[55] Furthermore, some areas of the body should not be injected at all.

When both central and attachment TrPs are present (see chapter 3), they tend to perpetuate each other, so both must be injected for lasting relief. After you receive TrP injections, you should go directly home and take it easy for a while. Your body needs some time to readjust.

Presently, insurance companies place arbitrary limits on TrP injections, if they cover them at all. The number of injections required depends on the patient's condition and the doctor's skill.[56] "The presence of concurrent fibromyalgia will increase the number of injections required and can justify recurrent injections every six to eight weeks since the fibromyalgia acts as a perpetuating factor that has no cure. Inactivating their TrPs can provide significant relief for many of these patients."[57]

Endnotes

1. Davies, H. T., I. K. Crombie, J. H. Brown, and C. Martin. 1997. Diminishing returns or appropriate treatment strategy?—an analysis of short-term outcomes after pain clinic treatment. *Pain* 70(2-3):203-208.

2. de Ridder, D., M. Depla, P. Severens, and M. Malsch. 1997. Beliefs on coping with illness: a consumer's perspective. *Soc Sci Med* 44(5):553-559.

3. Berman, B. M., J. P. Swyers, and J. Ezzo. 2000. The evidence for acupuncture as a treatment for rheumatologic conditions. *Rheum Dis Clin North Am* 26(1):103-115, ix-x.

4. Sandeberg, M., T. Lundeberg, and B. Gerdle. 1999. Manual acupuncture in fibromyalgia: a long-term pilot study. *J Musculoskel Pain* 6(4):39-58.

5. Deluze, C., L. Bosia, A. Zirbs, A. Chantraine, and T. L. Vischer. 1992. Electroacupuncture in fibromyalgia: results of a controlled trial. *BMJ* 305(6864)1249-1252.

6. Birch, S., and R. N. Jamison. 1998. Controlled trial of Japanese acupuncture for chronic myofascial neck pain: assessment of specific and nonspecific effects of treatment. *Clin J Pain* 14(3):248-255.

7. Cho, Z. H., S. C. Chung, J. P. Jones, J. B. Park, H. J. Park, H. J. Lee, et al. 1998. New findings of the correlation between acupoints and corresponding brain cortices using function MRI. *Proc Natl Acad Sci USA* 95(5):2670-2673.

8. Seem, M. 1993. *A New American Acupuncture: Acupuncture Osteopathy*. Boulder, CO: Blue Poppy Press.

9. Blunz, K. L., M. H. Rajwani, and R. C. Guerriero. 1997. The effectiveness of chiropractic management of fibromyalgia patients: a pilot study. *J Manipulative Physiol Ther* 20(6):389-399.

10. Hains, G., and F. Hains. 2000. A combined ischemic compression and spinal manipulation in the treatment of fibromyalgia: a preliminary estimate of dose and efficacy. *J Manipulative Physiol Ther* 23(4):225-230.

11. Nilsson, N., H. W. Christensen, J. Hartvigsen. 1997. The effect of spinal manipulation in the treatment of cervicogenic headache. *J Manipulative Physiol Ther* 20(5):326-330.

12. Skargren, E. I., B. E. Oberg, P. G. Carlsson, and M. Gade. 1997. Cost and effectiveness analysis of chiropractic and physiotherapy treatment for low back and neck pain. Six-month follow-up. *Spine* 22(18):2167-2177.

13. Triano, J. J., M. McGregor, and D. R. Skogsbergh. 1997. Use of chiropractic manipulation in lumbar rehabilitation. *J Rehabil Res Dev* 34(4):394-404.

14. Hawk, C., C. Long, and A. Azad. 1997. Chiropractic care for women with chronic pelvic pain: a prospective single-group intervention study. *J Manip Physiol Ther* 20(2):73-79.

15. Simons, D. G., J. G. Travell, and L. S. Simons. 1999. *Travell and Simons' Myofascial Pain and Dysfunction: The Trigger Point Manual, Vol. I*, Second edition. Baltimore: Williams and Wilkins, p. 117.

16. Gangi, S., and O. Johansson. 2000. A theoretical model based on mast cells and histamine to explain the recent proclaimed sensitivity to electric and/or magnetic fields in humans. *Med Hypos* 54(4):663-671.

17. Adey, W. R. 1993. Biological effects of electromagnetic fields. *J Cell Biochem* 51(4):410-416.

18. Giannini, A. J., D. A. Malone, A. Thaddeus, and J. Piotroski. 1995. The serotonin irritation syndrome. A new clinical entity? *J Clin Psych* 41(1):22-25.

19. Vallbona, C., C. F. Hazelwood, and G. Jurida. 1997. Response of pain to static magnetic fields in postpolio patients: a double-blind pilot study. *Arch Phys Med Rehabil* 78(11):1200-1203.

20. Burchard, J. F., D. H. Nguyen, L. Richard, S. N. Young, M. P. Heyes, and E. Block. 1998. Effects of electromagnetic fields on the levels of biogenic amine metabolites, quinolinic acid, and beta-endorphin in the cerebrospinal fluid of dairy cows. *Neurochem Res* 23(12):1527-1531.

21. Thoss, F., B. Bartsch, D. Tellschaft, and M. Thoss. 1999. Periodic inversion of the vertical component of the Earth's magnetic field influences fluctuation of visual sensitivity in humans. *Bioelectromagnetics* 20(7):459-461.

22. D'Andrea, J. A. 1999. Behavioral evaluation of microwave irradiation. *Bioelectromagnetics* Suppl 4:64-74.

23. Lai, H., and M. Carino. 1999. 60-Hz magnetic fields and central cholinergic activity: effects of exposure intensity and duration. *Bioelectromagnetics* 20(5):284-289.

24. Airaksinen, O., and P. J. Pontinen. 1992. Effects of electrical stimulation of myofascial trigger points with tension headache. *Acupunct Electrother Res* 17(4):285-290.

25. Hsueh, T-C., P. T. Cheng, T. S. Kuan, and C-Z. Hong. 1997. The immediate effectiveness of electrical nerve stimulation and electrical muscle stimulation on myofascial trigger points. *Am J Phys Med Rehabil* 76(6):471-476.

26. Kahn, J. 1994. Electrical modalities in the treatment of myofascial pain. In *Myofascial Pain and Fibromyalgia Trigger Point Management*. E. S. Rachlin, ed. St. Louis: Mosby.

27. Rachlin, E. S., ed. 1994. *Myofascial Pain and Fibromyalgia Trigger Point Management*. St. Louis: Mosby.

28. Chu, J. 2000. Early observation in radiculopathic pain control using electrodiagnostically derived new treatment techniques: automated twitch-obtaining intramuscular stimulation (ATOIMS) and electrical twitch-obtaining intramuscular stimulation. *Electromyogr Clin Neurophysiol* 40(4):195-204.

29. Travell, J., and D. Simons. 1983. *Myofascial Pain and Dysfunction: The Trigger Point Manual, Vol. I*. Baltimore: Williams and Wilkins. p. 27.

30. Travell, J., and D. Simons. 1992. *Myofascial Pain and Dysfunction: The Trigger Point Manual, Vol. Ii*. Baltimore: Williams and Wilkins. p. 128.

31. Liss, S., and B. Liss. 1996. Physiological and therapeutic effects of high frequency electrical pulses. *Integr Physiol Behavior Sci* 31(2):88-95.

32. Cassuto, J., S. Liss, and A. Bennett. 1993. The use of modulated energy carried on a high frequency wave for the relief of intractable pain. *Int J Clin Pharmacol Res* 13(4):239-241.

33. VanderArk, S. D., and D. Ely. 1992. Biochemical and galvanic skin responses to music stimuli by college students in biology and music. *Percept Mot Skills* 73(3 pt 2):1079-1090.

34. Hanna, J. L. 1995. The power of dance: health and healing. *J Altern Complement Med* 1(4):323-331.

35. Graham-Pole, J. 2000. *Illness and the Art of Creative Self-Expression*. Oakland, CA: New Harbinger.

36. Lange, K. 2000. Microvillar ion channels; cytoskeleton modulation of ion fluxes. *J Theor Biol* 206(4):561-584.

37. Chow, K., and W. L. Tung. 2000. Magnetic field exposure enhances DNA repair through the induction of DnaK/J Synthesis. *FEBS Lett* 478(1-2):133-136.

38. Collacott, E. A., J. T. Zimmerman, D. W. White, and J. P. Rindone. 2000. Bipolar permanent magnets for the treatment of chronic low back pain: a pilot study. *JAMA* 283(10):1322-1325.

39. Brown, C. S., N. Parker, F. Ling, and J. Wan. 2000. Effects of magnets on chronic pelvic pain. *Obstet Gynecol* 95(4 Suppl 1):S29.

40. Mooney, J., and F. M. Olbrechts. 1929. *The Swimmer Manuscript: Cherokee Sacred Formulas and Medicinal Prescriptions*. Washington, DC: Bureau of American Ethnology, Bulletin 99:62, 170-171, 180-184, 204-205.

41. McWhorter, J. H., and R. B. Davis. 1998. Cherokee prescriptions for acupressure and massage. *NCMJ* 59(6):368.

42. Keitel, W. 1999. [Occupational therapy in the diseases of the locomotor system]. *Z Arztl Fortbild Qualitatssich* 93(5):335-340. [German]

43. Simons, Travell, and Simons. 1999. *Op. cit.*

44. Rubenstein, S. 1990. The osteopathy alternative. *East West*, Dec, 45-49.

45. Flaws, Bob. 2000. *Curing Fibromyalgia Naturally with Chinese Medicine.* Boulder, CO: Blue Poppy Press.

46. *Ibid.*

47. Gerwin, R. D. 1999. Myofascial pain syndromes from trigger points. *Pain* 3:153-159.

48. Iwama, H., and Y. Akama. 2000. The superiority of water-diluted to 0.25% to neat 1% lidocaine for trigger-point injections in myofascial pain syndrome: A prospective, randomized, double-blind trial. *Anesth Analg* 91(2):408-409.

49. Simons, Travell, and Simons. 1999. *Op. cit.,* p 145.

50. *Ibid.*, p. 153.

51. *Ibid.*

52. Ishiura, S., I. Nonaka, and H. Sugita. 1986. Biochemical aspects of bupivicaine-induced acute muscle degradation. *J Cell Sci* 83:197-121.

53. Guttu, R. L., D. G. Page, and D. M. Laskin. 1990. Delayed healing of muscle after injection of bupivicaine and steroid. *Amm Dent* 49:5–8.

54. *Ibid.*, p.158.

55. *Ibid.*, p. 163.

56. *Ibid.*

57. *Ibid.*, p. 165.

CHAPTER 23

Nutrition: You Are What You Eat—Don't Be a Twinkie

Preventive medicine starts with what you put into your body; the food you eat, the air you breathe, and the water you drink. Life sends us a lot of mixed messages. Have you ever noticed those so-called "women's" magazines in the grocery? This week, one had luscious desserts all over the cover, with recipes inside. This magazine also had a test of your "fat IQ." I have a feeling that if you purchased the magazine, you failed the test.

Meal planning, food shopping, and food preparation take time. It's tempting to reach for fast, prepared food. Some of us have culinary skills that are not likely to turn out healthy, appetizing meals. Your gourmet fare may be limited to "Peanut Butter Angeli." When you read the ingredients in commercial peanut butter, it should give you pause. Sometimes the only reason that "peanuts" is listed as the first ingredient is that "sugar" is divided into several forms, such as corn syrup, molasses, sugar, honey, fructose, etc. Then come partially hydrogenated vegetable oils. Then when you prepare your sandwich you add more sugar in the form of jelly, and put that on bread (more partially hydrogenated vegetable oils and carbohydrates). In this chapter, you will learn why this kind of sandwich is a perpetuating factor. It is time to take a look at what you are eating, what you are absorbing, and ask yourself why you eat the way you do.

Cellular Factories and Adenosine Triphosphate

You need to know how your body creates the fuel it uses for energy. Did you ever wonder how that hamburger or pizza makes its way into your cells? There are no tiny cell teeth to chew up the ground beef and pepperoni. Neither are fruits and veggies shoveled into your cellular factories, which then release adenosine triphosphate (ATP) energy like water vapor from your mitochondrial smokestacks. The process is much more elegant and ever so much more complex. Many books are available to tell you how your food is actually digested. You probably learned about this in school. What happens in the cells is another matter. To produce energy, your cells must generate ATP. Adenosine triphosphate is the most common fuel that your body "burns" with oxygen (*oxidizes*) to produce energy (see chapter 1).

Your cells create most of the ATP inside the mitochondria, using a process called *oxidative physphorylation*. *Glycolysis*, another energy-generating process, occurs outside of the mitochondria, but still inside the cell. This area is called the *cytosol*. Mitochondria are, among other things, your intracellular energy factories. These factories have two membranes around them, and these membranes develop channels that open only in the presence of specific charged particles, called ions. Electrons and protons flow across the membranes by an exchange of ionic charge, which also results in shifts of acid-base ratios (pH), and concentrations of specific biochemicals. When you hear the doctors on TV shows shouting for "lytes," they are ordering a blood test for *electrolytes*, which are the electrically charged (ionic) amounts of specific minerals. These amounts, and their ratios, say a lot about what is going wrong in the body, and how to make it right again. It's all about balance.

For a proton, or positively charged particle, to enter an individual mitochondrion, it needs an enzyme escort. The mitochondrion gets the energy to make ATP from the movement of charged particles across the chemical and electrical interfaces. This is a complex process, and the ease with which it occurs depends on your general health, the health of the mitochondria, and the quality of the raw materials you supply. We are back to the basics: food, air, and water. The foods you eat can affect the rates at which your neurons synthesize and release neurotransmitters.[1] This process, as you have learned, is already out of balance in fibromyalgia (FMS).

Food Basics: A Pyramid Scheme?

Many of us have been taught about nutrition by learning the basic building blocks of the food pyramid. From what I have observed, many of us are building our food pyramids on shifting sand. Later in this chapter you will read about excess carbohydrate consumption and the special perils it can have to many of us. There are three basic types of nutrients; they are as follows:

- proteins, such as beef, fish, and poultry • fats, such as butter, cream, and vegetable oils • carbohydrates, such as vegetables, fruits, grains, pastas, and cereals

There are large variables in these food types. All fruits are not equal, for example, and neither are all vegetables or all grains. Some foods are misleading. For example, most cheeses are considered fat sources rather than protein sources. No, FMily. A baked potato topped with cheese is *not* a balanced meal.

Hal Blatman, M.D., a myofascial pain specialist from Cincinnati, Ohio, was kind enough to provide the following excerpt from his presentation at the Focus on Pain Seminar 2000.

Food can be a highly emotional issue. It can be a hard topic to approach logically, but your health requires that you do. Your state of health can often be described by a simple formula: $G - B + R = P$

G = good things you do for, and put into your body.

B = bad things you do for, and put into your body

R = reserve your body has left (what's present at birth minus what's been used)

P = pain and problems you are going to experience

In general, you come to see a doctor because you are dissatisfied with the "P" number. Theoretically, if you change the rest of the equation, your body can heal itself. There are some important but very simple rules to follow.

Rule 1. Do not put poison into your body. One example, avoid margarine: Bugs won't eat it and mold won't grow on it. What do these critters know that we don't? It will not support or sustain life. It is partially hydrogenated vegetable oil. Partially hydrogenated vegetable oil looks like cholesterol (which you need) and your body tries to put it into normal cholesterol processing. It can't. Partially hydrogenated oil is often hidden in foods like commercial peanut butter.

Fatty acid synthesis occurs in the cytosol—outside the mitochondrion but inside the cell. Your body can synthesize all the fatty acids it needs except for the essential, polyunsaturated fatty acids. Saturated, unsaturated, monosaturated, and polyunsaturated fatty acids refer to the molecular structure and chemical bonds in the fat. The nature of these bonds decides how they will be used in your body. Unsaturated fats are called that because they are capable of absorbing additional hydrogen ions. They are better for your health, but they pick up oxygen quickly and spoil rapidly. Saturated fats have all the spaces for hydrogen ions already full, so they last longer. The membranes in all of our cells are partly polyunsaturated fatty acids. Naturally occurring fatty acids are almost all in a configuration called "cis." "Trans"-fatty acids are produced when you heat "cis" fatty acids to a high temperature. The most common trans-fatty acids are margarine and vegetable shortening.

When you eat hydrogenated oil, cholesterol levels rise, and so does trans-fat. Trans-fat increases LDL cholesterol and reduces the level of HDL. Margarine and mayonnaise made from hydrogenated soybean oil often only lists saturated fat and not the trans-fat. The balance of fats affects the prostaglandin balance. Prostaglandins are quasi-hormones in the body that enable intracellular communication. The most serious danger of unhealthy fat is related to cell membrane composition. The cell membrane is largely made up of two layers of fat. These layers allow nutrients in and waste out. What do you want to be the building blocks of your cellular membranes? (I think I see a developing connection between the excess carbohydrates and trans-fatty acids in our diet and the increase in abdominal obesity, type II diabetes, and congestive heart disease.)

Aspartame is an excitotoxin. It readily crosses the blood/brain barrier, and can excite or stimulate the nerve cell to death. One theory is that the excitotoxic mechanisms underlie nerve tissue degeneration. When target neurons are overexcited, energy disturbance and pathobiochemical changes result in nerve cell death.[2]

Aspartame consumption may be a hazard because of its contribution to the formation of formaldehyde-like products. The amount of these chemicals in tissue proteins and nucleic acids coming from aspartame may be cumulative.[3] Research suggests that excitotoxins are important in the regulation of hormone secretion from the pituitary-thyroid axis.[4]

Rule 2. If you are going to run a racecar, you use 100+ octane fuel. The human body is a high performance machine. It does not run on low octane fuel like white sugar, white flour, and potatoes. One medium potato is like one half cup of sugar. Next lowest octane is wheat grain (bread, pasta). Soda can be devastating. Some sodas have ten teaspoons of sugar per can. Phosphates in soda deplete calcium, because your body uses its calcium to process phosphates.

Breakfast should be your *most nutritious* meal of the day. If you don't eat breakfast at all, your body goes to the cupboard at 9 A.M. and finds nothing. It doesn't know that lunch is coming in a few hours. It could be starving for days. It goes into starvation mode. It starts to eat muscle. You *need* to put something into your body for breakfast, and it should be something *good*.

Specialized mucosal cells lining your gut are responsible for making 95 percent of the serotonin in the body. Not much is made in the brain. Selective serotonin reuptake inhibitors (SSRIs) fool the body into thinking it has more serotonin, but that is like putting a bandage on a sore without treating it. The problem is that the gut is not making the serotonin in the first place.

Mucosal cells make immunoglobin A (IgA), responsible for the front line defense of the immune system. If they don't, white blood cells must compensate. The mucosal barrier keeps food, toxins, and waste from leaking from the colon. When these toxins leak, it causes even more work for the immune system. In leaky gut syndrome, the intestinal permeability barriers have been broken, intestinal mucosal cells have been injured, and the immune system is compromised. This leads to bacterial and toxin exposure.

Inside your belly are billions of critters. Good critters help digest food and make vitamins. Bad critters produce toxins that load the immune system, and they kill the good critters.

Rule 3. Feed the good critters like pet fish in a fish tank. Starve the bad critters so that they die.

This sounds simple, but it isn't. One problem is that the human body is a democracy. When we choose food, all our critters vote. If we haven't been taking care of ourselves, there are more bad critters than good critters, so we eat what *they* want. Good bacteria crave green, leafy vegetables. Bad bacteria want white flour and white sugar. Normal gut bacteria synthesize many vitamins and short chain fatty acids, degrade metabolic toxins, prevent colonization by pathogens, and stimulate maturation of normal immune response.

Improve your diet to promote your good critters and restore the integrity of your intestinal lining. Essential fatty acids function in cholesterol metabolism, hormone manufacture and regulation, and cell membrane syntheses. Think about fatty acid deficiency when you have abnormalities in these systems, such as hormone imbalance, cholesterol elevation, or chronic illness. Think of fatty acid balance, as well. Omega 6 and Omega 3 oil supplements and eating fish twice a week are helpful to restore bowel health. Lecithin, another good supplement, is part of the cell membrane, part of the protective sheath for brain, nerve cells, and muscle cells, and helps disperse fats for processing and removal. L-glutamine nourishes cells of intestinal mucosa, but you need to take it on an empty stomach to be more effective.

Many people with FMS and CMP have reflux and are put on H2 blockers. H2 blockers decrease the amount of acid in your stomach, and decrease your ability to digest proteins.

Eliminate bad critters. Discontinue eating foods to which you are allergic or sensitive. Replace digestive enzymes that may be insufficient in your body, and provide proper nutrients for cellular repair. Symptoms associated with increased bowel permeability include abdominal pain and distension, diarrhea, fatigue, malaise, joint pains, muscle pains, skin rashes, cognitive memory deficits, and feeling "toxic."

Leaky Gut Syndrome

One study found that 45 percent of FMS patients had circulating immunoglobin (IgM) antibodies against enterovirus compared to 10 percent in the control group. None of the fibromyalgia (FMS) patients had a history of recent gastrointestinal infection. The occurrence of IgM antibodies against enterovirus may indicate an abnormal immune response to prior or ongoing infection in some patients with FMS.[5] Or it may indicate leaky gut syndrome.

Many of us report intolerance to medications and responses to medications that are the reverse of typical side effects, in addition to food intolerance, multiple chemical sensitivities, and food cravings (usually for food that we should avoid). Leaky gut syndrome sets off a cascade, like a domino effect. Each domino sets off several more, which set off several more, and so forth. There are about 300 to 400 different species of bacteria in the small intestine. In this syndrome, some of these bacteria can get into abdominal lymph nodes, and travel from there to the liver where they produce toxins.[6] The cascade activates immune system and hormonal changes, which produce diffuse musculoskeletal and neuromuscular symptoms similar to those seen in FMS and CMP.

Lately, the current trend for a healthier diet has caused many people to eat high carbohydrate, low-fat diets. Fibromyalgia patients, who often have or are developing reactive hypoglycemia or insulin resistance, may have a problem metabolizing carbohydrates. For them, eating such a diet can lead to overweight and an inability to lose weight, fatigue, carbohydrate craving, and worsening of many FMS symptoms.

Carbohydrate Bombs: Are You at Ground Zero?

Carbohydrates come from plants. High-protein foods such as beef, pork, poultry, fish, cottage cheese, and tofu have negligible carbohydrates. *Carbohydrates stimulate insulin production.* Insulin enables blood sugar to move to our biochemical factories in the cells, and to be burned as fuel. If there is an excess of insulin and carbohydrate, the insulin allows this excess carbohydrate to be stored as fatty acids in fat cells. The excess insulin also *prevents the carbohydrates from being used as fuel.* This means that you not only gain weight as *fat,* you are also prevented from losing this fat because of the availability of excess carbohydrates.

Lynne August, M.D., is the Director and Nutritional Counselor at Health Equations in Vermont. She lists the following as symptoms of excess carbohydrate consumption: carbohydrate craving, excess body fat, high triglycerides/cholesterol, fluid retention, dry skin, brittle hair/nails, dry small stools, decreased memory and ability to concentrate, fatigue or dips in energy, grogginess when waking, headaches, mood swings/irritability, and sleep disturbances.

She has found that a high carbohydrate diet can contribute to allergies and to many disease processes. The ratios between certain minerals (and certain vitamins) are significant as well, and yet very few doctors run baseline vitamin and mineral analyses. Dr. August has developed a blood test profile, and written a book for physicians, to address this lack (see Appendix C: Reading List). The form of the minerals must also be checked. You need to know how much of a mineral is *ionized*, because that is the state in which they are functional. It is also important to study the anion gap (the ratio between sodium and potassium, chloride and CO_2, and calcium and phosphorus).

Reactive Hypoglycemia (RHG) and Insulin Resistance (IR)

There are a lot of references in this section, because far too many care providers refuse to believe that these conditions exist, in spite of all the research to the contrary. *Reactive* hypoglycemia is not the same as *fasting* hypoglycemia, which is the low blood sugar that occurs when you don't eat. Reactive hypoglycemia is not always picked up on routine medical tests. It usually occurs two to three hours after a high carbohydrate meal, overstimulating the release of insulin, which triggers a compensatory adrenaline response. Hypoglycemia also appears to induce abnormalities in decision-making processes,[7] and can contribute to fibrofog.

Some symptoms of hypoglycemia (tremulousness, palpitations, anxiety, sweating, hunger, paresthesias) are due to physiologic changes caused by the response of the autonomic nervous system. Other symptoms (confusion, sensation of warmth, weakness or fatigue, severe cognitive failure, seizure, coma) are the results of glucose deprivation in the brain.[8] Coexisting RHG makes treatment of FMS and chronic myofascial pain (CMP) extremely difficult. Myofascial TrP activity is so aggravated by it that it doesn't make sense to treat specific trigger points (TrPs) unless the hypoglycemia is also treated.[9]

When your body no longer responds appropriately to the insulin that you produce, you have developed insulin resistance (IR). Insulin resistance can have serious consequences. The hypothalamus becomes hypersensitive, keeping the pituitary and adrenal glands and the sympathetic nervous system on alert. This leads to endocrine dysfunction, insulin resistance, and other symptoms.[10]

Normal blood sugar levels that coexist with high insulin levels, obesity, or dysfunction in fat metabolism is a pre-hypoglycemic state that may be an early form of diabetes.[11] This would be a case of IR leading to RHG, instead of the other way around. Abdominal obesity, indicated by the fat pad over the belly, is a clinical marker of insulin resistance,[12] and is common in FMS. Abdominal obesity and neuroendocrine/HPA axis dysfunction are linked as predictors for disease.[13] A lax, pendulous abdomen is associated with certain TrPs.[14] People with insulin resistance have problems utilizing muscle glucose properly, and can't break up fat tissue in a normal manner.[15] Insulin resistance often occurs long before any symptoms appear.[16] It is important to develop life style changes, including healthy diet and exercise to help control this condition. Recent studies show that abdominal obesity (the fat pad on the belly) and insulin resistance are connected to hypothalamic-pituitary-adrenal axis dysfunction.[17]

One inexpensive over-the counter supplement that may help normalize the sensitivity of your body to insulin is the amino acid, taurine. Taurine is an amino acid that cats can't make themselves, so cat food has taurine added. This amino acid may help us to avoid the typical fibrofat belly pad, which is linked to insulin resistance.[18]

Dr. R. Paul St. Amand found that there is a large subset of fibromyalgia patients with reactive hypoglycemia. He calls this combination "fibroglycemia."[19] The symptoms he lists are: headaches, dizziness, irritability, chronic fatigue, depression, nervousness, difficulty with memory and concentration, nasal congestion, heavy dreaming, palpitations or heart pounding, tremor of the hands, day or night sweats, anxiety, leg cramps, numbness and tingling in the hands and/or feet, flushing, and a craving for carbohydrates and sweets. Most of these symptoms diminish five or ten minutes after eating sugar. Symptoms often worsen before menstrual periods and become severe after childbirth. When patients with "fibroglycemia" are put on a limited carbohydrate diet, they often feel a marked improvement after seven to ten days. But those are seven to ten very uncomfortable days. The headache and fatigue can be extreme, and if you are aware that sugar can ease the symptoms in the short term, you will be tempted to cheat. Caffeine must be avoided on this diet.

I use whey protein or egg white powder to help keep a good balance in my diet. I add the unflavored whey to some foods. It makes a great thickener in some recipes, for example, in vegetable puree soups with a chicken broth base. I make a "milk shake" using vanilla protein powder, frozen wild blueberries, and 2 percent milk. A little vanilla-flavored powder in applesauce can balance a meal that otherwise would be too low in protein.

It helps me to check the Zone recipe book (see Barry Sears in the Reading List). After I look at those recipes, it is easier for me to judge how much protein and carbohydrate to use. There is usually enough fat mixed in with the protein and carbohydrate. It is also important to know the glycemic index of your food intake, as well as the amounts of your carbohydrates and proteins.

The glycemic index measures how fast a food raises your blood sugar levels and how quickly your body responds. High glycemic index foods raise blood sugar quickly. The glycemic index of the food depends on the type of sugar in the carbohydrate; the amounts of fiber, protein, and fat in the food; and the method of cooking or processing.[20] Generally, the more fiber, protein, or fat in a food, the lower its glycemic index. Highly processed foods or foods high in refined sugars or flours typically have a high glycemic index.

Dr. Sears, the author of the Zone books, found that the best ratio for food balancing is 3 grams of protein to 4 grams of carbohydrate. Protein should comprise 30 percent of the diet, fats 30 percent, and carbohydrates 40 percent. Each time you eat either a meal or a snack, your food intake should match the 30/30/40 ratio, because every time you eat there is a hormonal response. You also need to adjust your caloric intake to meet the needs of your metabolism and the exercise you do. Once you are eating properly balanced and correct amounts of food, your food cravings will become less intense. Here are four things you can do to help modify your carbohydrate cravings:

Changing Your Eating Habits

1. Eat *moderate* amounts of fat. Fat will decrease the flow of carbohydrates into the bloodstream, and decrease carbohydrate craving.

2. Cut down on the amount of carbohydrates.

3. Eat protein as part of every meal and snack. It helps use up the fat stored in your body.

4. Exercise regularly, to decrease the amount of insulin in your blood.

If you decide to try the Zone balanced diet, when you start you may feel extremely fatigued and need to sleep a lot. Your body needs to rebalance, and it will. One study found that short-term exercise is even more effective than diet in enhancing insulin activity in individuals with abnormal glucose tolerance,[21] so don't neglect this important avenue for insulin control. Note that the balancing benefits of exercise can be wiped out if you drink a high-carbohydrate sports "energy" beverage to "recover" after exercising.

You may find it difficult to change your eating and drinking habits because they are hard-wired in your brain. To change your patterns, you need to modify your brain in at least three ways: the way it perceives stimuli, the basic way it responds to stimuli, and the way its many other systems *reinforce* the interactions between the first two.[22] For example, one way I have tricked my brain to be satisfied with less is to use smaller plates and smaller portions.

There is a difference between wanting food and being hungry. That sentence would be a good topic for a meditation. Explore that difference. Often people overeat to relieve stress. Eat only when you are hungry, and eat just enough to stop the hunger. If you have a problem with traditional breakfast foods, try eating a balanced, nutritional, nontraditional breakfast of foods you like. You may find that taking a walk before or after a meal aids your digestion and reduces stress. Learn to eat like a gourmet. Eat slowly, chew thoughtfully, and enjoy each bite. Eat less, but eat mindfully, and you will be satisfied.

Food Allergy/Intolerance

Food allergies and sensitivities differ in many ways from typical allergens that are inhaled into the respiratory system. Food allergies produce a wider range of symptoms, and some of these are emotional. Many of the common FMS symptoms, such as headaches, fatigue, fibrofog, mood swings, weight fluctuation, and insomnia, to name a few, can be caused or worsened by foods. Back in the days when certain foods were available only at specific times of the year, adverse reactions were more obvious. Now, food sensitivities often remain unsuspected because we eat the problem foods more often.

Which Foods Are Causing Your Allergies?

One of the many good reasons for keeping a journal is that you can include a food diary in your records. This should allow you to narrow the list of suspect foods. Then, eliminate suspect foods from your diet for a week or two. Later, return them to your diet, slowly, one at a time. If the symptom that you suspect to be caused by a food allergy recurs after you have first eliminated and then reintroduced a particular food, you have found your culprit. You may have a problem with more than one food. Note that it is common to crave foods to which you are allergic or sensitive. The most common food allergies and sensitivities occur with corn, wheat, fish, milk, nuts, and eggs.

If your body is intolerant of a food, you can usually eat a small amount without a reaction. If you are allergic to a food, however, even a tiny amount of it usually will trigger symptoms. If you are prone to headaches, avoid red wine, beer, caffeine, aged cheese, nuts, chocolate, and foods that are fermented, pickled, aged, or marinated. Sodium nitrates (found in bacon, cold cuts, hot dogs, and smoked foods), tyramine (found in aged cheese, chicken liver, overripe bananas, and avocados), and MSG are also common activators of headaches.

The top gas producers are milk and beans. Leading the list for heartburn are chocolate, fats, peppermint, garlic, onions, orange juice, hot sauce, tomatoes, coffee, and alcohol. Read labels. You will be surprised at some of the things found in foods. Restrict your diet to fresh, natural food grown without chemicals. Think about what you put into your mouth. Don't add toxins to an already toxic system.

Eating Wisely

Make regular shopping trips a high priority so that you will always have a good supply of healthy foods on hand. Make a food plan with a shopping list and take the list with you when shopping. Take time to cook good foods for yourself. Keep easy-to-fix, healthy foods on hand for the times when you are too busy to spend a lot of time cooking. When you cook, freeze the leftovers in meal-size containers. Identify several local restaurants where you can enjoy a healthy meal. Keep healthy snacks available. Don't buy junk food. Don't use food as a reward.

If your symptoms are very painful or your schedule is too hectic to shop, ask your supporters to pick up groceries for you when they pick up theirs. You can return the favor when you're able. If getting out is always difficult for you, contact a home health aid service in your area for grocery delivery service. In some areas, nutritious meals can be delivered to your home. The cost for such services is often small and/or on a sliding scale, depending on your income.

Refined Salt and Electrolyte Balance

Ionized mineral salts (sodium, potassium, etc.) in solution are called electrolytes. The correctly balanced exchange of electrolytic ions is what creates energy and allows information to flow properly between the body and mind. Your electrolytes must be in an ionized state to work for you, since charged ion exchange is how the body conducts its business. Refined salt, the type most people use, has had all of its trace minerals removed. Even commercial sea salt is refined, often with the use of intense heat. It then recrystallizes, but is missing most of the trace minerals. Moderate salt restriction aggravates both systemic and vascular insulin resistance.[23] We need salt, but we need the *right* kind of salt, with all the trace minerals still intact.

Dr. August recommends a special whole, sun dried, organic, and unrefined salt called Celtic Salt, which contains needed trace minerals (see the Grain and Salt Society in the "Products" section of Appendix A). She bases her nutritional supplement programs on a blood profile that she has developed. The patient's blood sample provides indications of the appropriate supplements necessary to restore and maintain balance.

Food Supplements

Diet and nutrition influence our state of mind. Even if we choose healthy foods, processing these foods can deplete needed vitamins. Vitamin and mineral *deficiencies* produce clear symptoms.

Vitamin and mineral *inadequacies* are not so easily detected. The "normal range" of vitamin values may have to be taken with a grain of (Celtic) salt. Is the "average" value the "optimum" value? If your body is stressed with chronic illness, you may have a much greater need for specific nutrients. "There is good reason to expect that serum vitamin levels within the normal range do not ensure optimal levels of nutrition."[24]

Vitamin and mineral insufficiency may be common perpetuating factors for both FMS and CMP.[25] When your body goes to the food cupboard and finds an inadequate amount of a vitamin or mineral, it has to make metabolic compensation.

One study found that nutritional supplements resulted in a reduction in initial symptom severity of FMS, with continued improvement in the period between initial assessment and the follow-up.[26] Doctor J. B. Eisinger found that vitamin B1 can help neurotransmitter dysfunction and the chronic pain of FMS,[27] and magnesium and selenium deficiency have been linked with muscle pain.[28]

The leaky gut syndrome, lack of adequate healthy food, metabolic dysfunction, increased metabolic requirement, increased excretion, increased destruction within the body, pregnancy and lactation, unbalanced diet, aging, smoking, and substance abuse can all contribute to vitamin or mineral inadequacy. Deficiency of some vitamins can contribute to decreased nutritional absorption.[29] Low "normal" levels of B1, B6, B12, and/or folic acid decrease the likelihood that any TrP therapy will be effective.[30] Complete information on specific vitamins and minerals, amino acids, and other supplements is beyond the scope of this book. Just some basics are presented here. There may be many other nutritional supplements helpful in specific cases of FMS and CMP. Remember, each one of us is unique in our needs.

The ABC's of FMS and CMP

You may have heard that B vitamins must be given in a complex form, that is, they should be taken together, rather than as single supplements. The reason for this is the interconnection and balancing act that is the story of the human body.

B1 (thiamin) is essential for normal cellular energy production, the conversion of glucose into energy, and it may be a factor in the energy crisis of TrPs. Inadequate thiamin may contribute to nocturnal calf cramps, edema, constipation, and fatigue. Tinnitus is sometimes helped by niacin and thiamin supplements. Heating can destroy thiamin. Thiamine absorption is impaired by alcohol, liver injury, magnesium deficiency, tannin in tea, and antacids, as well as by an enzyme that is found in many fish.

If you are taking diuretics, you may lose extra thiamin, which may affect your thyroid hormone level. David Simons found that when patients with low thiamine levels and evidence of low thyroid function are given supplemental thiamine, the hypothyroid symptoms may disappear. If you have thyroid insufficiency, even a small amount of thyroid may precipitate symptoms of acute thiamine deficiency, which may be misinterpreted as intolerance to the thyroid medication. The thiamine deficiency must be remedied first. Thyroid hormone levels may improve with the thiamin supplementation, without the need to add thyroid medication.

B2 (riboflavin) is important in growth and tissue repair; metabolism of carbohydrates, proteins, and fats, and adrenal gland function. Too much B2 interferes with the proper absorption of B1 and B6.

B3 (niacin) is important in cellular maintenance of the skin and the nerve and digestive systems. It helps convert food to energy, and functions in the synthesis of hormones, steroids, and fatty acids. B3 helps to protect against the effects of pollutants. It also helps your body eliminate them, and enhances peripheral circulation.

B5 (pantothenic acid) metabolizes carbohydrates, fats, and proteins. It takes part in the regulation of blood sugar levels and in nerve transmission.

B6 (pyridoxine) is a vital element in energy metabolism and nerve function, and is critical for the synthesis and/or metabolism of nearly all the neurotransmitters. Vitamin B6 is important in food metabolism, promotes nerve function, and supports the immune system. It may have antiseizure effects. B6 deficiency results in reduced absorption and storage of B12, increased excretion of vitamin C, and blocked niacin synthesis. B6 acts with vitamin E to control the metabolism of unsaturated fats, and with vitamin C in tyrosine metabolism. It is also important in amino acid metabolism. B6 insufficiency is common in the elderly and in women taking oral estrogen or cortisone. There is considerable variance among patients in their need for B6.

B7 (biotin) is important in food metabolism and in cellular energy production. B7 strengthens hair and nails.

B9 (folic acid) is critical to brain function. Folate insufficiency is the most common vitamin insufficiency, and is likely to perpetuate TrPs.[31] People with folic acid deficiency tire easily, sleep poorly, and feel discouraged and depressed. Folic acid deficiency can also contribute to constipation, diffuse muscular pain, restless legs, low basal temperature, and a sensation of always feeling cold.

B12 (cobalamin) and folic acid often work together. B12 deficiency, which can lead to irreversible neurological damage, can be masked if you have too much folic acid. Both of these vitamins are required for DNA and fatty acid synthesis. A deficiency of B12 will increase the energy problems experienced in CMP. Vitamin B12 inadequacy is common in people with blood sugar irregularities and in those over the age of fifty.

Vitamin A is an antioxidant and aids night vision. It is an important factor in tissue health (especially tissue linings in areas like the gut), and in the immune system. Your body makes vitamin A out of beta-carotene. Beta-carotene is less toxic than vitamin A, and you get the same benefits from taking it.

Vitamin C is an essential vitamin cofactor in many enzymatic reactions, including synthesis of the neurotransmitters norepinephrine and serotonin. Vitamin C can prevent some postexercise soreness and stiffness, and it prevents some bruising. It helps other vitamins to function, and contributes to the overall stress response of the body. It may help diarrhea caused by food allergy,[32] and may decrease toxicity and TrP irritability caused by chronic infection. People who are ill have a greater tolerance for vitamin C than healthy individuals do.[33] The need for vitamin C may be much greater if you take aspirin, estrogen, or if you smoke. Your body eliminates vitamin C, even in large doses, in twelve hours. Time-release vitamin C is eliminated in sixteen hours. For these reasons it is better to take smaller doses of vitamin C, twelve hours apart, than to take one larger tablet.

Vitamin D boosts calcium and phosphorus absorption.

Vitamin E is an antioxidant and is crucial to healthy cell membranes, immune and endocrine systems, and the sex organs. It protects lung tissue from pollutants, and may reduce PMS and muscle cramps.[34]

Minerals and trace elements are important for health. Iron, calcium, potassium, and magnesium are needed for normal muscle function. A deficiency of these minerals tends to increase the irritability of myofascial TrPs.

Calcium is necessary for the release of acetylcholine at the nerve terminal and for the excitation-contraction mechanism of the actin and myosin filaments.

Chromium is involved in blood sugar regulation.

Iodine may relieve fibrocystic breast pain.[35]

Iron provides the oxygen to hemoglobin and myoglobin.

Manganese is vital for the normal function of brain, reproduction, and glucose metabolism.

Magnesium is crucial to the workings of muscles and to electrical stability in cellular tissue. It is used in the metabolism of glucose, nerve conduction, the production of adenosine triphosphate (ATP), and the maintenance of membrane integrity.

Potassium is needed for neurotransmitter function. A diet high in fat, refined sugar, and oversalted food can lead to potassium deficiency. Diarrhea, laxatives, and some diuretics increase potassium loss.

There are a great many trace minerals, and we don't know what all of their functions are, nor what our needs are for them. One study showed calcium and magnesium supplementation might be a beneficial complementary treatment for FMS.[36] We are in need of more research to be done on nutrients. I consider Celtic salt my trace mineral "insurance policy."

Nutritionists are learning more and more about the short- and long-term effects of a diet high in refined, processed, and artificial chemical-laden foods. The preliminary indications are that many of us are junk-food junkies, and we have to clean up our act before we are going to feel better. Several classes of drugs increase our need for vitamins, as does the leaky gut syndrome. Some doctors use short-term intravenous minerals and vitamins for patients with leaky gut syndrome, to enable healing to begin. Some of these supplements are given through IV infusions (IV drip) and not injected as a bolus (all at once). Digestive enzymes may be taken *with* food to help digestion, or *without* food to help digest any food residue.

How much of a vitamin or mineral do you need? Dr. Blatman warns that the level of a specific vitamin or mineral may be the limiting step in a critical cellular process. If you don't have enough of a vitamin or mineral to enable a certain process to take place, the process doesn't happen, happens incompletely, or happens at a slower rate. We need whatever it takes so that the biochemical processes requiring this substance are not limited. A vitamin or mineral inadequacy implies that there is a rate-limiting step present in a critical cellular process.

Too many critics of food supplements charge that when you take supplements, all you get is very expensive urine. Ingesting a sufficient amount of supplements to satisfy the "rate-limiting step" concept means that *some* of the supplement, the excess, will be excreted in the urine.

Many prescription medications are used to help the body compensate for inadequate nutrition or to treat nutrition-related illness. These medications are more expensive than nutritional supplements. I agree with Dr. Blatman. Nutritional supplementation makes sense. You must be careful, however, to take the supplements that *you* need. Some vitamins and minerals can be harmful if taken in excess. Consult a medical care provider who knows this topic thoroughly and can get your blood tested.

It is difficult to get insurance companies to reimburse you for food supplements. You need a doctor who knows that many of us with chronic conditions have vitamin and mineral insufficiencies and absorption problems. Then, the doctor must write a prescription for what you need. At that point, you may still have to argue with your insurance company. The references we've provided in this book may help you win that argument.

The Water of Life

Water is one of the most important substances that you take into your body. Most of us don't drink enough water and the water we drink may not be healthy. Most drinking water is not tested very well, and is certainly not tested for every possible pollutant. Look into good filtration systems at least for your drinking and cooking needs.

We are polluting our world. Researchers have found that a large number of the man-made chemicals that we have released into the environment, as well as a few natural ones, have the potential to disrupt the endocrine systems of many animals, including humans. Among these are persistent compounds that include some pesticides, industrial chemicals, and other synthetic compounds. These compounds already affect many wildlife populations. There are many possible routes of exposure, and it's very difficult to work out which are the main ones. These biochemical and chemical substances are often concentrated in fat.[37] Be very careful what fats you eat. You may be consuming more than you know.

Diet is a crucial factor in treating FMS and CMP effectively. Improper diet is also implicated in many allergies and diseases. In these days of fast food, sticking to a healthy diet is very hard, but it can pay off in reduction of symptoms, increased vitality, and an overall sense of wellness.

Endnotes

1. Wurtman, R. J. 1983. Behavioral effects of nutrients. *Lancet* 1(8334):1145-1147.

2. Vecsei, L., G. Dibo, and C. Kiss. 1998. Neurotoxins and neurodegenerative disorders. *Neurotoxicology* 19(4-5):511-514.

3. Trocho, C., R. Pardo, I. Rafecas, J. Virgili, X. Remesar, A. Fernandez-Lopez, et al. 1998. Formaldehyde derived from dietary aspartame binds to tissue components in vivo. *Life Sci* 63(5):337-349.

4. Alfonso, M., R. Duran, and M. C. Arufe. 2000. Effects of excitatory amino acids on serum TSH and thyroid hormone levels in freely moving rats. *Horm Res* 54(2):78-83.

5. Wittrup, I. H., A. Wiik, and B. Danneskiold-Samsoe. 1999. Antibody profile in patients with fibromyalgia compared to healthy controls. *J Musculoskel Pain* 7(1-2):273-277.

6. Gershon, M. D. 1998. *The Second Brain.* New York: HarperCollins.

7. Blackman, J. D., V. L. Towle, G. F. Lewis, J. P. Spire, and K. S. Polonsky. 1990. Hypoglycemic thresholds for cognitive dysfunction in humans. *Diabetes* 39(7):828-835.

8. Cryer, P. E. 1999. Symptoms of hypoglycemia, thresholds for their occurrence, and hypoglycemia unawareness. *Endocrinol Metab Clin North Am* 28(3):495-500, v-vi.

9. Simons, D. G. 1988. Myofascial pain syndrome due to trigger points. In *Rehabilitation Medicine.* J. Goodgold, ed. St Louis: Mosby, pp. 686-732.

10. Bjorntorp, P., G. Holm, and R. Rosamund. 1999. Hypothalamus arousal, insulin resistance and Type 2 diabetes mellitus. *Diabet Med* 16(5):373-383.

11. Ionescu-Tirgoviste, C. 1998. Proposal for a new classification of diabetes mellitus. *Rom J Intern Med* 36(1-2):121-134.

12. Grundy, S. M. 1999. Hypertriglyceridemia, insulin resistance, and metabolic syndrome. *Am J Cardiol* 83(9B):25F-29F.

13. Bjorntorp, P., and R. Rosmond. 2000. The metabolic syndrome—a neuroendocrine disorder? *Br J Nutr* 83 (Suppl 1):S49-57.

14. Simons, D. G., J. G. Travell, and L. S. Simons. 1999. *Travell and Simons' Myofascial Pain and Dysfunction: The Trigger Point Manual.* Second edition. Baltimore: Williams and Wilkins.

15. Abbasi, F., T. McLaughlin, C. Lamendola, and G. M. Reaven. 2000. Insulin regulation of plasma free fatty acid concentrations is abnormal in healthy subjects with muscle insulin resistance. *Metabolism* 49(2):151-154.

16. Rao, G. 2001. Insulin resistance syndrome. *Am Fam Physician* 63(6):1159-1163, 1165-1166.]

17. Pasquali, R., and V. Vicennati. 2000. The abdominal obesity phenotype and insulin resistance are associated with abnormalities of the hypothalamic-pituitary-adrenal axis in humans. *Horm Metab Res* 32(11-12): 521-525.]

18. Anuradha, C. V., and S. D. Balakrishnan. 1999. Taurine attenuates hypertension and improves insulin sensitivity in the fructose-fed rat, an animal model of insulin resistance. *Can J Physiol Pharmacol* 77(10:749-754.

19. St. Amand, R. P., and C. C. Marek. 1999. *What Your Doctor May Not Tell You About Fibromyalgia*. New York: Warner Books.

20. Daoust, J., and G. Daoust. 1996. *Fat Burning Nutrition: The Dietary Hormonal Connection to Permanent Weight Loss and Better Health*. Del Mar, CA: Wharton Publishing.

21. Arciero, P. J., M. D. Vukovich, J. O. Holloszy, S. B. Racette, and W. M. Kohrt. 1999. Comparison of short-term diet and exercise on insulin action in individuals with abnormal glucose tolerance. *J Appl Physiol* 86(6):1930-1935.

22. Austin, J. H. 1999. *Zen and the Brain*. Cambridge, MA: MIT Press.

23. Feldman, R. D., and N. D. Schmidt. 1999. Moderate dietary salt restriction increases vascular and systemic insulin resistance. *Am J Hypertens* 12(6):643-647.

24. Simons, Travell, and Simons. 1999. *Op. cit.*, p. 188.

25. *Ibid.*

26. Dykman, K. D., C. Tone, C. Ford, and R. A. Dykman. 1998. The effects of nutritional supplements on the symptoms of fibromyalgia and chronic fatigue syndrome. *Integr Physiol Behav Sci* 33(1):61-71.

27. Eisinger, J. B. 1998. Alcohol, thiamin and fibromyalgia. *J Am Col Nutri* 17(3):300-303.

28. Eisinger, J. B., A. Plantamura, P. A. Marie, and T. Ayavou. 1994. Selenium and magnesium status and fibromyalgia. *Magnes Res* 7(3-4):285-288.

29. Simons, Travell, and Simons. 1999. *Op. cit.*, p. 189.

30. *Ibid.*

31. *Ibid.*

32. *Ibid.*, p. 205.

33. *Ibid.*, p. 207.

34. Hendler, S. S. 1991. *The Doctors' Vitamin and Mineral Encyclopedia*. New York: Simon and Schuster.

35. *Ibid.*

36. Ng, S. Y. 1999. Hair calcium and magnesium levels in patients with fibromyalgia: a case center study. *J Manipulative Physiol Ther* 22(9):586-593.

37. Cadbury D. 1997. *Altering Eden: The Feminization of Nature*. New York: St. Martin's Press.

CHAPTER 24

Your Healing Team

Some doctors consider patients with fibromyalgia (FMS) and chronic myofascial pain (CMP) as "difficult." Patients often carry with them the frustration of years of attempts to get medical professionals to take them seriously. Their neurotransmitters are dysregulated, so they may be tearful, defensive, hypersensitive, or even hostile, with sudden mood shifts. They are often in great pain and, in past experiences with the medical establishment, they may have been ridiculed and abused.

Patients are genuinely disturbed that their bodies are not performing up to par; while at the same time, their family, friends, and employers are placing demands on them that can't be met. Lack of understanding about the neurophysiology of chronic pain syndromes and the advent of evidence-based medicine has often resulted in insufficient care for patients who need help.[1]

Doctors need to meet their patients with sincere compassion and understanding, and a desire to understand the cause of the pain. They need to be comfortable developing a partnership with you and the rest of your medical team. If they can't do this, they should not be treating patients with FMS and CMP. It is acceptable to refer these patients to a doctor who can and will treat these conditions. It is not acceptable to see these patients, take their money, and then treat them with lack of respect and understanding.

Much of this nonprofessional attitude on the part of medical personnel is due to their lack of training. "[M]uscles in general and trigger points (TrPs) in particular receive little attention as a major source of pain and dysfunction in modern medical school teaching and in medical textbooks."[2] Doctors must *know* how to examine patients for CMP. If your muscles are weak, your doctor must understand why they are weak, and not just start you on a strengthening program. If you have myofascial TrPs, a strengthening program could be a recipe for disaster.

It is unethical for a doctor to give you a diagnosis of FMS and then say, "There is no cure. Learn to live with it. Good-bye." Jan Dommerholt, Director of Rehabilitation who works with Dr. Robert Gerwin (see chapter 15), says that doctors who have this attitude have patients with "iatrogenically-maintained FMS." The doctor is a perpetuating factor. One of the keys to FMS symptom relief is your physician's willingness to try new strategies if the current ones don't work for you.[3] There is a lot that can be done to improve quality of life, and care providers must be willing to provide care that will do that. This includes investigating perpetuating factors and teaching healthy lifestyle changes and ways to improve and maintain function. When the diagnosis is given, hope must be given, as well. "Following a structured program for assessment and treatment, most people with FMS can experience substantial improvement in the quality of their life."[4]

Many patients don't describe all of their symptoms to their doctors because they sense the doctor's disbelief. In our culture many people expect physicians to see all and to know all, which is a recipe for trouble for both doctor and patient.

For those of us who have FMS or CMP, there are only three kinds of doctors. The ones who already *know* how to diagnose and treat FMS and CMP, the ones who are willing to *learn* about FMS and CMP, and our *former* doctors. Don't expect your doctor to know everything, but do expect your doctor to tell you when he or she doesn't have an answer. Don't expect overnight relief. There is no "quick fix." Do expect your doctor to look at the materials you bring in, if they are reasonably concise, referenced, and pertinent. This is why I wrote, "What Everyone on Your Medical Team Should Know," in *The Fibromyalgia Advocate*,[5] and included specific handouts for each member of your medical team. I hoped to whet the appetite for knowledge. Once a doctor recognizes that FMS and CMP are real and common conditions, and that there is research available, true medical education can begin.

Why You Need a Medical "Team"

Your needs may be different from another patient with FMS and/or CMP, so your team will be made up of different types of specialists. Research has shown the need for a multidiciplinary team to manage complex chronic pain conditions as the following extracts testify:

> Frequently, clinicians incorrectly diagnose patients and resulting treatments are ineffective, which may promote the development of chronic pain. The treatment of nociceptive pain should be multimodal and involve spinal manipulation, muscle lengthening/stretching, trigger point therapy, rehabilitation exercises, electrical modalities, a variety of nutritional factors, and mental/emotional support.[6]

> An outpatient interdisciplinary treatment program was effective in reducing many FMS symptoms. Treatment gains tended to be maintained for at least six months. There were large individual differences in response to treatment. Identification of subgroups of FMS patients and their specific clinical characteristics may be useful for maximizing treatment efficacy.[7]

> Treatment of chronic pain is most successful when it is approached in a multidisciplinary fashion with the focus not only on treatment of underlying etiology, but also on the secondary impacts of pain on the patient's life. The management of chronic pain requires special expertise. Treatment of chronic pain includes a variety of medications, psychological support, and rehabilitation.[8]

There was a woman who was stationed overseas. Janet Travell had treated her for about eight years before Janet stopped seeing patients. This woman wanted to come back to the States to be treated by me as a successor to Janet. Before seeing Janet, she had had about fifteen years of unrelenting muscular pain. Janet had actually given her two hours, which stretched to three. Two hours just to hear the story, and then an hour to be looked at.

And at the end of all this, the patient broke down and said, "I'm sorry to have taken your time because I know you can't help me." Janet put her hand on the patient's hand and said, "I know what you have and I can help you." And that was the beginning of healing. Being in the presence of someone who knew what she had gave her confidence."

—From Robert Gerwin, M.D., neurologist, Bethesda, MD, organizer of Focus on Pain Travell Seminars

All FMS patients require three components to their treatment: (1) improvement of sleep by means of appropriate medications, (2) aerobic exercises that help combat depression and improve the emptying of the muscles of noxious catabolites, and (3) direct treatment of soft-tissue problems. Physical therapy methods are helpful but because wide areas of the body are involved, myotherapy may be more effective. Currently, FMS is basically a management problem with a great deal of trial and error. This is no different from the majority of medical problems that we can manage but not cure.[9]

Your Part in the Team

It is important for you to learn about the relationship between TrPs and CMP. Then, you can demand that your medical care team become at least as well informed. Make sure your medical care team understands that these are physical ailments. The constant effort of dealing with pain has reduced your physical activity, limited your social activity, impaired your sleep, caused loss or change of your family role, and perhaps been responsible for loss or change of your job. These changes alone can cause emotional turmoil. It is clearly true that some of us also have emotional problems, and these can worsen the physical symptoms of FMS and CMP. These emotional issues must be dealt with, but the physical needs must be met as well.

Your doctor may need your help in finding your perpetuating factors—those factors that reinforce, aggravate, and continue the conditions that sustain your TrPs. Your doctor and/or bodyworker needs to uncover factors like skeletal defects, but you can help by becoming more aware of how you move through your life.

It is important that everyone on your medical care team understands that regaining function is very important for your quality of life, but it isn't the only thing that is important. Quality of life is crucial. It's a great goal to be able to return to work, and to have meaningful employment, but it is not sufficient that your life be productive. You deserve to be happy as well. Sustainable work is work that doesn't leave you shaking and in tears from the pain, unable to cook or eat dinner. Working one day shouldn't cause total collapse the next day.

As a rule, when you visit your doctor, it is usually because of a specific symptom. Often, that symptom is pain. Doctors often want you to relate your pain to other experiences. A scale that rates pain from 1 to 10 doesn't do the job. Numbers are meaningless when discussing pain levels, except to give an idea as to what you are experiencing in relation to what you have previously experienced. The scale numbers 1 to 10 mean different things to different people. Many women can describe the pain they feel as worse than labor pains. Other people can say their pain is worse than a third-degree burn, or a heart attack, or whatever they have experienced in the past. Comparison helps.

You must be honest with your health care team. When you decide on a regimen, it is up to you to see it through. That means lifestyle changes, including diet and exercise, regular hours for sleep, mindwork, and whatever else it takes. If you aren't doing your part, you can't look to your health care team to "fix" it. Medications alone won't do it, and bodywork you have done to you by others won't do it alone either. The most important member of your medical team is *you*.

Your Primary Care Physician

If you have FMS or CMP, finding a primary care physician may be difficult. If you already have an excellent physician, and she or he knows little or nothing about FMS and CMP but is willing to learn, stay with that doctor and provide her or him with as much information as you can find. Your doctor can always become educated. But learning to be compassionate is something else.[10]

You may need to travel to find a doctor who is experienced in these conditions who can evaluate you and then set up a chronic pain management plan for you and your doctor to follow.

A good doctor works for *you*, not for the insurance company or your employer. Your doctor's most important task is to help you find the guidance and tools you need to manage your condition. To do that effectively, your doctor must know the direction in which to go. Someone on the Internet once posted this message: "I'm teaching a course in FMS. Translation: I have a new doctor." Add CMP, and that phrase all too often describes the situation very clearly.

To test for FMS, doctors need to take a good history, and look for signs of bodywide allodynia and sleep disturbance, especially lack of restorative sleep. They also have to test for eleven of eighteen tender points, using 4 kg pressure. This is the pressure it takes to cause the doctor's fingernail to whiten. In one study, very few physicians were able to estimate even close to 4 kg pressure. Most of the results were widely scattered. If your doctor is unsure about the pressure to apply to your body, there is a pressure threshold meter that can be used for routine diagnosis of FMS. The tissue compliance meter is a handheld, mechanical instrument that measures soft-tissue consistency objectively and quantitatively.[11] Dr. Robert Gerwin has created a wonderful video series for your physician to learn how to diagnose myofascial TrPs (see Appendix C). It is very thorough. He also has hands-on training available, organized with the physician's busy schedule in mind. Continuing medical education credits are available for physicians, dentists, and bodyworkers who take these courses. There is no excuse for not getting up to speed.

What to Look for in a Primary Care Physician

When choosing your primary care physician, whether that person is an allopathic Medical Doctor (M.D.), a Doctor of Osteopathy (D.O.), a Doctor of Chiropractic (D.C.), or a Doctor of Naturopathy (N.D.), you'll want someone who is willing to work with chronic pain conditions. Perhaps the most important criterion, though, is finding someone you can trust and who trusts you. You'll want someone who believes FMS and CMP are real conditions, who will keep current on therapies and research, and who will treat you in accordance with the most up-to-date information. Janet Travell said that above all, doctors must believe that their patients hurt as much and in the way that they say they do. She speaks of the "mystery of history," and says that to take a good history, the physician must first be willing to believe the patient.

Medicine is a service occupation. You hire a doctor and his or her staff to help in your care. You are the employer in this unwritten contract. If there is a problem, speak up. You need a doctor who knows how to listen and how to communicate and will take the time to do both. Your doctor should be your consultant and your partner.

There are some who thought they had a doctor who understood and was sympathetic to their needs. When they obtained copies of their medical records, however, they found out that their doctors had been clueless all along. They saw entries in their medical logs that had no resemblance to what they remembered. Their doctors had been acting sympathetic, but had been writing words like "neurotic," "hypochondriac," and "psychosomatic." One doctor wrote, "She wants to try all that crazy New-Age bodywork." One doctor referred his patient to seven different specialists, and then accused the man of "doctor shopping." Most of these people were able to find better doctors, but not all were able to get the harmful words erased from their medical records. They are still paying for their former doctors' lack of knowledge.

Because FMS and CMP do not respond to cookbook medicine (there is no one cause, and no one treatment), you need a doctor who knows how to work with a health care team, who communicates with them regularly, and receives their communications with interest. Your primary care physician needs to understand the basic concepts of FMS, CMP, and chronic pain states.

Finding a good doctor is more difficult than just finding a doctor you like. Ask your friends for recommendations. Talk to the people in your support group.

One way to ensure that you make the right decision is to schedule a compatibility interview with any potential doctor, during which you describe your previous bad (or good) experiences with health care providers; find out whether the doctor is comfortable dealing with FMS and CMP; and discuss important health care options and lifestyle choices. Here are some questions you might ask:

1. When are the best times to reach you?

2. What are the best ways to get in touch with you?

3. Are you willing to talk with and work with other family members or supporters?

4. Who will be available to answer questions when you're not available?

5. What kind of health care program do you recommend?

6. What is your opinion about alternative, noninvasive treatments?

7. Are you willing to work with other health care professionals in determining the most appropriate treatment for me? If not, why not?

8. Are you comfortable dealing with chronic pain conditions? What is your assessment of the importance of pain control?

9. Are you comfortable dealing with patients who are educated about their conditions and manage their own health care?

10. Will you be comfortable if I want a second opinion?

Don't expect a doctor to read tons of information you bring in to the office. Don't drop off huge medical books and expect your doctor to read them. Do expect openness to well-referenced, scholarly, concise, and current material.

The Good Doctor Checklist

The following characteristics are typical of good medical practitioners. How does your doctor rate? If s/he does not rate high, perhaps it's time to discuss these issues with your doctor and/or to seek out a new one.

A good doctor:

- Believes that steps can be taken to relieve your symptoms. • Accepts FMS and CMP as legitimate medical conditions. • Enforces your self-esteem rather than diminishing it. • Listens well. • Believes you. • Is knowledgeable and sympathetic to those with FMS and CMP. • Is willing to advocate for you within reason. • Is trustworthy. • Permits you to bring a family member or friend along on visits. • Encourages you during a visit to ask the questions that might be bothering you. • Encourages you to ask for explanations if you don't understand what you're being told. • Allows you to disagree. • Is honest with you about your diagnosis. • Supplies willingly copies of your test results. • Accepts that you may bring lists of questions, a tape recorder, and so on to office visits. • Shows interest in and, within reason, reads what you bring in concerning FMS and CMP.

The Initial Visit

A thorough medical evaluation begins with the doctor taking a careful medical history. This includes a completely frank discussion of all symptoms, even those that seem irrelevant or unimportant. The physician you choose for this examination needs to be sensitive, compassionate, and willing to listen to and address your concerns. You need to feel comfortable, safe, and validated during the examination. The examination for FMS and CMP *demands* physical palpation, as well as a detailed history. Palpation is a time-consuming art that is not well honed in many practitioners. This must change.

Palpating TrPs can cause severe pain for days. Your doctor should examine a muscle for TrPs only if s/he is going to treat that muscle afterwards. You may need additional pain medication before and after the exam. If there is a myotherapist working with your doctor, Spray and Stretch treatment can be very beneficial at this time. Plan on taking it easy for the rest of that day and evening, with frequent stretching, and be sure to drink extra water.

For your initial evaluation, gather the information specified below:

- A detailed list all medications, vitamins, and health care preparations you are using for any reason, and their dosages.

- A detailed, thorough medical history of yourself and your family. For example, you may remember your mother talking about her thyroid disorder or your early growing pains, or your Uncle Jake's description of his diabetes or his lapses of memory. For help in compiling this history, talk with family members.

- A list describing changes in your appetite, diet, weight, sleep patterns, sexual interest, ability to concentrate, memory, and bowel and/or urinary habits.

- A detailed list of your symptoms, when you last had them, and for how long. Include what helps and what makes them worse.

- A detailed list of any recent stressful life events, such as the loss of a loved one, job changes or problems, family problems, or moving.

- A detailed account of your diet, use of caffeine-containing substances (coffee, tea, chocolate, soft drinks), use of alcohol, and any smoking habits.

If your doctor advises particular medications, diet, exercise programs, or other courses of treatment, you have a responsibility to investigate every aspect of this recommendation thoroughly. Only then will you be able to determine whether it is something you are willing and able to do, what might stand in the way of your ability to implement this treatment, whether there are possible side effects, and so on. This will give you more information on which to base questions to ask your doctor.

Test Results

Ask your doctor to explain your test results and what they indicate relative to your overall health. Education is an important part of assuming responsibility for your own health. The more you know, the better your decisions will be.

Ask for copies of all of your test results. You may not understand what they mean (most of us don't), but these copies should be in your possession. You then can make your records available to other health care providers, eliminating the need for expensive duplication of tests or lengthy time delays while new testing is completed. Your doctor may be willing to forward test results to other members of your health care team. These records also provide an accurate history of changes you undergo through the years.

Repeat Visits: What You Need to Do

When a new symptom occurs, don't automatically assume that FMS or CMP has caused it. It may be caused by another illness. It is wise to have a complete physical examination periodically so that your primary care physician can monitor your progress. Keep communication lines open between all the members of your medical team.

Be clear about your problems with function. Tell your doctor whether you are having difficulty brushing your teeth, taking a bath/shower, grocery shopping, handling change, writing, brushing your hair, walking, lifting, climbing stairs, getting dressed, picking up children, driving, exercising, eating, making love, and so on. Be specific in describing your symptoms and in how they disrupt your life.

Many people find it helpful to make lists of questions before going to see their doctors. Here are some questions you may want to ask:

- What do my symptoms mean? • Could these symptoms be side effects of my medications? • What is the purpose of the test you're recommending, and why is it necessary? • What are the risks involved in the treatment you're prescribing? • Do I have any other options? • Do I have to limit my activities during this treatment?

During your office visit, take notes. Make sure you understand what is said to you. If you don't, get clarification. You may have memory and cognitive deficits, so take a tape recorder, or ask for detailed instructions in writing.

What You Don't Need

In many cases of long-undiagnosed chronic pain syndromes, the doctor shoulders the burden of convincing the patient that the condition is treatable. Often, for patients who have FMS or CMP, it is the other way around. You don't need doctors who won't listen and/or won't believe you. You certainly don't need doctors who blame you for your symptoms. This is inappropriate, abusive behavior. If your self-esteem is already low, this attitude can destroy what little you have left.

Does your doctor seem cold, abrupt, or too busy to talk? Are you afraid of or intimidated by your doctor? If you are assertive, does your doctor become impatient with you? Has your doctor ever said, "I don't want to hear that," when you say you aren't doing well? Has your doctor yelled at you or belittled you? If you answered yes to any of these questions, you have a problem. Everybody has a bad day, but abusive behavior is never appropriate and should not be tolerated.

I would like to address our medical care providers. For years, some of you (let's be honest—many of you) have been saying that FMS and/or myofascial pain don't exist. There is no shame in admitting you were wrong. There is no penalty involved if you now admit that these conditions do exist. There is a great penalty for your patients if you don't, and it is not one that they have to pay.

The documentation is here, so your patients will find doctors who *will* support them. For those of you who still insist that there is no such thing as myofascial pain or FMS, there is only one thing to say. Goodbye. Don't accept patients with these diagnoses. Send us to doctors who can help us improve our quality of life, and return us to the highest level of function we can achieve.

If you have had many misunderstandings with your doctor, or bad experiences with other health care providers, you may want to visit your doctor with someone who can run interference for you. This person should be able to supply details when you forget, be knowledgeable about FMS and CMP, know what questions you want to ask, and be willing to ask them if you become too stressed or forget to ask them.

Some primary care doctors can't wait to refer chronic pain patients to other doctors. It's appropriate to send these patients to a pain management specialist for assessment and stabilization if that specialist has an adequate background in the treatment of FMS and CMP. It is inappropriate for the primary care doctor to expect that pain management specialist to become that patient's primary care provider.

The primary care physician must be willing to take over the maintenance of chronic pain patients once the pain specialist has decided on a pain regimen. This includes maintaining the appropriate medications.

The Medication Issue

When chronic pain patients ask for pain medication, they are often treated like drug addicts. However, if you have FMS and CMP, before you begin to understand what is going on in your body and mind, and sometimes even after, you most likely have no way of knowing when you're going to experience extra pain. If you have to beg for pain medication, this situation is compounded by guilt. Sometimes you're placed in this uncomfortable position by a gatekeeper, a receptionist or nurse who asks questions like, "What, you need more pills? Why, we gave you ten only a few weeks ago!"

Studies show that many doctors are unaware of current knowledge in pain management. This may cause you to receive less than optimal care, due to your doctor's unwarranted fear that you will become an addict if s/he prescribes opioids for chronic nonmalignant pain.[12] Certainly, your doctor should check you carefully if you suddenly need a great deal more medication. There may be another reason for your pain. But, often, doctors have been on the receiving end of a "narcotics" education that is just plain wrong.

As one patient put it, "Sometimes I feel the doctor is blaming me for my illness, that I must not be following each and every instruction as stated. I can't help it if his suggestions don't work. I know fibromyalgia is not easy to treat. I don't want to get high. I just want to feel as normal as possible."

What Your Doctor Needs from You

Here are some guidelines for developing a good relationship with your doctor:

- Be reasonable. Your doctor has many patients.

- Don't expect a cure.

- Don't expect handholding. (That's what support groups, friends, and family are for.)

- Don't waste your doctor's time with irrelevant talk.

- Write questions in advance and have them ready for the doctor at your visit.

- Be honest with your doctor. If you aren't going to comply with a treatment or medication regimen, say so. Perhaps there are alternatives.

- Repeat back what you hear in case of any misunderstanding. For example: "Did you mean for me to take this three times a day only while I'm awake, or three times in a twenty-four-hour day?

- Listening goes both ways. You are paying for your doctor's advice, so listen well.

- If your doctor recommends a treatment program, share your concerns, but remember that *you* decide. Don't change a treatment plan on your own; communicate with your doctor.

The cost of medical care is an issue for many of us. Discuss this concern with your health care providers. They may be able to steer you to programs that assume some or all of the costs of your treatment or medications.

Other Members of Your Healing Team

A physiatrist (fizz-ee-at-trist, or fizz-eye-at-trist) is probably the most logical specialist to treat CMP until the field of myofascial medicine is organized. Physiatrists specialize in physical medicine and rehabilitation. They help you restore as much physical function as is possible. If you have FMS as well, your physiatrist may want to call in an endocrinologist and a neurologist, too. Note that expertise in a specific specialty is no guarantee that a doctor understands FMS and CMP. Furthermore, the lack of a specialty is no sign that the doctor doesn't understand the two conditions. There may be general practitioners who can help you. I have known some great physiatrists who understood both FMS and CMP, and I have also met some who didn't know a TrP from a Shasta daisy. Make sure that your doctors have well-used copies of the *Trigger Point Manuals*.

Your Bodywork Therapist

Some of the most important people in your life are your bodyworkers, who may or may not have a degree in physical therapy. Some people have more than one bodyworker and receive a different type of bodywork from each. It is vital that you find the best and the most appropriate therapists for yourself. The proper physical therapy for arthritis, for example, is not interchangeable with FMS or CMP care.

If you have FMS, find a bodyworker who is knowledgeable about it, who is comfortable dealing with it, and who understands your pain. If you have CMP, if possible, find a certified myofascial TrP therapist close by, or at least someone who is *very* familiar with the *Trigger Point Manuals*.

Travell and Simons have made it abundantly clear that weight training and work hardening programs should not be used on people with TrPs, although they *may* be appropriate for *some* people who have *only* FMS, if the work level is started *very* low.

For those with TrPs, pain and muscle tightness will grow progressively worse if inappropriate therapy continues. When their grip strength finally gives out, weights may be strapped to their wrists. When patients refuse (rightfully) to continue the program, the health care team may even blame them for being noncompliant, and the insurance company may refuse to pay. This is intolerable. If you have TrPs, you must also avoid the use of cool swimming pools, which may chill your muscles, may cause cramping, and will aggravate your TrPs.

Insurance companies must learn that a physical therapy degree does not confer automatic knowledge of TrPs. Certified myotherapists have that training. Schools that teach physical therapy need to understand that they *must* teach their students about myofascial TrPs for their care to be effective for myofascial pain.

Psychological Support

It is inappropriate for a primary care physician to expect a psychiatrist to assume chronic pain management. Nonetheless, there are some types of psychological and psychiatric support that can greatly aid some patients with FMS and CMP. There are many types of psychological support, such as marriage counseling, pastoral counseling, vocational counseling, and social work. Which areas in your life need help the most? Find someone who would best fill your needs. Make sure that whomever you find is educated about the cognitive aspects of FMS.[13]

Team Healing

How do you get your care providers to work as a team? Sharing communications is one way. You are the manager. Write a letter of intent and make copies for each member of your team. List all members, and clearly explain: These people are my healing team. Explain the part each one plays. Let them know your total plan for health maintenance. Include your pharmacist, dentist, spiritual advisor, etc. Get team members accustomed to the idea that they should send copies of relevant reports to each other. Let them know that *you* would like a copy of all reports. Keep a copy of this letter for your files. Get your team used to communications with you and with each other. Remind them they are part of a team—*your* team.

Pain Clinics

When it comes to FMS and CMP, pain clinics offer a mixed bag. Some are good, some are bad, and some are downright ugly. Some pain clinic personnel know little about FMS and CMP. How can you tell? If your doctor wants you to attend one, ask to first speak to some people who have been through the program at the recommended clinic. Make sure these patients are people with FMS and CMP. Stay away from pain clinics that:

- Insist you sign a promise that you will not acknowledge pain

- Are organized like military boot camps

- Don't understand the nature of FMS and CMP (i.e., think they are the same or that they don't exist)

- Will not allow you to mention pain to relatives or companions during your treatment

- Want your relatives and companions to sign an agreement to disregard your pain

- Insist that you discontinue all medications

Some pain clinics are great for evaluation and stabilization. Some take in people who are hurting and actually provide some help. And some pain clinics have actually disabled people who have come to them for help.

Joint Dysfunction, FMS, and CMP

Too often, the lack of basic training in FMS and CMP leads not only to inappropriate physical therapy, but also to inappropriate procedures. Some of these cause irreversible damage. Surgery is one of the most detrimental of these practices. It has its place, certainly, but unless there is an obvious perpetuating factor, such as an operable tumor, that place is not in the treatment of FMS and CMP.

Joint dysfunction and TrPs may exist independently, or they may coexist, feeding on one another. If they coexist, both conditions must be treated. It is important to discover which one is the origin of the majority of the pain, and try noninvasive therapies first. The tendency is to focus on the abnormality that is easily seen and then ascribe the patient's condition to it. If the patient has a bulging disc or degenerative joint disease and the real source of the problem is sought, found, and cured, no change has taken place in the imaging study at all.[14]

Treating the Patient, Not the X-Ray

Your medical team members must be willing to treat *you*, and not your X-ray or other tests. This means that they need the training to realize that most "disc" problems do not require surgery. The next section was written by my friend, the late Ken Hoelscher (M.D., physiatrist), on the subject of disc surgery. Like me, Ken spent a lot of his time answering Internet questions. He gave me permission to include this excerpt in this new edition, and hoped that it would enlighten some medical team members.

About one-fourth of the population without any known back problems or complaints of back or buttocks pain has a herniated disc (medically called herniated nucleus propulsus, or HNP). Not a *bulging* disc but an absolute *herniation*. . . . One of the best studies I've come across was by Dr. S. W. Wiesel, an orthopedic surgeon who teaches at both Georgetown and GW medical schools.[15] Dr. Wiesel noted the following:

> "Spinal disease was identified in an average of 19.5% of the (nonsymptomatic) under 40-year-olds, and it was a case of HNP in every instance. In the over 40-year-old age group, there was an average of 50% abnormal findings. . . . So every disc definitely doesn't require surgery. In fact, the great majority don't."

The Saal brothers are affiliated with the Stanford University Medical Center, Menlo Park, CA 94025. They offered a choice to patients with HNPs who were definitely and severely symptomatic: buttocks pain shooting down the back of the leg into the heel or toe or both. They *could* have had surgery, and all were unquestionably cases in which even the most conservative M.D. would not question the judgment call. Or, they could be treated conservatively by a program of, essentially, "If it hurts, don't do it." Medications were available, but for the most part they simply were encouraged to be active to the point of pain, to avoid painful positions or situations, but to be as active as their HNPs would permit. At the end of six months, about half were completely without symptoms. At the end of five years, the status of the surgically treated group and the nonsurgical group were virtually *identical*.

The human body is a self-healing machine, in most cases, which has resources we have yet to dream of, and we shouldn't sell it short by thinking some M.D. has to go charging in on a white HMO card and save us from ourselves. Steroid injections will suppress local inflammation temporarily. If the cause isn't corrected, the inflammation will recur. More steroid shots over a period of time will only damage the associated ligaments.

—Ken, a physiatrist from Syracuse, New York

I looked up these articles. In one[16] I found the conclusion that "cervical disc herniations can be successfully managed with aggressive nonsurgical treatment," with "high patient satisfaction." In another,[17] "Successful outcomes were achieved in 50 of the 52 (96%) nonoperatively treated patients. A subcategory of patients with extruded nuclear fragments had an 87% success rate. Ninety-two percent of the overall study population was able to return to work."

As much as it grieves me to know that this is the last writing we will do "together," I know Ken is smiling from Above, knowing that his words may still be keeping readers from unnecessary surgery. Here are two more excerpts from medical journal articles that reinforce the argument for conservative treatment:

> Conservative chiropractic treatment may provide an effective therapeutic intervention in selected cases of cervical disc protrusion. Instrument-delivered adjustments may provide benefit in cases in which manual manipulation causes an exacerbation of the symptoms or is contraindicated altogether.[18]

> The lumbar muscles, especially the multifidi, are a largely neglected source of pain and vertebral joint dysfunction. Even those with extrusion of disc material are responsive to manual reduction.[19]

Always find out your noninvasive options, and if you have been considering disc surgery, ask your doctor to review the journal articles cited above, as well as relevant paragraphs from chapter 7.

The quality of your rapport with your healing team will have a direct impact on the quality of your life. It's worth your time and effort to set up a coordinated team, and to do your part to help the relationship work as smoothly as possible. Both your state of health and your peace of mind will benefit.

Endnotes

1. Thorson, K. 1999. Is fibromyalgia a distinct clinical entity? The patient's evidence. *Baillieres Best Pract Res Clin Rheumatol* 13(3):463-467.

2. Simons, D. G., J. G. Travell, and L. S. Simons. 1999. *Travell and Simons' Myofascial Pain and Dysfunction: The Trigger Point Manual*. Second edition. Baltimore: Williams and Wilkins.

3. Millea, P. J., and R. L. Holloway. 2000. Treating fibromyalgia. *Am Fam Physician* 62(7):1575-1582, 1587.

4. Hall, S. 1999. Common pain scenarios. *Aust Fam Physician* 28(1):31-35.

5. Starlanyl, D. 1998. *The Fibromyalgia Advocate*: Oakland, CA: New Harbinger Publications.

6. Seaman, D. R., and C. Cleveland III. 1999. Spinal pain syndromes: nociceptive, neuropathic, and psychologic mechanisms. *J Manipulative Physiol Ther* 22(7):458-472.

7. Turk, D. C., A. Okifuji, J. D. Sinclair, and T. W. Starz. 1998. Interdisciplinary treatment for fibromyalgia syndrome: clinical and statistical significance. *Arthritis Care Res* 11(3):186-195.

8. Russo, C. M., and W. G. Brose. 1998. Chronic pain. *Annu Rev Med* 49:123-133.

9. Zohn, D. A. 1997. Relationship of joint dysfunction and soft-tissue problems. *Physical Medicine and Rehabilitation Clinics of North Am* 8(1):69-86.

10. Spiro, H. 1992. What is empathy and can it be taught? *Ann Intern Med* 116(10):843-846.

11. Fischer, A. A. 1997. New developments in diagnosis of myofascial pain and fibromyalgia. *Phys Med and Rehab Clin of N Am* 8(1):1-21

12. Lebovits, A. H., I. Florence, R. Bathina, V. Hunko, M. T. Fox, and C. Y. Bramble. 1997. Pain knowledge and attitudes of healthcare providers: practice characteristic differences. *Clin J Pain* 13(3):237-243.

13. Starlanyl. 1998. *Op. cit.* See the section "What Your Mental Health Worker Should Know."

14. Zohn, D. A. 1997. Relationship of joint dysfunction and soft-tissue problems. *Phys Med Rehab Clin North Am* 8(1):69-86.

15. Wiesel, S. W. 1984. A study of computer-assisted tomography. I. The incidence of positive CAT scans in an asymptomatic group of patients. *Spine* 9(6):549-551.

16. Saal, J. S., J. A. Saal, and E. F. Yurth. 1996. Nonoperative management of herniated cervical intervertebral disc with radiculopathy. *Spine* 21(16):1877-1883.

17. Saal, J. A. 1990. Dynamic muscular stabilization in the nonoperative treatment of lumbar pain syndromes. *Orthop Rev* 19(8):691-700.

18. Polkinghorn, B. S. 1998. Treatment of cervical disc protrusions via instrumental chiropractic adjustment. *J Manipulative Physiol Ther* 21(2):114-121.

19. Schneider, M. J. 1991. The traction methods of Cox and Leander: the neglected role of the multifidus muscle in low back pain. *Chiro Tech* 3(3):109-115.

CHAPTER 25

Support Structures

A structured support system is essential to optimize the quality of your life. Healthy people can afford to take more casual approaches to arranging support, but for those of us with chronic pain, a casual approach is a recipe for trouble. If you pay no attention to establishing a support system, you may find yourself without help when you really need it. Develop a support system that ensures you will always have support when you are in "flare," when you need encouragement, or when you just need companionship. However, developing such a system is often not easy for those who have chronic pain conditions like fibromyalgia (FMS) and chronic myofascial pain (CMP).

Issues in Developing a Strong Support System

There are many issues that make it difficult for people with FMS and CMP to find and keep strong support, even in our families. Several of them are listed here along with some possible solutions. If your problem is not listed here, do some creative problem solving. Ask yourself, "How could I do, manage, or handle this in a different way so that it does not make it difficult for others to be supportive of me?" You could ask some others, such as family members and health care providers, to help you find solutions that will work for you and those who care about you.

Problem: Others don't understand what you are going through. They may get irritated because you spend so much time going to health care appointments and taking care of yourself.

Possible solutions:

1. Hold meetings with family members and other supporters, describe to them what you are experiencing and how it is affecting you and your life. Tell them what you are doing to help yourself feel better.

2. Educate them about FMS and CMP. Share this book and other resources with them. Invite them to attend workshops and informational meetings with you. Introduce them to informative Web sites.

3. Ask them to go with you to health care appointments to increase their understanding of FMS and CMP, what you need to do to help yourself, and how they can be helpful.

4. Attend a support group for people with FMS and CMP and/or other chronic pain conditions. You can find listings for these groups in your local newspaper. At these groups you will meet people who are experiencing what you are experiencing and can understand better than anyone else. These people often become the very best supporters. You can also ask any of your current supporters to go to these meetings with you.

Problem: You are often moody, irritable, depressed, and generally "just hard to get along with."

Possible Solutions:

1. Do everything you can to relieve the pain and other symptoms—keep up with your health care appointments, medications, and therapies (it is hard to be supportive of someone who is not doing his or her part in trying to feel better).

2. Be aware of the effect you are having on others, and work to control those behaviors that make it difficult for others to be with you and support you.

3. Use "I" statements like "I feel grumpy" instead of accusatory statements like "Your cheerfulness is driving me mad."

4. When you are feeling moody, irritable, depressed, and "hard to get along with," do something you know will help you to feel better such as listening to some of your favorite music, watching a video that makes you laugh, reading something that is funny or inspirational, or petting your cat for a while. Make a list of things that help you feel better when you are "grumpy" and post it in a convenient place for easy referral.

5. Being low in complex carbohydrate intake can cause irritability. Determine whether this is an issue for you.

6. Consider taking antidepressant medication.

Problem: You may be very needy and demanding. Taking responsibility for your care may overwhelm others and may keep them from doing the things they want to be doing.

Possible solutions:

1. Have at least five supporters (including family members and friends) so that no one person has to do everything for you that you need to have done. Often people will say things like, "I have my spouse," or "I have my daughter so I don't need anyone else." These close family members can become overwhelmed, too. They need time to take care of themselves and to do the things they want to do. If they don't get this time, they may become very resentful.

2. Call a meeting of your family members and other supporters to discuss what it is you need and how that can be managed, so no one will feel overwhelmed.

3. Avoid always asking the same person for help.

4. Take really good care of yourself. Do whatever you can do to avoid "flare" so you can do more to take care of yourself.

Problem: Your ability to be involved in certain enjoyable activities with others may be limited.

Possible solutions:

1. Make a list of activities you can do with others to make up for those you cannot. For instance, while you may not be able to play softball, hike, or even work in the family garden, you may be able to join others in going for a walk, doing some bird or animal watching, watching

videos, going to the movies, attending a concert or art show, discussing a current issue. Share the list of things you can do with your supporters. Let them select the activities they would like to do with you and set up a schedule to make it happen.

2. Watch for "windows of opportunity" when you feel well enough to do those activities with others that you normally can't do. Then do it, being very careful not to overdo.

Assessing Your Current Support System

A good rule of thumb is to have at least five reliable friends or family members (or FMily members from fibromyalgia support groups) whom you can call on when you need support. Each of us needs different kinds of support from our supporters. Some supporters may be able to provide help like cooking the meals and cleaning the house, while others might be good listeners and assist you in making plans for your care. Others might attend church with you each week or go with you to the movies.

In general, supporters are people who:

- you enjoy being with • you choose to spend time with when you want to relax and have a good time • you turn to when you need someone to talk to • you can turn to for help in decision making • you depend on for assistance with the tasks of daily living and special health care needs that have become impossible for you

Good supporters allow you the space to change, grow, make decisions, and even to make your own mistakes. They allow you to express your feelings and emotions and your needs and wants. You don't want them to have all the answers, and they don't want or expect you to have all the answers for them.

Your supporters need to be educated about fibromyalgia (FMS), chronic myofascial pain syndrome (CMP), and related issues. In addition, you need to know about any issues that are important to them. For instance, if a supporter is diabetic, make it a point to learn about that illness and how it impacts on your supporter's life.

Perhaps the most valuable trait of a good supporter is the ability to listen without judging, criticizing, or giving advice. A good supporter lets you freely express all of your feelings and emotions. Your supporters will be people you like, respect, and trust, with whom you share common interests and rapport, and with whom you can share anything. *You and your supporters need to have an understanding of mutual respect for each other's confidentiality.*

Supporters should also be people who can count on you when they need a friend. If they don't often ask you for assistance or support, then do something nice for them so they will know how much you appreciate them. One of the nicest things you can do for them is to listen to them when they have something to share.

When you begin your journey on the road to healing, you may not have five supporters. Family members and friends who had supported you in the past may have distanced themselves as your needs intensified. Most of the people you consider your supporters may be health care providers. While health care providers are often excellent supporters, they can't be available to you all the time or for certain activities, and they may, at any time, change jobs or move away. It is best to develop a strong system of "natural supports" like family members and friends who are more readily accessible.

Who do you consider to be your supporters right now? Who do you reach out to when you are having a hard time? If you live with others, like a spouse, adult children, or housemates, you may or may not consider them to be supporters. Perhaps you have friends, neighbors, coworkers, and colleagues who you consider to be your supporters. *Make a list of these supporters with their phone numbers. Post it near your phone.* You could also include health care providers on this list.

This list is important as it is often difficult to remember your supporters and look up their phone numbers when you are having a hard time. *Are there five really good supporters who meet your needs for support on this list? If not, how many more do you need to meet that goal?*

Building a Support System

Developing supportive relationships doesn't just happen. Most of us have to work on developing and maintaining supportive relationships all our lives. You must choose your supporters yourself. No one else can determine who should be your supporters. Supporters have to be people with whom you feel absolutely comfortable. You may want to ask someone who already is a supporter to help you find other supporters but the choice is always yours. Begin looking for support close to or at home. Remember, your supporters will need guidance from you in how to give you the kind of support that you need.

Family: Are there some family members who might be good supporters whom you have not called upon in the past? These could be family members in your household like adult children or a spouse. Or they could be family members who do not live with you like aunts, uncles, cousins, parents, or grandparents.

Acquaintances: Do you have some acquaintances whom you like who might be able to fill a more supportive role? Perhaps some people you knew in the past, present or past coworkers, even people you grew up or went to school with. It could be someone with whom you do volunteer work or a person who attends your church or a special interest group. Use your local newspaper as a guide for finding out about groups and events in your community that you could attend to make new friends while doing something you enjoy.

Support groups: Fibromyalgia and chronic myofascial pain support groups are excellent places to find supporters. In these groups you become acquainted with people who can really understand what you are going through because they have already experienced or are going through very similar life experiences themselves. One woman told me that, "The daily grind of FMS and CMP was wearing me down. Then, I met someone at a support group meeting. After that, I met one of her friends. Before we knew it, we had a support network. I feel so much better knowing that I can give help as well as get help. It feels so good to be able to be useful again."

Try new things: In order to make new friends, you may have to do some things you don't usually do. In the process you may find that you like or enjoy doing these new activities. For instance, you may never have gone to formal religious services. If it feels right to you, try attending one. You may wish to try several different houses of worship. If one feels like a good fit for you, go back several more times. You may want to attend regularly and become a member. You may meet some people there who will become your friends and possibly even supporters. Or, you might register for an adult education class to learn something new. At the class you may meet one or several people with whom you feel a stronger connection. You could join a women's group or men's group, a group for single parents, a bird-watchers group, or a group of gourmet cooks. There are many options and opportunities. Become aware of what is happening in your community and try going to things that interest you. If it feels right, go again and again.

If you cannot work, check out volunteer activities where you can meet other people with similar interests. It is important to be careful not to overwork or to become involved in tasks that might worsen your symptoms. Most communities have a clearinghouse for potential volunteers. Check it out. Make sure the people you will be assisting understand your limitations.

How Do People Become Supporters?

When you've talked with the same person several times at a support group or at some other shared activity, you may decide to exchange phone numbers. After several conversations, you may want to do something special together like going out to lunch or a movie. The relationship may become more and more supportive as you get to know each other, or it may not, depending on how you and the other person feel.

When you are sure that both of you feel comfortable together, and you are talking with each other about more personal matters, you may want to tell that person more about your condition. If that person is interested in your condition and is curious about how you manage, you might ask whether he or she is willing to become one of your supporters. (Don't do this until you know the person very well. When you do ask for support, explain in detail what you want and need from your supporters.) Tell the person that, in return, you will be their supporter, doing your best to provide for them all that you expect of them. (It must be very clear that you are requesting a two-way, or mutual, relationship.)

Tell the person that you have several supporters and that it is not necessary for any individual supporter to be available for you at all times. At any given time, supporters will have excellent reasons why they are unavailable, including work responsibilities, family responsibilities, other plans, illness, or vacations. And they may not be comfortable cleaning or doing heavy work. Make it clear that you expect your supporters to set limits on how they can be supportive. If you ask a supporter for company or assistance and that person says he or she is unavailable, respect that response and find someone else to meet your needs. This keeps supporters from becoming burned out, and keeps you from interfering with their lives.

Keeping Your Support System Strong

Let your supporters regularly know what you want and need from them. For instance, you might say, "Today, I just need you to listen to me while I vent and express my angry feelings. Then I want to figure out this situation for myself." Another time you might say, "Today, I'd like some feedback and advice. I also need a reality check." Being absolutely clear in stating your needs is the best way to get what you need for yourself.

If possible, spend as much time focusing on your supporters' needs as they spend focusing on yours. Using the peer counseling structure described later in this chapter is a good way to ensure that you both receive equal time to be heard. You may want, and ask for, your supporters to work with you in deciding the next best step to take in a difficult situation. Then, when you have figured out what to do, your supporters can assist you in taking that step. Your supporters provide sympathy and encouragement when you need it. You, in turn, offer sympathy and encouragement to them when they need it.

Don't give up on supporters immediately if they criticize, judge, and/or advise you without having been asked to do so. First, explain to them what it is you want and need as well as what you don't want. Then, see if they can support you in the way you described. Many people are not accustomed to listening to someone talk without commenting. They feel that if you say something, it's their job to respond by telling you whether you are right or wrong and what you should do about it. But, if you state your wishes clearly, eventually most people can learn how to listen without feeling the need to respond immediately.

If you note early warning signs of a flare coming your way (see chapter 13), contact supporters and schedule time with them. Also, when you have a crisis, such as the loss of a job or a disagreement with a family member, plan time for additional support. Then you will have someone to listen, to help you make decisions, and to help you take any necessary action.

You don't want to wear out the people you've chosen to support you. In addition to making the support relationship one of give-and-take, you can take the following actions to keep the relationship in balance.

- Support your own good health: Others will enjoy being supportive of you if you do everything you can to keep yourself as healthy as possible, using the strategies you learn from this book, other resource books, your health care team, and others who have either FMS or CMP or both.

- If you have a hard time making and keeping friends, ask your health care provider or others you respect and trust if you have social habits or behaviors that others might find offensive. Are you too loud, too pushy, too negative? Listen to what they say without getting angry or becoming defensive. Ask others to verify these opinions. If you do have such habits, work with a counselor, your health care team, and friends to rid yourself of these habits. Admitting to others that you are working on eliminating these behaviors may be difficult. It will take work. You will need support while you do it.

- Delegate responsibility. If you are having a really hard time with fibrofog, flare, or depression and are unable to make decisions for yourself, you may need members of your support team to make decisions for you. For this reason, it's important for at least two supporters to know which treatments are all right with you and work well for you, and which treatments are either unacceptable or have not worked for you in the past. They need to know what procedures are necessary to get you help, if and when you are unable to seek help for yourself.

- Arrange meetings. You may want to arrange meetings between your key supporters and your health care team members when you are well. Then, if they need to contact each other when you are having a hard time, they will already be acquainted. Let supporters know who your health care professionals are, what roles they play in your life, and how they can be contacted. This makes it possible for you to get help fast when you need it. At these meetings you can explain what you want from your supporters, describe and explain the symptoms that indicate when you are having an especially hard time, and let supporters know what your health care team members would like them to do about it. This is also a good time for members of your support system to get each other's phone numbers and the phone numbers of your health care providers so they can coordinate efforts if necessary. Invite your support team members to a local support group meeting.

- Plan on enjoyment. Most of the time you spend with your supporters should be focused on enjoying each other's company and having a good time; in other words, being friends. It is just as important to be there for each other in the good times as it is in the more difficult times.

- Plan ahead for phone calls. Ask your supporters what time of day they prefer for receiving phone calls. Avoid late night or early morning calls unless you have a true emergency. The person you call at 8 A.M. may have fallen asleep only a few minutes ago.

- Keep a list. Make a list of your support team members with their phone numbers. As you implement the strategies described in this chapter and gain new supporters, update your list. The time when it is hardest to remember who your supporters are is also the time when you most need to reach out to them. Have copies of the list by your phones, on your bedside table, in your journal, and in your pocket or purse.

- Assess the appropriateness of the support for which you are asking. Have you been using your professional health care team as moral support? Is this kind of support appropriate if you have a mental health counselor, psychologist, or psychiatrist? Frequent calls to members of your health care team when you need attention or reassurance is not appropriate. Calling too often for moral support is a good way to trigger "burnout" in your health care providers; it leaves your doctor, physical therapist, or other care providers feeling very frustrated. If you have a psychologist, social worker, or other counselor, you may want to talk to that person about this problem. He or she can help you set up a healthy support system.

- Avoid dropping in on your friends and supporters. Call them before you stop by to make sure that it is a good time to visit.

Tips for Supporters

If you are a supporter, and all of us are, there are some very important things you need to remember. Always:

- Take good care of yourself. • Make sure *you* have plenty of support. • Listen, but put realistic boundaries around the time you have available. You don't have to listen for hours on end when you need to get some rest or have other things you must do. Tell the person you are supporting how much time you have to listen, and then return to your other activities. • Be supportive whether or not the person you are supporting is able to take your advice.

Avoid:

- Trying to rescue or fix the person you are supporting. • Doing things for the person you are supporting that he or she can easily do. • Assuming you know what the other person wants or needs. Ask before taking any action! • Doing things for the person you are supporting that you don't really want to do. • Overwhelming the person you are supporting with comments, ideas, and suggestions—just one or several is plenty.
- Nagging. Nagging never helps.

Being in a Committed Relationship

When you have a chronic pain condition, your spouse or partner is especially vulnerable to stress caused by the changes in your family role. Often your significant other is the one who has to take over many of your responsibilities, as well as taking on the role of primary care giver for you. It isn't easy for anyone to see you in pain, and feel helpless to make it better. Many things may be a turn-off—coughing, choking, and gagging are not exactly romantic.

Your spouse may come from a family where problems were dealt with by being ignored. This may be the case when your spouse is the child of an alcoholic. Your illness may be the spur that makes or breaks your relationship. A marriage counselor may be the saving grace and the helper you need to get through the transition in your relationship.

All chronic illness stresses marriage, even the best of marriages. You need to keep your lines of communication open. Give your partner some time off. You can use this space, too, to develop and be your own person. The most profound changes that chronic pain conditions can bring may be the deepening and enriching of your relationship.

If your spouse or partner is an active part of your support structure, this may ease your symptoms and moderate the negative effects of your lower activity level.[1]

The following suggestions will help to keep your relationship strong. They may even help improve how unsettled couples deal with troubling issues.

- Be honest with your partner about how you are feeling (without whining). If you are not feeling well or you are experiencing severe pain, let her or him know what you are doing to help yourself and how they could be helpful and supportive.

- Talk openly with your partner about your needs and expectations. Give your partner the opportunity to determine those needs and expectations he or she can meet, and find other people to take care of those needs that your partner can't fulfill.

- You both may be feeling emotions like grief, sadness, depression, and anger or you may both feel overwhelmed. Be aware of each other's feelings and talk about them openly. Peer counseling with each other may be helpful for working through these feelings.

- Get outside help when necessary—don't expect your partner to do everything.

- Keep your support system strong. Ask your other supporters for help and support on a regular basis.

- Encourage and support your partner to take good care of him or herself, to do the things he or she likes to do, to pursue new or special interests, and to spend time with the people he or she enjoys.

- Plan special times together on a regular basis. Perhaps you could set aside one evening or day a week to "go on a date," to do something special that both of you enjoy. You each could take turns being the person who decides what you will do. For instance, you could go out to dinner, have a picnic by a bubbling stream, attend a movie or a play, go for a drive to an interesting place, or play some board games. Take vacations together, relax at a beautiful place you both enjoy.

- Take some time off away from each other—an occasional vacation, a whole day, or an afternoon or evening to do something enjoyable and special. By talking honestly about both of your needs, you can determine how often and how long these times should be.

- Spend time doing things that you enjoy doing alone.

- Let your partner know as often as possible how much you appreciate all he or she does for you. Say "Thank you" and "I love you" often. Reinforce this with hugs and other kinds of warm physical contact.

- When talking with your partner about how you are feeling use "I" statements like, "I feel grumpy and out of sorts today," or "I wish this pain would go away," instead of accusatory statements like, "You make me feel really badly," or "This pain is all *your* fault."

- You may be so good at hiding your pain that your partner may forget you have it and its associated limitations. Avoid becoming upset if this occurs. Gently remind your partner of how you are feeling, the things you need to do to help yourself, and the things you can and cannot do.

- Couples counseling may be helpful in addressing these issues. If your partner doesn't feel comfortable going to see a counselor, go by yourself and share the counselor's suggestions with your partner.

Assistance from Your Partner

It is an added bonus if your partner can learn to help with your therapy. If possible, make your partner a part of your healing. This will give you a chance at closeness you would otherwise miss. You can take walks and talk together. You can exercise together. Eat healthy together.

If you can, teach your partner a way of doing trigger point (TrP) acupressure on you that won't increase your soreness too much. Teach him or her to feel gently for the TrPs. If your muscles are very tight, your partner may not be able to feel the lumps under your hardened myofascia. This is probably an indication that you need electrical stimulation, myofascial bodywork, and/or attention to perpetuating factors before you can begin acupressure.

In severe cases, a light stroking touch may be all that you can tolerate. Ask your partner to gently brush his or her fingers over the top of your skin, softly stroking and hardly touching the surface. This can work soothing wonders on your head and neck.

Don't have your partner use acupressure on the tender points of FMS (see chapter 1), acupressure will not help these points. Trigger points caused by myofascial pain syndrome (see chapter 3), however, respond well to acupressure, but, unfortunately, it is easy to overdo. Have your partner start gently, so that you won't be sore the next day. Experiment, find what works best for you. When you feel better, be sure to return the favor using very light strokes. This form of bodywork is very relaxing and will please your partner. Mutual massage in this manner can help the two of you to bond more deeply. Gentle touching is very good for strengthening emotional ties.

Peer Counseling

Many people have found peer counseling to be a useful self-help technique that helps them to deal with the ongoing pain and frustration of FMS and CMP. Peer counseling builds relationships by assuring mutuality while providing opportunities for expression that relieve stress and support positive action and change.

In a peer counseling session, two people who are mutually supportive spend a previously agreed upon amount of time together, dividing the time equally, paying attention to each other's issues, needs, triumphs, and distresses. Sessions usually last one hour but they can be shorter or longer. Half of the time is spent addressing one person's issues while the other person listens, pays attention, and provides support. Then, they switch roles for the other half of the time. There is an ongoing agreement of complete confidentiality—anything shared during a session is not allowed to be shared with others. Judging, criticizing, and giving advice are also not permitted.

Sessions should take place in a comfortable, quiet atmosphere where there will be no interruptions or distractions, and where the matters discussed during the session cannot be overheard by others. Disconnect the phone, turn off the radio and television, and do whatever is necessary to eliminate other distractions. Although most people prefer sessions where they meet in person, peer counseling also can be conducted over the phone when necessary.

The content of the session is determined by the person who is talking. This person can use the time however he or she wants. The session may include eager talk, tears, crying, trembling, perspiration, indignant storming, laughter, reluctant talk, yawning, singing, or punching a pillow. A session does not always deal with emotional issues. For example, the person whose turn it is may want to spend the time planning how to carry out his or her life goals. The only thing that is not okay is hurting the listener. The person who listens and pays attention needs to do only that—be an attentive and supportive listener. Full control must remain at all times with the talker.

The Peer-Counseling Process

1. Find someone with whom you feel comfortable, someone you think you will be able to listen and pay attention to, as well as being someone you would trust to listen and pay attention to you.

2. When you have found that person, agree to exchange time listening to each other on a regular basis (daily, weekly, biweekly).

3. Agree on the amount of time to exchange. That time can vary from week to week to week. It may be five minutes over the phone or one hour for each person, or anything in between.

4. Find an environment where you will not be disturbed; take the phone off the hook, or have your calls held; find a childcare person or a baby-sitting cooperative to watch your child during your peer-counseling sessions.

5. As the listener, listen intently. Keep your focus on the talker and do not think about your own problems until it is your turn to speak.

6. As the talker, trust the listener by sharing all that you can about yourself. Say what you really think as much as you can.

7. As the talker, bring up and work on whatever you think will help you most. Take charge of your own time. Bring your watch to the session or an alarm clock. Be aware when your time is up and it is time to switch roles. Do not depend upon the listener to tell you that your time is up.

8. It is a good idea to start sessions by recounting something good that happened in the past week. End sessions by sharing something you are looking forward to. This technique will color your sessions with positive feelings for both the past and the future.

You may want to build time into your life for regular, ongoing peer counseling sessions. For instance, you may want to spend every Friday from 1 to 2 P.M. in the afternoon doing peer counseling with a supporter. This kind of structure helps to assure ongoing use of this valuable technique.

More About Support Groups

Support groups are wonderful places to make new, understanding friends. They provide an opportunity for you to be with people who have similar problems and issues, people who understand and can be supportive. You can form long-lasting friendships, or perhaps even find a life partner. New members of support groups for people with chronic pain conditions often express their relief at finally having found others who understand and believe in them. Communication is easy in a support group because you all share the common experience of dealing with FMS and CMP. Participants validate their common experiences while sharing information and giving feedback and support.

Finding a Support Group

There may be FMS and CMP or chronic pain support groups in your area. As a rule, they are listed in the community calendar section of your newspaper. Your local hospital, health agency, or health care professionals also may refer you to local support groups. After you find a support group, attend their meetings several times before making your decision about whether it is the right one for you. Every group can have an "off night" where people just don't get along with each other.

There may not be a specific FMS and/or CMP support group in your area. If that is the case, then you may need to start your own. This is easier to do than it sounds. Many national newsletters and organizations have informational packets that can help you start a group (see Resources). When starting a support group, it is helpful to have a physician, nurse practitioner, physician's assistant, or other professional associated with your group who can function as an ongoing resource for information.

The first time you hold a support group meeting can be scary. Spend the first part of the meeting having all those who are present give their names and say a little about themselves. That helps to get things going. To break the ice, you can start with yourself. Assure participants that they can come or go as they choose, they can stay seated or to get up and stretch, and that they can share or remain silent. Group members must agree at the onset that personal information shared at the group will remain confidential. In addition, group members should agree not to divulge to anyone outside the group any information about who attends the group. Support groups are about acceptance and empowerment. No criticizing or judging is allowed. Expression of emotion is encouraged.

Allow some social time to discuss what has helped others and what has not helped, and time to discuss individual problems and possible solutions. Simple, healthy refreshments help ease the process of people getting to know each other. Spread out the group's workload as much as possible. Find an assistant leader to chair some of the meetings, and to be there when you can't attend. Solicit help from volunteers for copying handouts, arranging for refreshments, and taking care of other details.

Your group may decide to have to guest speakers or educational programs. Possible topics include: hypnosis, massage, acupuncture, chiropractic treatment, medications, well-spouse support, easy cooking, FMS and CMP and the family, how to deal with insurance companies, and exercises. You may want to have an informational packet for people attending the group for the first time containing basic informational handouts and specific information about the group. Take time at the beginning of the meeting to get acquainted with any newcomers, so that they feel welcomed and comfortable.

Put some fun in to your support group. This can be especially important in times of extra stress, like the holidays. As part of our January FMS and CMP support group meeting, we have a gift swap. This is our notice:

> The Gift Exchange! Bring in something that may have use for someone else, but not for you. In an effort to declutter your life and have some fun, people are asked to bring something to swap. Don't buy anything. It does not have to be new. It needn't be a holiday gift. Please don't wrap it. The catch: you bring something, you take something else back home!

In February, we have a picnic, complete with tropical T-shirts under parkas, luau music, and lots of laughter and friendly support.

Your Rights and Your Support System

The following list of actual rights compared to traditional assumptions is from *The Relaxation & Stress Reduction Workbook*.[2] Use this list as a general guide for dealing with people in your life on a day-to-day basis.

Traditional Assumption: It is selfish to put your needs before others.

Actual Right: You have the right to put yourself first.

Traditional Assumption: It is shameful to make mistakes.

Actual Right: You have the right to make mistakes.

Traditional Assumption: If you can't convince others that your feelings are reasonable, then your feelings must be wrong, or maybe you are going crazy.

Actual Right: You have the right to be the final judge of your feelings and to accept them as legitimate.

Traditional Assumption: You should respect the views of others, especially if they are in a position of authority.

Actual Right: You have the right to form and voice your own opinions and convictions.

Traditional Assumption: You should always try to be logical and consistent.

Actual Right: You have the right to change your mind or decide on a different course of action.

Traditional Assumption: You should be flexible and adjust to unpleasant circumstances. Others have good reasons for their actions, and it's not polite to question them.

Actual Right: You have the right to protest unfair treatment or criticism.

Traditional Assumption: You should never interrupt people. Asking questions reveals your stupidity to others.

Actual Right: You have the right to interrupt people in order to ask for clarification.

Traditional Assumption: Things can always get even worse than they are now; don't rock the boat.

Actual Right: You have the right to negotiate for change.

Traditional Assumption: You shouldn't take up others' valuable time with your own problems.

Actual Right: You have the right to ask for help or emotional support.

Traditional Assumption: People don't want to hear that you feel bad, so keep it to yourself.

Actual Right: You have the right to feel and express pain.

Traditional Assumption: When someone takes the time to give you advice, you should take it very seriously. They are often right.

Actual Right: You have the right to ignore the advice of others.

Traditional Assumption: Knowing that you did something well is its own reward. People don't like show-offs. Successful people are secretly disliked and envied. Be modest when complimented.

Actual Right: You have the right to receive formal recognition for your work and achievements.

Traditional Assumption: You should always try to accommodate others. If you don't, they won't be there when you need them.

Actual Right: You have the right to say "No."

Traditional Assumption: Don't be antisocial. People are going to think you don't like them if you say you'd rather be alone instead of with them.

Actual Right: You have the right to be alone.

Traditional Assumption: You should always have a good reason for what you feel and do.

Actual Right: You have the right not to have to justify yourself to others.

Traditional Assumption: When someone is in trouble, you should help them.

Actual Right: You have the right not to take responsibility for someone else's problem.

Traditional Assumption: You should be sensitive to the needs and wishes of others, even when they are unable to tell you what they want.

Actual Right: You have the right not to have to anticipate others' needs and wishes.

Traditional Assumption: It's always a good policy to stay on people's good side.

Actual Right: You have the right not to worry about the goodwill of others.

Traditional Assumption: It's not nice to put people off. If questioned, give an answer.

Actual Right: You have the right to choose not to respond to a question or situation.

Endnotes

1. Goldberg, G. M., R. D. Kerns, and R. Rosenberg. 1993. Pain-relevant support as a buffer from depression among chronic pain patients low in instrumental activity. *Clin J Pain* 9(1):34-40.

2. Davis, M., E. Eshelman, and M. McKay. 1995. *The Relaxation & Stress Reduction Workbook*. Oakland, CA: New Harbinger Publications.

CHAPTER 26

At Work and at Home: Making Your Life Easier

There are many things you can do to make your home life easier for yourself and for those with whom you live. This chapter is a collection of some of the things that people who have fibromyalgia (FMS), chronic myofascial pain (CMP), or other chronic pain conditions have found to be helpful. You have probably discovered other helpful items or ways to do things for yourself by trial and error. You thought about the problems you were having and came up with some possible solutions, tried them, used those that worked well, and discarded the others. Here are three examples of helpful solutions that may be of use to you. Take what you can use and discard the rest.

Problem: You are not able take care of certain household responsibilities.

Possible Solutions:

- Identify those household responsibilities you can do so that you can still do your part. For instance, you may not be able to do heavy-duty chores like vacuuming, mopping, and scrubbing, but you may be able to do the laundry (provided you have an automatic washer and dryer), wash and dry the dishes, light dusting, and some cooking. Then, have a meeting with the members of your household, explain to them the things you can do and those you can't, and ask others to do the things you cannot do.

- If possible, hire someone to come in and do the difficult household chores. If money is an issue, consider hiring responsible teens, who usually will work for less money than an adult supporting a household; they can do a good job. Or barter with friends—they do for you what you can't do, and you do for them some of the things you are able to do. Perhaps there is an organization in your community that provides this service on a sliding scale basis or free.

- Live in a space that requires minimal care or where some care is provided, such as a condominium where the exterior is maintained without your help.

Problem: You have stopped working. Other family members are resentful because you can no longer make a financial contribution to the household's expenses.

Possible solutions:

- Apply for disability payments. See chapter 27.

- Check out possible part-time work options or different kinds of work that might be possible for you to do, given your symptoms.

- Let others know how much you appreciate their financial support. Assure them that you are doing everything you can to relieve your symptoms so that you can carry your share of the financial load again.

- Do whatever you are capable of doing to relieve the household duties of family members who provide financial support.

Problem: You live alone. Living alone can be especially challenging if you are dealing with FMS and/or CMP.

Possible solutions:

- Work on keeping your support system strong.

- Live in a place that is easy to clean and maintain, where you can move around easily (few stairs), and is close to public transportation.

- Hire someone to help you with household tasks or take advantage of free services that may be available in your area.

- Invite your supporters to your home often to share potluck meals, games, video watching, and other activities.

- Consider getting a dog, cat, or some other pet.

In the process of figuring out what works for you, use these problem-solving techniques, along with other ideas in this chapter and the following set of rules for survival.

Surviving the Game of Life with FMS and/or CMP

Simplify. Keep your household tasks as simple as possible. Analyze how you do things and see if there are easier ways that might be less stressful and/or painful. For instance, bed-making is often a frustrating task. Tucking in the sheets under the mattress can be enough to cut the skin around your cuticles. Wear gloves. If you have particular trigger points (TrPs), folding sheets can be agonizing. But if you strip a bed, wash the sheets, and put them back on, you don't need to fold at all. Janet Travell suggested trying to make your bed on your knees. That would help the folks who have only back and arm TrPs, but if you have bodywide TrPs, it's murder. Get a nice comforter instead. It works very well for hiding the evidence of a messy bed. Whatever you do, find the easiest way to do it.

Delegate. Is there something that must be done that you no longer can do because it has become so painful? You may be able to delegate the task. Ask someone else to do it. It may take time to teach someone else how to do it, but once you do delegate the task, you may wonder why you struggled with it for so long. Have weekly meetings with family members to divide up chores. You may want to have a rotating chore chart so that everything gets done and no one gets stuck doing the same chore over and over again.

Little children love to help. If you have no children of your own, borrow some. If you can't afford to pay for help from older children, perhaps you can trade with them by supplying tutoring. More often than not, there is a way to work these things out.

Set limits. When a relative or friend places unreasonable demands on your time and energy, use the experience as a chance to practice your skills at deciding what you can and cannot do, and to educate the other person about what you are experiencing. Give the other person options. For example, you might say, "You know, Aunt Tillie, I have fibromyalgia and chronic myofascial pain. I am quite limited in what I can do. I can either take you food shopping or out to dinner. Which would you prefer?" When possible, use either/or choices when confronted with too much to do. Say "No" when you have to, gently, and perhaps with regrets, but firmly nevertheless.

Pace yourself. Organize your day so you have time to rest. Try not to do more than one activity, in any small time period, that requires using a particular set of movements or muscle groups. For example, if you must climb steps, allow yourself some time to recover after climbing them.

Give yourself permission to admit that you have a medical condition. For example, rather than doing all the housecleaning, yard work, or similar types of physical activity in one long day, break up your tasks and do what needs to be done over several days. Listen to your body; when it tells you that you have been doing something long enough, stop. Use a little more than what feels like half of your energy at one time, as if you could do twice as much—if you absolutely had to. This provides you with a reserve. Don't wait until you have reached your limit and then collapse; you must learn to say "No" to yourself and others.

Modify. You can modify your home and change your habits to be as fibro-friendly as possible. For example, you can organize your closet so that coordinated tops and bottoms of outfits are on the same hanger. When you hang your shirts up, you can button them in advance, except for the top two buttons. That way, you can pull them over your head and not have to fumble with the buttons (if that is easier for you). You can buy shoes with Velcro closings so you don't have to struggle with shoelaces, or use elastic laces.

You can also modify your kitchen. Consider not using the higher storage cabinets if you must reach or climb something to access them. Keep your kitchen stocked with paper plates and plastic utensils for those times when your grip strength isn't great and doing the dishes is hard for you.

Find alternatives. One woman in our support group was always upset at the holidays. Each of her children said they wanted her to slow down and take it easy. But each child also said, "The holidays wouldn't be the holidays without your_____." One child wanted chocolate chip cookies made from scratch, another wanted upside-down pineapple cake. One daughter said she waited all year for the special bread that was based on her great-great-grandmother's recipes. But this grandmother had no energy left to enjoy the festivities. By the time her family sat down to their holiday dinner, she was exhausted.

But last year she did enjoy the holidays. She followed the advice of some of the women in her support group and made booklets of her favorite recipes. She gave them to her children as gifts, along with little stories of her childhood and theirs, complete with pictures. It was now time, she explained, for them to learn how to make those wonderful treats, and she would help with the tasting. Now she can enjoy herself during the holidays, and her children have priceless heirlooms.

Adjust your point of view. Think of your to-do list as a tool that helps you achieve your goals, not as a set of chores. Try to respond to the relentless grind of your illness as a never-ending challenge. For example, one woman says that she often feels as if she is living inside a maze. Mazes are used as endurance tests and as amusing puzzles and pastimes. Its all in your point of view. How you look at it can influence how you deal with it.

Delete. Whenever you are faced with a routine task you loathe doing, re-evaluate the task. Sometimes it isn't necessary. If ironing is painful for you and washing things out by hand is no fun, you can simply decide not to do those chores anymore! Just put your clothes into the washer, dry them, and wear them. Many synthetic fabrics do not need ironing. If you cannot stand wearing anything but cotton, try to find the crinkly kind of cotton that doesn't need to be pressed. And, if you have to wear a wrinkled garment, probably no one will notice. And if they do, so what?

Be Assertive. Prepare statements like the following to use when you are working with others:

- Because of my illness, I can only do so many things per day.

- I can't do what you asked me to do because that would push me beyond my physical limits right now. Is there an alternative you can suggest?

Develop a list like this one to keep your house guests (and family) from making extra work for you:

- If you sleep on it, make it up. • If you wear it, hang it up. • If you drop it, pick it up. • If you put it down, put it away. • If you eat out of it, wash it, or put it in the dishwasher. • If you make a mess, clean it up. • If you open it, close it. • If you use the last of it, replace it. • If you borrow it, put it back where it belongs. • If it rings, answer it. • If it cries, love it. • If you don't know what to do, ask.

Educate your guests. Teach your visitors about FMS and CMP. Send them some handouts ahead of the time they are expected to arrive for their visit. Let your guests know you need pure water, time for rest, walks, meals at certain hours with certain types of foods, and what you can and cannot do. Don't sacrifice your exercise, medications, therapy, or other healing routines. You may have to pay for the extra trauma of a visit or trip anyway, but buy it as cheaply as you can. Ask guests to reschedule their visit if they have a cold or some other contagious illness. If you are going for a visit, you can do the same. Send your hosts a handout indicating your special needs.

Relieving fatigue. The fatigue of FMS and CMP is often overwhelming; it may be the main symptom interfering with your ability to function in your family role. As an example, a woman once said to me, "I have a choice today, I can either wash my hair or unload the dishwasher. Everything takes more time for me. Some days, even the effort of breathing can cause me to be short of breath!" Fatigue can affect your ability to function in a big way. It's a sign you need to stop the world and get off for a while. Rest, take a walk, laugh, play. Make sure to schedule time for doing the things you do to enjoy your life.

Save your energy. Listen to your body. Avoid tasks that stress your body. Make your work easier. Plan ahead, simplify, use short cuts, labor-saving devices, self-help devices, organize, ask for help. And don't forget to save some of your precious energy for fun.

Sleep. Do everything you can to improve the quality and quantity of your sleep. Have a family meeting to discuss this issue. It is in your family's interest that they help you with this.

Often authorities advise people who can't sleep to avoid taking naps during the day. You may find, however, that a short nap during the day is essential to your functioning. Go with what works for you. If you're not sleeping at night, avoiding rest during the day may squelch the only sleep you can get.

One reader reported that the only decent sleep she ever got was on the sofa in the afternoon. She tossed and turned all night long in her bed. Her mattress was a superfirm type, touted as healthy. Her sofa was very soft. She also used a cervical pillow. (It had taken her several tries to find one that worked for her.) She used a sofa cushion as a pillow when she napped, the kind with a button in the middle. She put her head in the depression the button made, and she had neck support. Without her cervical pillow and soft sofa, she couldn't sleep. With them, she could.

Because of neck muscle tightness and range-of-motion restriction, many people with FMS or CMP find it very difficult to locate a cervical pillow to support their necks properly. When such pillows fit, they can be lifesavers. If they don't fit, your misery will be compounded. Check with your chiropractor, physical therapist, or hospital supply shop. They will often let you buy one on a trial basis, if you don't remove the plastic.

Make meal preparation easy. The fatigue associated with FMS or CMP may last a long time or a short time, and you never know when it may strike. Be prepared. Have easy to prepare foods and extra meals in the freezer or on the shelf that can be prepared by other family members. A microwave oven can be a lifesaver for a family when one person is experiencing chronic pain and others are busy with school, work, and other obligations. It can also help to minimize cleanup. Pre-cut dinners, such as stir-fry (in a microwave or frying pan with little oil or butter), casseroles, pot pies, and salads are good. Many things can be made ahead and heated later in the microwave, so you can clean up the preparation dishes and lessen dinnertime stress.

Meal preparation is another place where you can get help from family members. Even small children can set the table and prepare simple foods. Healthy take-out sometimes may be the only solution if you are having a hard time and there is no one to help.

Chairs that work for you One of the most common perpetuating factors of TrPs is the poorly designed chair. Check your chairs. See chapter 7.

Helpful Hints to Make Life at Home Easier

There are some simple things you can do to improve the quality of your home life. These ideas have come from FMily members everywhere.

- For extra warmth, use grain-filled small pillows covered with flannel, heated in the microwave. They will stay warm for hours, providing relaxing warmth to painful areas. Chill them in the freezer and they make good ice packs. You can also fill a knee sock with grain and do the same: knot the toe end, fill, and knot the other end. Just don't get it wet.

- Get up slowly and deliberately after lying down or sitting.

- If you get the chills, put on a warm hat, even in the house.

- Keep your personal telephone book on a hook next to the phone for easy access.

- Use the automatic redial on your phone. Think of using a phone with memory numbers for people you call frequently, as well as for emergency calls.

- The next time you buy a car, look for comfort. Choose power steering, cruise control, adjustable seats, and air-conditioning. Avoid deep bucket seats.

- Use felt tip pens for writing. They are easier on the hands.

- Look for special garden tools that have bent handles for easier use. Find ways you can cultivate your health by cultivating a few plants. Don't be too ambitious; start small.

- Ask your optician to help you find frames for your glasses that aren't too tight but won't slide down your nose. Consider using a tube or chain holder to keep your glasses around your neck when you aren't wearing them.

- Put your keys on a large key chain that is easy to find. The kinds that can be hooked onto a belt or belt loop are especially handy.

- Keep several sets of ear plugs by the bed. If you can't sleep at night because of noise, or if you haven't slept well and don't have to get up at a certain time, use them to cut down on sensory overload. Keep at least three sets in case you drop any when fumbling for them at night.

Clothing Hints

- Sit when you are dressing, especially when putting on socks, stockings, and shoes.

- Avoid buying garments that need hand-washing and/or ironing as much as possible.

- Check your closets. Rid yourself of tight, constricting clothes.

- Dress for comfort. Wear loose, well-made clothes with pockets for handkerchiefs and medications. Elasticized waists can be very comfortable.

- Check tag sales and garage sales for comfortable clothing so you can keep extras handy.

- Cut the labels out of your clothes to avoid scratches and cuts.

- A fanny pack may be more useful than a pocketbook and will hurt your body less.

Housework Hints

How you feel about housecleaning is all in the way you look at it. Once you've attained your FMS/CMP degree, you are intelligent enough not to be a slave to old habits. *A little disorder in the house is good for the soul. It says that you have more important things to do—like taking care of yourself.*

- When your daily chore list looks too formidable, see what can wait until next week, or next month, or can be deleted altogether. Don't overload tomorrow.

- Get a soft, new paintbrush to clean pleated shades and knickknacks (or better yet, give the "heirlooms" away as presents).

- Organize your work areas with lightweight items placed higher than heavy items.

- Close all doors and drawers when they aren't in active use.

- Make sure rugs are anchored on pads that prevent slipping.

- If you need to do a task that might involve climbing or reaching, wait until a friend is there with you, in case you fall. Better yet, ask the friend to do it.

- Use thinner, cheaper washcloths. They are easier to wring out.

- Keep pathways and stairways free of clutter.

- You can save trips up and down the stairs by reserving a spot, close to the stairs, to stack things that need to go up the stairs, another for things going down, and carrying them when you absolutely have to make the climb up or down.

- Hire household help if possible, especially for large tasks like window cleaning. You may be able to find a high school student who won't charge a lot willing to clean or do lawn care in the summertime.

- Do necessary chores while listening to inspirational, positive-thinking tapes or novels on tape. Dust off your mind while you dust your shelves. Check your library for tape selections.

- There are self-help kitchen aids such as jar openers, sharp knives, scissors, loop handles, and others. Ask your library, medical supply store, or an occupational therapist for information.

- Get into the habit of returning everything to its place after you use it. You will be amazed at how much this can simplify your life.

Kitchen Hints

- When you need to replace kitchen equipment, purchase easy-to-grasp utensils and bowls with nonskid bases. Request them as gifts.

- At the grocery, buy smaller, easier to handle sizes of the products you use. Consider using a grocery scooter on bad days. Even if you are only picking up a few things at the grocery, use a cart. A cart is also great to lean against while you are waiting on line for the cashier at the supermarket. Wet your fingers to open plastic produce bags at the grocery. That makes it easier to separate the two sides. Ask the person bagging the groceries to carry them to the car for you. Ask a family member or neighbor to carry your groceries into the house for you.

- Open plastic bags with scissors. Keep several pairs of scissors in a handy location.

- Carry a container of good spring water around with you. In the summer keep a small plastic jar partially filled with water in the freezer. Then, when you need a cool drink, you can just fill it with water and it will be the right temperature. The new bottle tops with straws make for easy drinking and fewer spills.

- Consider buying a commercial ingredient mixer that you don't have to hold.

- Keep insulated rubber gloves handy for when you must handle cold things. Use insulated oven mitts when carrying freezer items.

- Rather than grating cheddar cheese for cooking, freeze it in portion size. After it is defrosted, the cheese will crumble readily.

- Paper plates are light and they don't break. Find some that are relatively sturdy and environmentally friendly.

- Some salad forks, pickle, or junior forks are much lighter than regular forks and are easier to lift and use.

- Boil water in the microwave, and leave the door closed for a few minutes. You can then clean the microwave with a paper towel.

- Put your toaster on a metal tray. The crumbs will be easier to clean.

- Spray furniture wax on your stainless steel sinks and appliances. Things won't stick to them as easily.

There are many ways that you can improve your home and family life. Because some of the options are costly, like new mattresses and chairs, you may have to prioritize your needs, making allowances for financial restraints. However, some improvements can have such a dramatic effect on your wellness and your ability to participate in your family's life that you may decide to use a credit card to make your purchases.

Chapter 27

Ability and Disability

Fibromyalgia (FMS) and chronic myofascial pain (CMP) may force you to make major changes in your job or career. Perhaps you have had to cut back hours, modify your responsibilities, or change jobs entirely. You may have lost jobs because they were not appropriate to your special needs. These circumstances can be especially hard if, as many people do, you depend on your job or career for self-identity, respect, and esteem as well as for your income. The pressure is further increased if you are the sole support for yourself and your family. If you have increased work-loss time, your employer may feel burdened by this extra cost. Your job itself may be a basic part of your health problem by causing increased physical and mental stress that worsens your symptoms.

Although having a job may seem like a major problem, it can also be part of your solution. A job keeps your mind off your problems and gives you healthy ways to interact with other people and be accepted as you are. This chapter will encourage you take a closer look at your job, examine how it affects your life, and help you make some decisions to improve or change difficult work situations. It will also guide you through the process of getting disability benefits for the short or long term if that becomes necessary.

Risks in the Workplace

Injuries and disorders caused by overexertion and repetitive motion (formerly known as "work-related musculoskeletal disorders" and now called "occupational myalgias") are the leading causes of Worker's Compensation cases in the United States.[1]

One study[2] has shown that these injuries can be extremely expensive if they are not treated appropriately. The treatment usually includes job-related changes. Many things can contribute to these injuries, including repetition, awkward postures, excessive production rates or durations, and inadequate breaks. This study shows that these injuries often have a positive outcome when these factors are appropriately evaluated and addressed. Your doctor must do what is necessary to ensure that you get support from your employer to modify the perpetuating factors you may be facing in your workplace environment.

There are some common workplace activities that are known to aggravate FMS and/or CMP. Review the following list and check off anything that is an issue for you. Write down any other activities that are part of your job that may cause or worsen your symptoms.

- prolonged repetitive motion • maintaining one position for long periods of time
- extended hours (with FMS and CMP it is difficult to work for long periods) • heavy

lifting, or lifting and bending • high stress • keyboard too high or too low • poor equipment that makes it harder for you to do your job • poor or no seating • limited breaks

If the source of strain is not obvious, describe your work situation to your bodyworker. He or she can help you to identify those activities, movements, and stressors that are likely to overload your muscles with trigger points (TrPs). As you become aware of them, note them in your journal. Record any movement at work that increases your pain. You and your bodyworker, working together, usually can figure out what is causing your problem.

What Can You Do to Create Needed Change?

One study showed that most women with FMS and CMP have limitations in their ability to work, but they can continue to work at a level matching their ability if they can get the adjustments in the workplace they need.[3] These adjustments should be made as soon as possible.

In another study, 55 percent of those with FMS and CMP had continued to work, but most of them were working shorter hours and had changed their jobs.[4] Tasks such as carrying and holding objects were often the most difficult. Their symptoms had had a profound influence in their lives. Most of the patients in the study had changed their habits and life routines because of FMS and CMP.

You may need to do some creative thinking to find solutions to workplace problems. The following is a list of possible strategies for creating workplace changes. Check off those you think apply to your situation:

- Your bodyworker may be able to teach you how to avoid or modify movement or perform a particular task without aggravating any TrPs.

- Make a list of activities that are less aggravating to FMS and CMP than other activities. For example, walking on a level surface, some types of teaching, light desk work, and light sedentary occupations that allow varied tasks and changing positions. Then work with your coworkers or supervisor to figure out how you can begin to focus on the types of work that are less physically stressful to you.

- Break down big tasks and projects into small pieces that feel "do-able."

- Before you begin to do a task, ask yourself if there is an easier way to do it.

- Focus on how much you've accomplished rather than on how much you still have to get done.

- Avoid comparing yourself with others or focusing on your failures.

- Educate your supervisors about your medical condition(s) in writing, especially if you are taking medication or have symptoms that can have an impact on your job. (Note that some symptoms of FMS and CMP can be mistaken for drug or alcohol abuse symptoms. This makes it even more important to educate your supervisors.)

- Notice the time of day when you feel most energetic and clearheaded. If possible, tackle your more difficult jobs during those hours.

- Don't work through your breaks, lunch periods, or after hours. Use that time to do simple relaxation or deep breathing exercises, take a walk, do something you enjoy, or chat with a supporter.

- Set your priorities. Focus your energy where it can be used most effectively.

- Keep lists of what you need to do, and keep them where you will find them when you need them.

- Ask your bodyworker for some exercises you can do at work that will help you to avoid muscle strain.

- If possible, end each day by writing out a list of the tasks that you want to tackle the next day. That will give you a head start on tomorrow. Then, leave your list and your worries on your desk for the day, and go home.

- Use a freezer at work to store gel packs (or bring your own cooler) to use while you are working and find an outlet to plug in your heating pad near your workstation.

- What you wear to work can make a big difference in your comfort level. You may need to keep three sizes of clothing at work to accommodate body swelling and shrinking. Soft slippers and adjustable (Velcro) flexible sandals are helpful for those days when your feet swell. Avoid wearing constricting clothing that worsens pain. If your wardrobe money is limited, check out tag and rummage sales and used clothing stores. It hurts less when you spill indelible ink on a pair of pants that cost only a dollar.

- Some of the survival skills discussed in chapter 26 may help you in your workplace as well.

- Laugh whenever you can. Laughter boosts your immune system and lowers your blood pressure.

Optimizing Your Workstation

If you have FMS and CMP, working at a desk or some kind of machine, especially a computer, can be a real challenge. Using the following techniques might mean the difference between success at your job and hopeless frustration.

- When you talk to someone, turn your chair to face that person so that you don't have to twist your body.

- Keep work close to your body, with your upper arms held vertically. This is especially difficult for people with short upper arms. People with short upper arms do not fit on regular chairs. They have to lean to one side to use the armrests. This places strain on the muscles and can aggravate, perpetuate, and even initiate TrPs. If you do have short upper arms, find a comfortable chair, or adjust your chair to work for you. You may need to bring in foam rubber pads or sponges to tape to the chair arms to elevate them to a height more suitable for your needs. The pads or sponges make a soft resting place for the arms. Discuss this problem with your supervisor or your physical therapist. She or he may have some other suggestions for you.

- If you have TrPs, it is important to get up to stand and stretch every twenty minutes. Set a timer. Flex your fingers. Check to see that your shoulders aren't hunching. Move your head and neck around and do circular eye exercises (see chapter 19). This helps to avoid eyestrain.

- Use health aids like back supports, elastic supports, armrests, and wrist rests to help you do your work comfortably.

- Place soft pads under your keyboard, fax, and other electronic devices to absorb the noise they produce.

- If you spend a lot of time on the phone, get a speaker phone to avoid neck and arm strain. Avoid hunching your shoulder to cradle the phone receiver to your ear.

- Arrange your workstation so that the tools you use most frequently are the most convenient to reach.

- Make sure your computer screen is 18 to 30 inches from your eyes, about an arm's length. If you are farsighted and use reading glasses, when working at your computer you may need a pair that is a lower strength because your eyes are farther from the screen than from other written materials. Ask your eye doctor.

- Make sure your chair does not compress your circulation. The chair seat must not compress your hamstring muscles. Fit your hand under your hamstrings when you sit. If your hand doesn't fit, you need a footrest (see chapter 7).

- If you get shin-splint pain, try a triangular- or wedge-shaped footrest. Place the footrest with the point toward you. A large ring-binder can function as a footrest if need be.

- If you must make a presentation and are having a problem with dry throat, keep a supply of pure, room temperature water close by. Adding a lemon or lime twist will make it more refreshing.

Keyboard/Mouse Issues

People with FMS and CMP often struggle with their inability to type or use a keyboard as efficiently as they feel they should. One hand doesn't work as fast as the other, and each finger may work at a different speed. Your typing speed may vary widely from day to day. Fortunately, there are ways to make your life easier and your typing better whether you use a keyboard or a mouse.

- Make sure that your fingernails are short. The tips of your fingers should be able to touch the keys on the keyboard.

- A product called Hand-eze can be very helpful for keeping your hands in good shape. These fingerless gloves are available from a company called Dome (see Resources). They are made of a special type of Lycra that support and massage your hands. These gloves must fit your hands very well. The company will send you a form to size your hands properly, before you order a pair.

- Use wrist rests to rest your hands when you are not typing. Develop the habit of keeping your hands off the wrist rest when you aren't resting them. Using the wrist rest while you type puts your hands in a position that is not ergonomically correct.

- If using a mouse is hard for you, mouse alternatives, such as trackballs, Glidepoint, touch pads, or a graphic tablet may be the answer. Try them out before making a purchase to be sure they will really be helpful to you; you may lack the fine motor control some of them require. Note that Microsoft products have key commands for almost everything you need to do.

- Use a scanner to avoid having to type in new data. Investigate copyholders, pen expanders, and other health aids.

Here are some rules to follow to maximize your keyboard and mouse abilities:

- Keep your wrists straight and held in a neutral position, not bent up, down, or to either side.

- Don't stretch your fingers to reach for faraway keys—stretch your arm to put your fingers within reach.

- Keep your fingers curved as you type, with your thumb relaxed.

- Drop your arms and shake your fingers occasionally.

- If you are using a mouse, hold it loosely, and don't rest your arm on the surface while you work the mouse.

- Use your entire arm—not just your hand—to move the mouse.

- Check out the lighting at your workstation. Be sure to keep glare away from your screen. Adjust your screen brightness or contrast for better viewing.

Environmental Issues in the Workplace

Everyone needs and deserves a workplace where there are few interruptions, that is quiet, smoke-free, with clean air and adequate, well-positioned lighting. These amenities are especially important if you have FMS and CMP. You may find the hum of fluorescent lights unbearable. An air compressor can give you such a headache you may have to go home. When your neurotransmitters are not functioning properly, normal office noises can make you feel very anxious and irritable. Odors from chemicals and solvents may worsen your symptoms and make it impossible for you to work. Lack of exposure to outdoor light may make you tired and depressed. What is merely annoying or even unnoticeable for others may be intolerable for you. How can you solve these kinds of environmental problems?

First, you can ask your supervisor or employer to make the needed modifications. Then, if you can, have the annoyance moved, eliminated, or modified. Finally, if the necessary changes affect other employees, you may need to educate them about your special needs and let them know how these changes will also benefit them.

Your Employer

Your best option for working successfully with your employer is to establish an open and honest relationship based on mutual respect. Keep your employer advised of any circumstances that may affect your ability to do the job for which your were hired. Keep your employer's needs in mind as well as your own as you work to find solutions to problems that will allow everyone's needs to be met. Also, become familiar with your company's disability plan so you will know what you are talking about and what rights you have when you talk to your employer.

If you are changing jobs, consider telling your prospective employers what you will need by way of special accommodations. You can decide to tell a prospective employer about your special needs before or after you are hired. By making a very careful job choice, however, you may find that special accommodations are not necessary.

The Americans with Disabilities Act

The Americans with Disabilities Act of 1992 (ADA) guarantees equal opportunity to people with disabilities in the areas of employment, state and local government services, public accommodations, and telecommunications. It also states that employers must make reasonable accommodations both for apparent and nonapparent disabilities. If you are in a situation in which your health affects your ability to do your job, or changes to your job will be necessary to protect your health, notify your employer. If you feel that FMS or CMP is affecting your work situation or your ability to be employed, contact the National Institute on Disability and Rehabilitation (see Resources). This institute provides a resource guide that contains information on a variety of ADA materials, including guides, manuals, publications, training programs, and technical assistance programs. For a free booklet on ADA, contact the Office of Equal Employment Opportunity (see Resources.)

Your Coworkers

Other employees may become resentful if they see that you are receiving special accommodations. They will be more understanding and accepting if they understand exactly why you need these accommodations. Be as open as you can with them when describing FMS and CMP. Educate them about what you can and cannot do. When they understand the pain you deal with, they will be hard-pressed to be jealous of your accommodations. It is likely that you will find they know others who experience these same symptoms, or perhaps they have some themselves. Some visible reminders of your disability may help ease the situation. Let them see when you are using gel packs or a heating pad. Let them know what your wrist rest or support is for.

Avoid unhealthy workplace dynamics. Stay out of the competitions that can develop between coworkers. Avoid listening to gossip or spreading rumors. Don't allow yourself to be exploited or harassed. Just do your own job as well as you can. Encourage healthy office dynamics by showing a healthy appreciation for the aid you receive from others and praise coworkers for the good work they do.

Time for a Change?

Due to the nature of your job, you may not be able to modify your work situation to suit your physical needs. For instance, if your job requires heavy lifting, there may not be anything your employer can do to accommodate your condition. It may not be possible for you to keep a job that requires you to enter data eight hours a day. You may need to find a different job. An occupational therapist can help you in making this decision. Ask your doctor for a referral.

When making decisions about work and career, consider the fact that many people with disabilities are able to use the skills they acquired in dealing with their disorders to develop careers in special education, support, counseling, advocacy, and administration. Their life experiences make them especially effective in these roles.

Many people have found that creative job development (which in many cases means self-employment) is the best way to meet their needs for flexible scheduling, low stress, private space, and creativity in their careers. When you have created your own job, you can take a break when you need it. You can schedule your work to meet your personal needs. Your new career, directed only by you, will make good use of your abilities and creativity. Both of the authors of this book have done just that.

Answering the following questions will help you to decide whether you need to make a job change:

1. What do you value about your job?

2. What would you like to change about your job?

3. What jobs have you enjoyed in the past?

4. What are your favorite hobbies and activities?

5. Could you turn these into a job?

6. What skills do you have? (You may have skills that you don't even know are valuable. Take an inventory of them all.)

7. Are you satisfied with your current work or career?

8. Does your work enhance your health?

9. Would you like to pursue a different career, one that matches your special needs, interests, and abilities?

10. What would such a job be like? How would you spend your day?

11. Would you need more education or training to get such a job? If so, where could you get that training? How much would it cost? (Make a few phone calls.) How could you make it happen?

Take advantage of all of the resources available to you to find a job that is right for you or to assist and support you in creating a career for yourself. Contact the Department of Labor at http://safetynet.doleta/gov/career.htm for comprehensive information, or ask your local librarian for help.

Vocational Rehabilitation

The federal government, in cooperation with state governments, has set up a nationwide system of vocational rehabilitation services. These services provide various kinds of vocational assistance and support to people with disabilities. To access the assistance, you don't need to wait until you know exactly what it is you want to do. If jobs or careers are an issue for you, establish your connection with your local or state vocational rehabilitation services right away. They have a wide variety of resources available to guide and assist you in all phases of career development, and they can help you develop a step-by-step approach to achieving your goals. If you don't think they are giving you the help and support you need, don't hesitate to tell them. Ask them if there is any way that you can work together to get what it is that you feel you need. Note that to receive services, you may have to present medical documents or a statement from your physician verifying your condition. Contact http://votech.about.com or your local librarian for more information.

Employment and Training Services

States are federally mandated to provide individuals with free employment and training services, such as aptitude testing, job screening, job referrals, placements, and vocational counseling. These offices have comprehensive listings of local area employment opportunities. They can also refer you to other agencies when necessary. You can find your local employment and training office in the Yellow Pages of the phone book under Employment Agencies.

Small Business Development Centers

Each state has federal and state funded Small Business Centers that provide in-depth counseling assistance at no cost to people starting new businesses, and/or to existing firms. The centers' services include comprehensive resource referral libraries. They sponsor workshops on a variety of business-related topics. Call your State Small Business Administration Office, listed in your phone book under United States Government, for more information.

Office of Economic Development

Many larger towns and regions have offices of economic development that provide a range of services to businesses. Check the phone book to find such offices in your area. You can try looking under your state listing in the white pages. For example, Vermont lists this as the Office of Economic Opportunity. Sometimes it is listed under the county or region. If you have trouble locating an office, ask your local librarian to help you.

Libraries

Libraries are an excellent source of information to use in your job development plan. They are great for finding educational facilities and programs, career ideas, organizations, corporations, and how-to references. Your librarian can guide you to the proper resources.

Education and Training

If you're planning to change jobs, you may need to return to school. Returning to school at any level can be useful, exciting, and challenging, whether it to finish high school or to obtain a graduate degree. To make it work for you, here are some things you can do:

- Develop a Wellness Recovery Action Plan for managing your symptoms and use this plan daily. It is the best way to keep your symptoms from worsening and making it hard for you to do the things you want to do. See chapter 16.

- A good support network, both personal and professional, will increase your chances of achieving a successful educational experience. See chapter 25.

- Many schools have an Office of Disability Support Services (ODSS). Visit that office. You may need documentation (such as a medical report) of your disability to present to the ODSS before you can make use of their services.

Hints for Ensuring Success

- Before you return to college, contact the college's financial aid officer for information on the financial scholarships that might be available. When all other resources have been exhausted, you may be eligible for financial assistance from the Department of Vocational Rehabilitation. This assistance could help you to finance your education.

- For the first several semesters, carry a reduced number of classes until you become acclimated to the new environment and lifestyle.

- Become familiar with the resources on your campus. There may be a learning center or its equivalent that will assist you in sharpening your study skills and also may provide tutoring services. Some counseling centers provide support groups for students returning to campus after a long absence.

- If your disability prevents you from repaying student loans, contact the lender immediately and request a medical deferment. Note that granting deferment of your payments is not automatic. You must continue to make payments until you are notified that the deferment has been processed and approved. If you do not continue payments, you may be in default. Once your loan is in default, it can be very difficult to change that status.

- If you have to leave school for any reason, be sure to withdraw officially so that you do not fail your classes by default. For some classes, you may be able to have the designation "Incomplete" recorded as your grade, thereby earning the right to complete the course requirements at a later date.

When You Can't Work

As much as you may want to work, there may be either short or long periods of time when you cannot work at all or cannot do the kind of work you enjoy, are trained to do, or where you have the most experience. The stress of working when you are in severe pain can worsen your symptoms. Your ability to work may be affected by the severity of your symptoms, perpetuating factors, and coexisting conditions. Also, you may need time away from work to do the things you must do to relieve your symptoms—that is, to employ the kinds of strategies described in this book. Your inability to work can be an enormous hardship if you have to support yourself, or if you are responsible for providing all or part of the income for others. In 1989, Dr. Frederick Wolfe found that 30 percent of all fibromyalgia (FMS) patients surveyed had changed jobs because of FMS, 17 percent could not work at all, and 54 percent had problems performing daily functions.[5]

This section of the chapter will give you some basic information on applying for benefits and possible sources of income and services. This will be only the beginning of your search for help. Benefits programs vary in from state to state and often change. The ability to secure benefits also depends on your current circumstances, which also may change, making you either eligible or ineligible for specific programs. You will need to read the recommended booklets and check out related Web sites in the Resource section. You will have to make a lot of phone calls and may even have to undergo some personal interviews in your search for help. These may be difficult. Get help and assistance from your supporters.

Applying for Benefits: General Information

When you are applying for benefits, do your best to provide the most complete and accurate information possible. Ask the agency to which you are applying for assistance. If, due to the severity of your condition, applying for these benefits is hard for you, ask one or several of your supporters for assistance.

Be aware that you may be denied benefits. You may even be denied benefits more than once. If that happens, don't give up. Be persistent. Call the agency and asked them why they refused you. Then, based on their response, reapply. You may have to get a lawyer to plead your case. If you can't afford a lawyer, call the governor's office in your state and ask how you can obtain legal aid either free or at low cost. You could also write or call the offices of your state or federal legislators for assistance—especially if you do not receive responses in a timely manner. The legislators want your vote and often members of their staffs will be glad to help you. Remember, you deserve these benefits. Advocate for yourself until you receive them.

Note that there are many people in decision-making positions who are ignorant about the unique issues faced by people with FMS and CMP. They may even deny that FMS or CMP exist. You might encounter this problem over and over again, so be prepared. Here are three ways to combat this ignorance:

1. Never allow anyone to tell you that FMS and CMP are not real, or that you have no right to services and benefits.

2. Keep a file of credible information that describes FMS and CMP. Give copies of this information to people who need to learn more about FMS and CMP or those who deny the existence of these debilitating illnesses.

3. Keep your self-esteem intact. Keep reminding yourself that you are a very valuable and special person who deserves the best that life has to offer. If keeping your self-esteem high is an issue for you, refer to self-help books on how to build self-esteem and do the suggested activities regularly.

The following information is usually requested by agencies. Before you begin your search for assistance and/or benefits, compile all of this information and keep it together in one place for easy access as you may need to refer to it frequently:

> • social security card and/or social security number • photo identification • evidence of your financial situation and proof of any income • name, address, and phone number of your landlord • proof of rent and utility payments • registration and titles for all vehicles that you own • bank statements • copies of all your medical records (you have a right to these copies at a reasonable cost) • worksheet describing functional difficulties (see the end of this chapter) • Fibromyalgia and Myofascial Pain Syndrome Functional Questionnaire (see end of this chapter)

Qualifying for Benefits

To determine whether you can qualify for benefit or assistance programs, you first must establish whether you meet the particular agency's definition of disabled. In most cases, you must be incapable of performing any work, although this rule has some flexibility if you are over the age of fifty.

When applying for benefits, your case will be greatly enhanced if you have a report from your employer or previous employer that describes your past work performance (prior to FMS and CMP) and what you are currently able to do. For example, the report might say:

> Patient's previous job required climbing three flights of stairs, sitting at a computer for eight hours a day, coordinating company payroll and complex mathematical analyses. Periodically required to lift up to 10 pounds. Patient now requires frequent shifts of position, approximately every 15 minutes, and requires varying muscle function groups. Cognitive deficits include inability to handle simple checkbook balancing, short-term memory loss, and failure of grip strength. Muscle weakness includes buckling ankles and loss of positional sense. Patient has limited range of motion, loss of time sense, and currently is unable to drive or take public transportation. Cannot work.

You may need to see several physicians before you obtain a diagnosis of FMS and/or CMP. You tell the doctors that you are in pain, but where is the proof? Your tests results are normal. Research now indicates that certain patients are predisposed to get FMS and CMP,[6] but some doctors don't even believe that FMS and CMP are real illnesses and others know very little about it. You may be told it is "all in your head" or that you have "emotional problems." Clearly, more education is needed and you may have to do the educating.

When you speak to your doctor or attorney, describe the ratio of your good days to bad days. Mention fluctuations in the level of your pain. Describe exactly what it is you are experiencing. Explain everything. Be sure that your explanation includes the following information:

- what you used to be able to do

- what you can do now

- what you cannot do now

- how you have had to modify your lifestyle to accommodate your condition

Use simple language and assume that wherever it is possible to misunderstand, everything will be misunderstood. You may find that your descriptions of your symptoms are challenged because the symptoms are "transient" (they come and go). Officials often find it very difficult to grasp the concept of variable symptoms. Persist!

In order to use your medical records as proof of your need for disability benefits, the records will have to be very specific. When you are choosing your medical team, make sure your key player, your primary physician, is caring, careful, and articulate in keeping records. Your doctor should *specify* all of your pain symptoms and then list the specific factors or activities that would cause these symptoms to worsen. A complete report, if supported by a good medical record, need be only two to three pages long. Receiving disability benefits depends on how well your doctors document your case and how much they know about how they have to document it for you to become eligible for benefits.

Fibromyalgia and CMP are not on the SCI's List of Impairments. The SSA List of Impairments lists the conditions that are so *severe* that the people who have those conditions are *automatically* considered disabled. You can find this list in *Disability Evaluation Under Social Security* (The Blue Book), which contains the medical criteria that SSA uses to determine disability. It is intended primarily for physicians and other health professionals. This 205-page book can be obtained free of charge. Send your request by mail, fax, or phone to SSA:

Social Security Administration
Public Information Distribution Center
P. O. Box 17743
Fax: 410-965-0696
Phone: 410-965-0945

It can also be found at http://www.ssa.gov

The impairment of FMS and CMP vary too much from person to person to have them on an automatic disability impairment list. Many people with FMS and/or CMP are not disabled. Disability for FMS and CMP will have to be decided on a person-by-person basis. Some people who are granted disability benefits may find that with time off to pay attention to perpetuating factors and to create the proper support systems, they eventually will be able to resume a modified work schedule

When you try to qualify for benefits, always be prepared for difficult or unexpected situations. For example, one man in Maine was receiving disability payments, but he was filmed working in his garden and his benefits were canceled. His doctors had to write many letters to the state office explaining that they had prescribed yard work for him as a form of exercise. His ability to do a few hours of gardening a week did not translate into being able to work nine-hour shifts in a hospital (his previous job). This man fought to have his benefits reinstated and he won.

One person on the Internet commented that, like the rest of society, most people with FMS and CMP are hard workers. They enjoy doing a good job and they don't seek help until there is no other recourse. They are then treated as if they are trying to take advantage of the system. These problems should no longer exist. Dr. Mark Pelligrino[7] says that FMS and CMP are recognized by the courts, Worker's Compensation, and Social Security as bona-fide medical conditions. One long-term (eight year) follow-up study reported that for fibromyalgia, the symptoms remained stable over the years, with muscle function markedly reduced. It also reported that the condition had and continues to have a marked impact on work capacity.[8] Another study[9] administered a Quality of Life test scale to women with fibromyalgia, insulin-dependent diabetes, chronic obstructive pulmonary disease, osteoarthritis, rheumatoid arthritis, and permanent ostomies, and to a control group. The fibromyalgia patients consistently scored among the lowest in all measurements.

This isn't much comfort, but based on Internet communications, it appears that in other nations, the requirements for disability eligibility for FMS and CMP are just as biased and illogical as they are in the United States.

Starting the Claim Filing Process

Start the process of applying for benefits by filing claims with the agencies you feel would be most likely to give you the needed assistance, i.e., SSI or SSDI, Worker's Compensation, etc. These agencies are described later in this chapter. My vocational rehabilitation counselor guided me in this process, so you might look there for help. You could also reach out to your state agency of protection and advocacy. Every state has one of these agencies as mandated by the federal government. You can get the phone number for this agency by contacting the office of the governor in your state. Processes for filing these claims vary from state to state, agency to agency, and from person to person depending on your circumstances.

The agency to which you apply will need to know the nature of your medical condition; your physician's (or physicians') name(s), address(es), and telephone numbers; your job background and education. When you call, if an interview is required, the agency will set up an appointment for you. They will also send you a packet with information and forms.

You must make the agency understand what kind of problems you have. Describe your problems with fingering, dexterity, depth perception, changing vision, sensitivity to fumes and dust, movement, lifting, ability to concentrate, and any other issues that affect your ability to work. Use the Fibromyalgia and Myofascial Pain Syndrome Functional Questionnaire at the end of this chapter as a guide.

The Forms

There will be many forms for you to fill out. If writing is extremely painful for you, ask a family member or someone among your supporters to do the writing for you. Some of the forms will seem irrelevant or biased against people with chronic pain. That is why the Fibromyalgia and Myofascial Pain Syndrome Functional Questionnaire form at the end of this chapter is so important to you. The questions on this form are meaningful for the person with FMS and/or CMP. You are usually allowed to add many pages of comments, but sometimes agencies process only the information that is included on their forms.

The Interview

Always bring a tape recorder to all of your personal interviews and record the meeting, whether it is an initial interview, a follow-up interview, or an appeal for your claim. Your interviewers will probably tell you that you can have copies of their tapes, but they may take a long time getting them to you.

In the interview, "tell it like it is." Be clear about the extent of your disability and describe how it affects your ability to work. Be clear, straightforward, and to the point. Provide good examples but don't overwhelm or bore the interviewer with irrelevant information.

Sometimes these interviews can be very demoralizing or demeaning. Try not to get upset. If you get upset or are rude to the interviewer, that may affect your case adversely. Try to keep your emotions under control until you get home and have a long cry, or can talk about your feelings with your family or pound your pillows.

The Review Process

When you first file a claim for benefits it sets off an in-depth investigation of your problem and disabilities. The investigation will include checking out your medical history, the initial description of your condition, including your capacity for lifting, walking, standing, and sitting; your job history, the date you last worked, and a description of your past work. You will also need to show proof of citizenship and your insurance status.

You will be examined by a physician working for the Disability Determination Service, which is a branch of the Social Security Administration (SSA). You may find that you must wait a long time before you can see the doctor. The examination is brief and you may find that your medical records are not available for review by the SSA's physician. To avoid this problem, request your records from your physician as soon as you know you will need them. Make as many follow-up calls as necessary to obtain them. You have a legal right to obtain copies of all your records.

Insurance doctors are the doctors that the insurance company calls in to verify your claim of disability. They are well paid by the insurance companies, but they may not know a thing about either FMS or CMP. A number of insurance doctors have licenses to practice in ten or more states so they can work for insurance companies. That means they may be biased. It is also important for you to know that the physician-reviewer who is a part of the SSA's reviewing team is usually not a practicing physician and may know little or nothing about FMS or CMP.

After this initial examination and review, it may take six to eight months for you to receive a response from the agency to which you applied. Ask your congressperson to request that this process be speeded up for you, especially if you are dependent on these benefits for basic necessities.

If Your Claim Is Denied

Be prepared: Initial applications for disability benefits are routinely denied. Apply again and again until you are accepted. Hire a disability lawyer through your local legal aid organization, if there is one available. Note that, if you receive a denial, the letter will usually offer suggestions for alternative work that might be available for you. These suggestions may have no relation to your work history or ability to work. You don't have to act on them.

If your first claim filing is denied, you must make an appeal to the SSA within sixty days of the denial mailing. This appeal is called a Request for Reconsideration. *The SSA will not hear your appeal if it is filed late.* You can file it at the SSA District Office or through an attorney who deals with these cases. The attorney will usually charge 25 percent of your back pay benefits from six months after the first date that you reported yourself as unable to work. (You are not entitled to Social Security Disability (SSD) benefits for the first six months of your disability. However, unemployment benefits may be available to help you get through this hard time.)

Your claim may be denied two times. At the time of the second denial, you must file a Request for Hearing within sixty days.

This will result in a trial by a judge, usually within four months. You must be sure that the lawyer you pick is a specialist in SSD and/or Supplemental Security Insurance (SSI) and that he or she knows something about FMS and CMP, or is willing to learn. You and your physician may be asked to testify. Some people have indicated that their references were not even contacted. The key to the hearing is a comprehensive medical chart and report. Your physician must be familiar with the SSA Listing of Impairments.

As mentioned earlier, there is no specific SSI listing for FMS or CMP. Sometimes, you have to utilize other listings, since you may have many of the criteria for a psychiatric or other disability evaluation. In your detailed medical records, your doctor must record your adaptive reactions, physical limits, and dysfunctions, in addition to your medical signs and symptoms. Ask your doctor to be well prepared. Give him or her any information that you think will be pertinent to your case.

Every patient visit to the doctor should result in entries concerning physical capacities (verified with measured weights); timed durations for sitting, standing, and walking (by history); the nature, location, and intensity of pain (by history); psychosocial and adaptive behavior, including the ability to interact appropriately with others, follow instructions, adhere to a regular schedule; and the entire complex of depressive symptoms.

If the judge rules that you are not disabled, you may appeal to the Appeals Council within sixty days after the judge's ruling. Their decision, usually reached within seven months, almost always agrees with the judge. You can appeal this decision by filing suit in the U.S. District Court. (Note that an attorney handling this type of case must be licensed to appear before a U.S. District Court.) Usually, the District Court will return the matter for a new hearing (this hearing is called a remand). The remand is based on the initial application.

As you can see, this can be a long and very difficult process. Be persistent. As you make your way through this unwieldy system, you are paving the way to an easier path for those who follow.

Finding Benefits and Services in Your Area

In order to find the services and benefits that are available to you, you will have to do some research and take some action—usually this means making a lot of phone calls. If someone tells you that you have reached the wrong office, ask them whom to call. Keep calling and following up on contacts until you find the help you need. If your symptoms make it impossible for you to do this for yourself, ask someone else to do it for you. When you know what it is that you need (financial support, help with medical bills, health care services, grocery money, etc.), use the following list to help you find the available help:

- Call your state governor's office or hot line.

- Contact community action agencies and offices of health and human services.

- Look at the listings in the front of your phone book for places you can go to for help.

- Check out the listings in your phone book under U.S. Government, for your state, county, city, or town.

- Ask the reference librarian at your library for help.

- Watch your newspaper for articles about organizations that might be helpful to you.

- Ask your health care providers and other people dealing with FMS and CMP for information and advice.

- See the Resources section at the end of this book in Appendix A.

Emergency or Short-Term Assistance

While you are waiting to get long-term benefits, you may need emergency or short-term assistance, or assistance to meet specific needs. This can be a long and arduous process, especially when your symptoms are worse than usual, you are in "flare," you are being trained to do another kind of work, or when you need to take time from work to do the things you need to do to relieve your symptoms. While you will have to do some research to find appropriate sources of help, some possibilities include the following:

Financial Assistance

Temporary Assistance for Needy Families is a program that provides short-term financial assistance to families in need. (This program may have different names in different states.) The amount of payment depends on the parameters of the program, your needs, and your circumstances. Emergency assistance is often available from organizations in your community like churches, shelters, and community action organizations. The amount and availability of this assistance varies widely from place to place.

Unemployment Insurance

Unemployment insurance is available under certain circumstances and for a specific length of time after you have been laid off from a job. It provides regular cash payments while you try to find another job—in this case a job that you could do in spite of your symptoms. The amount of money you receive from this source will depend on the wages you have earned in the past, and how long you have worked. This kind of insurance payment varies from state to state.

Worker's Compensation

Worker's Compensation may be available to you if your FMS and CMP was triggered by a work-related injury or illness. Again, the availability and extent of these benefits vary from place to place.

Food

You may be eligible for federally issued food stamps that can be used to purchase food. There are some restrictions on their use and they won't cover all of your grocery purchases. You also may be eligible to receive one or two meals a day through a "Meals on Wheels" program.

Housing

There are some federal and state programs that can provide short- and long-term housing aid and rent subsidies. Check this out with your local social service agencies. Look in the Yellow Pages under social services.

Utilities

Some states provide assistance in purchasing heating fuel and in making other utility payments.

Transportation

Many community action agencies provide inexpensive bus services or have volunteer drivers who can drive you to health care appointments or to shop.

Personal Help with Daily Life

There are agencies that will help you with household chores and personal care. The cost may be covered by health care programs. Sliding scale fees based on income are sometimes an option. These programs have different names in different localities, but are commonly known as home health care agencies. Your physician can provide you with information on these programs in your area.

Medical Assistance

Medicaid. This federal program provides payments for health care services to people who meet certain criteria for inclusion in the program. It is available to some people with low incomes who have disabilities. Contact your local or state welfare office for information.

MediCare. This federal program provides medical insurance to people who have been approved for Social Security insurance payments and for those who are eligible for Social Security Disability benefits, and for all people who are over the age of sixty-five.

Health Clinics

Many communities have free or low cost clinics where you can receive health care services. Check your phone book for listings.

Free or Reduced Cost Medications

Some pharmaceutical companies give medications to doctors for patients who cannot afford to buy them. For more information go to the Web site www.phrma.org and put the word "patients" in the Search box at the upper left. This will take you to a list of links for specific medications and pharmaceutical companies that have programs that may help you get that specific medication. Or call 202-835-3400. There is also an organization called The Medicine Program that will help you access needed medications if you have no insurance coverage for medications, don't qualify for government programs that provide for medications, or have a low income. You can visit their Web site at www.themedicineprogram.com/info.html, or call 573-996-7300.

Long-term Assistance

It is wise to begin applying for long-term disability benefits as soon as you find you are unable to work, even if you are hoping to get back to work very soon. This is because the process for securing such aid can be long and difficult, and if you can't get back to work for some time, or if you need retraining for a new kind of work, there is a good chance that receiving these benefits will be very helpful to you.

Social Security Disability Insurance (SSD)

Social Security Disability Insurance provides benefits to workers under the age of sixty-five who can no longer work, and for people who have reduced incomes due to a disability. In order to qualify you must have a disability that prevents you from working that is expected to last at least twelve months, and that you have earned credits for a certain amount of time worked previous to applying. For additional information, contact your local Social Security Administration Office, visit their Web site at www.ssa.gov, and for specific information for people with FMS and CMP go to www.ssas.com. For an attorney to help you file for these benefits, call 800-431-2804 or visit the Web site at www.nosscr.org.

Supplemental Security Income (SSI)

Supplemental Security Income (SSI) is a federal needs-based disability program for people who are disabled according to the Social Security Administration definition and who have limited income and resources. You do not need any work credits to receive these benefits. For further information contact your local Social Security Administration.

Describing Functional Difficulties

Use the following worksheet to help you gather the information you must provide to the agency to which you are applying for disability benefits:

1. Are any of the following functions disrupted by your condition? If so, describe how they are disrupted:

   - Breathing • Eating • Dressing • Walking • Hygiene • Bathing • Bowel and Bladder Control • Grooming • Communicating • Standing • Sitting • Sleeping • Lifting

2. Do you use assistive devices? If so, which ones, how do you use them, and what do you use them for?

3. Which of the following activities are influenced by your illness? How are they affected? Describe.

   - Writing • Reading • Meal preparation • Shopping • Doing laundry • Climbing stairs • Telephoning • Taking medicine • Managing money • Working • Traveling • Dealing with people • Hearing • Seeing • Speaking • Using your hands

Fibromyalgia and Myofascial Pain Functional Questionnaire

The Fibromyalgia and Myofascial Pain Functional Questionnaire was modified from the Fibromyalgia Impact Assessment Form developed by J. Mason and others.[10] It was created to fill the need for a meaningful form to show specific disabilities common to people with FMS and/or CMP. Filling out copies of this form with your doctors may make the difference between receiving or being denied disability benefits.

Fibromyalgia and Myofascial Pain Functional Questionnaire[11]

To: _____

Re: _____ (Name of patient)

_____ (Social Security Number)

Please answer the following:

1. Nature, frequency, and length of contact with your patient:

_____

_____

2. Does your patient meet the American Rheumatological Association clinical testing criteria for fibromyalgia? _____ Yes _____ No

3. List any other diagnosed impairments or coexisting conditions:

_____

_____

4. Prognosis: _____

_____

5. Have your patient's impairments lasted or can they be expected to last at least 12 months? _____ Yes _____ No

6. Identify the clinical findings, laboratory and test results that show your patient's medical impairments: _____

_____

7. Identify all of your patient's symptoms:

_____ Multiple tender points	_____ Numbness and tingling
_____ Nonrestorative sleep	_____ Sicca symptoms
_____ Chronic fatigue	_____ Raynaud's phenomenon
_____ Morning stiffness	_____ Dysmenorrhea
_____ Subjective swelling	_____ Anxiety
_____ Irritable bowel syndrome	_____ Panic attacks
_____ Depression	_____ Frequent severe headaches
_____ Mitral valve prolapse	_____ Female urethral syndrome
_____ Hypothyroidism	_____ Premenstrual syndrome
_____ Vestibular dysfunction	_____ Carpal tunnel syndrome
_____ Lack of coordination	_____ Chronic fatigue syndrome
_____ Cognitive impairment*	_____ TMJ dysfunction
_____ Multiple trigger points	_____ Myofascial pain syndrome

_____ Difficulty communicating   _____ Dizziness

_____ Balance problems   _____ Headaches/migraines

_____ Shortness of breath   _____ Multiple chemical sensitivity

_____ Stress incontinence   _____ Free-floating anxiety

_____ Mood swings   _____ Unaccountable irritability

_____ Sensitivity to cold, heat, humidity, noise, light

_____ Problems climbing or going up/down stairs

*Explain nature of cognitive impairment(s) by circling those that apply: trouble concentrating, inability to get known words out, visual perception problems, short-term memory impairment, fugue states (staring into space before brain can function), inability to deal with multiple sensory stimuli, difficulty multitasking, other:

_____

8. If your patient has pain:

   a) Identify the location of pain, including, where appropriate, an indication of affected areas:

   _____ Lumbosacral spine   _____ Thoracic spine   _____ Head

   _____ Face   _____ Cervical spine   _____ Chest

	Right	Left	Bilateral
_____ Shoulders	_____	_____	_____
_____ Arms	_____	_____	_____
_____ Hands/fingers	_____	_____	_____
_____ Hips	_____	_____	_____
_____ Legs	_____	_____	_____
_____ Knees/ankles/feet	_____	_____	_____

   b) Describe the nature, frequency, and severity of your patient's pain:

   _____

   _____

   c) Identify any factors that precipitate pain:

   _____ Changing weather   _____ Fatigue   _____ Movement/overuse

   _____ Stress   _____ Hormonal changes   _____ Cold   _____ Heat

   _____ Humidity   _____ Static position   _____ Allergy

   _____ Other _____

9. Is your patient a malingerer?   _____ Yes   _____ No

10. Do emotional factors contribute to the severity of your patient's symptoms and functional limitations?   _____ Yes   _____ No

11. Are your patient's physical impairments plus any emotional impairments reasonably consistent with symptoms and functional limitations described in this evaluation? ___Yes ___No

12. How often is your patient's experience of pain sufficiently severe to interfere with attention and concentration?

_____ Never _____ Seldom _____ Often _____ Frequently _____ Constantly

13. To what degree is your patient limited in the ability to deal with work stress?

_____ No limitation _____ Slight limitation _____ Moderate limitation

_____ Marked limitation _____ Severe limitation

14. Identify the side effects of any medication that may have implications for working, e.g., dizziness, drowsiness, stomach upset, etc: _____

_____

15. As a result of your patient's impairments, estimate your patient's functional limitations if your patient were placed in a competitive work situation:

a) How many city blocks can your patient walk without rest or severe pain? _____
   Comment _____

b) Please circle the hours and/or minutes that your patient can continually sit and stand at one time without experiencing delayed onset symptoms:

Sit   Stand/walk

_____ _____ Less than 2 hours

_____ _____ About 2 hours

_____ _____ About 4 hours

_____ _____ At least 6 hours

c) Does your patient need to include periods of walking during an 8-hour day? _____ Yes _____ No _____ Cannot work 8-hr day

d) Does your patient need a job that permits shifting positions at will from sitting, standing, or walking? _____ Yes _____ No

e) Will your patient sometimes need to lie down at unpredictable intervals during a work shift? _____ Yes _____ No

f) With prolonged sitting, should your patient's legs be elevated? _____ Yes _____ No _____ Cannot tolerate prolonged sitting

g) While engaged in occasional standing/walking, must your patient use a cane or other assistive device? _____ Yes _____ No

h) How many pounds can your patient carry in a competitive work situation without suffering delayed onset symptoms?

	Never	Occasionally	Frequently
_____ Less than 10 lbs	_____	_____	_____
_____ 10 lbs	_____	_____	_____
_____ 20 lbs	_____	_____	_____
_____ 50 lbs	_____	_____	_____

In an average workday, "occasionally" means less than one-third of a workday, "frequently" means between one-third to two-thirds of the workday.

i) Does your patient have any significant limitations in reaching, handling or fingering? _____ Yes _____ No

If yes, please indicate the percentage of time during a workday on a competitive job that your patient can use hands/fingers/arms for the following repetitive activities:

HANDS (grasp, turn, twist objects) Right _____ % Left _____ %

FINGERS (fine manipulation) Right _____ % Left _____ %

ARMS (reaching incl. overhead) Right _____ % Left _____ %

j) Does your patient have difficulties with fine motor control? _____ Yes _____ No

16. On average, how often do you anticipate that your patient's impairments and treatment or treatments would cause the patient to be absent from work?

_____ Never _____ Less than once a month

_____ About twice a month _____ About three times a month

_____ About once a month _____ More than three times a month

17. Please describe any other limitations that would affect this patient's ability to work at a regular job on a sustained basis: _____

_____

_____

18. Does your patient have: (Y or N)

_____ nausea _____ cramps _____ buckling ankles

_____ buckling knees _____ leg cramps _____ sciatica _____ muscle twitching

_____ anxiety _____ lack of endurance _____ handwriting difficulties?

Date: _____ Signed: _____

Print/type name: _____

Address: _____

Endnotes

1. Keyserling, W. M. 2000. Workplace risk factors and occupational musculoskeletal disorders, Part 1: A review of biomechanical and psychophysical research on risk factors associated with low-back pain. *AIHAJ (A Journal for the Science of Occupational and Environmental Health and Safety)* 61(1):39-50.

2. Yassi, A. 2000. Work-related musculoskeletal disorders. *Curr Opin Rheumatol* 12(2):124-130.

3. Henriksson, C., and G. Liedberg. 2000. Factors of importance for work disability in women with fibromyalgia. *J Rheumatol* 27(5):1271-1276.

4. Henriksson, C., I. Gundmark, A. Bengtsson, and A. C. Ek. 1992. Living with fibromyalgia: consequences for everyday life. *Clin J Pain* 8(2):138-144.

5. Wolfe, F. 1989. Fibromyalgia: the clinical syndrome. *Rheum Dis Clin N Am* 15(1):1-18.

6. Pellegrino, M. J., G. W. Waylonis, and A. Sommer. 1989. Familial occurrence of primary fibromyalgia. *Arch Phys Med Rehabil* 70(1):61-63.

7. Pellegrino, M. J. 1993. *Fibromyalgia: Managing the Pain.* Columbus, OH: Anadem Publishing.

8. Bengtsson, A. E., Backman, B. Lindblom, and T. Skogh. 1994. Long-term follow-up of fibromyalgia patients: clinical symptoms, muscular function, laboratory tests—an eight-year comparison study. *J Musculoskel Pain* 2(2):67-80.

9. Burckardt, C. S., S. R. Clark, and R. M. Bennett. 1993. Fibromyalgia and quality of life: a comparative analysis. *J Rheumatol* 20(3):475-479

10. Mason, J., S. L. Silverman, and A. L. Weaver. 1991. Fibromyalgia Impact Assessment Form. *Arth Care Res* 4:523.

11. Starlanyl, D. 1998. *The Fibromyalgia Advocate.* Oakland, CA: New Harbinger Publications.

CHAPTER 28

Opening Doors

You may find it difficult to get what you need and deserve in order to deal with fibromyalgia (FMS) and/or chronic myofascial pain (CMP). When you have invisible chronic illnesses that are not well understood, sometimes your rights are violated. You have special issues and needs that others do not have, and you deserve to get those needs met. Having your needs met can be the essential difference between disability and ability.

Your medical team is made up of professionals, not deities. You have a right to information. You have a right to know what your test results are, what they mean, and how you are progressing (or why not). You have a right to discuss options and to have a say in your treatment plans. You have a right to judge whether a medication or therapy works for you, and a right to ask for alternatives. Communication should flow both ways. Chronic invisible illness may have closed some doors for you. It's time to open others. Some days I feel that I am fighting the entire world. Then I look at what others have done, and at all the marvelous newsletters that are now available to us (see Resources). None of us is fighting alone. We can take a lot of heart and a lot of hope in that. When one door closes, you can open another one.

When a doctor says, "I don't believe in FMS and CMP, that's your cue to say, 'Thanks for your time, Doctor, and goodbye.'" It's hard enough to deal with a disability that people can't see. When your doctor won't listen, doesn't know, and won't learn, it's time to find a new doctor. One person wrote, "My doctor says I should be happy that my arm goes numb, because when it's numb it doesn't hurt; so I should quit bothering him about it." I wonder what, or who, is numb here? That's abuse and neglect. Even an HMO can't insist on sending you to a doctor who is unable to diagnose and/or manage your conditions. They must pay for someone who is. Trying to force the issue may mean a battle. I can't prevent that, but I have tried to give you the ammunition you need to win such battles.

Being able to get to physical therapy, feed yourself, and take care of your own needs does not mean that you can work a forty-hour week in a construction firm. Even taking telephone calls might leave you relatively immobile, and thus worsen your trigger points (TrPs), unless your employer is willing to make structural accommodations to your needs. Your employer must be able to respond to your need for flexibility and make the necessary accommodations for you to do your job. Otherwise, it's discrimination. This is also true if you cannot get doctor referrals, the tests you need, or the therapy you need to regain as much of your ability to function as you can.

Authority figures and other persons of importance may make comments like these to you:

- You look fine to me. Why can't you work forty hours a week?

Janet Travell Story

I watched Dr. Janet Travell examine and treat a young dentist who had been in pain for three years. His pain had driven him to close his practice the year before. Dr. Travell was an unforgettable sight. She looked little more than five feet tall, with body contours that suggested her eighty-eight years had taken their toll. Her white hair was straight, and she wore blue tennis shoes; she teetered as she moved. She seemed to fatigue easily, so she braced herself against the treatment table as she moved around it. But whatever she may have lost to time physically it was not reflected in her mental functions. She emphasized the value of carefully eliciting a pertinent medical history from the patient. What impressed me most was the way she went after perpetuating factors. I thought of a prized police dog sniffing out drugs—nothing seemed to escape her.

She took a couple of yellow sponges from a bag. They were the kind you might use to clean kitchen counters. Dr. Travell put them under the dentist's elbows so he could rest them on the sponges and relax his muscles. She encouraged the audience to recommend to their

- Why can't you walk two flights upstairs to attend class?

- Why do you need weekly physical therapy appointments?

- Why do you need disability payments?

- Why should *you* have a special chair?

- Stay at your desk. Your fidgeting gets me nervous.

- I know somebody who had fibromyalgia, and she took this health food drink, and it cured her overnight.

- It looks like fat to me. Lose some weight. You're just out of shape.

- If you *really* cared, you'd remember.

- If you saw an expert on this, you'd get better.

To counteract these hurtful and damaging remarks you must be able to advocate for yourself. This process is covered thoroughly in *The Fibromyalgia Advocate*.[1] This chapter describes some general steps that you can take to open new doors.

Believe in Yourself

What do you do when your body and mind seem to be fighting you every step of the way? Negotiate a peace settlement. Find out what they need. *You must believe in your own worth.* If you have the low self-esteem that is so common to people with chronic illnesses, you need to work on changing your attitude, or you will not be able to negotiate successfully to meet your needs. Keep a special affirmation in your heart, one that works for you. These may help:

- I am worth the effort it takes to advocate for myself and protect my rights.

- I am a child of God. I walk in the Light. I can do this.

- I am entitled to my rights, and will be guided through this.

- My needs are real, and I will find the help I require to get my needs met.

- I am on the right path. I will find the right door. All will be well.

Create a statement proclaiming your own worth that feels right to you and repeat it when you need strength. I wear my polar bear shirt when I have to deal with problem issues, because bears are symbols of strength and perseverance. Find what works for you. Spend time with people who affirm and validate you. Avoid people who are judgmental and critical.

There are many good books available to teach you how to raise your self-esteem. One of the best is *Self-Esteem*.[2] It is small and useful to carry with you when you are going to face a challenge.

Know Your Rights

Everyone is entitled to equality under the law. Some people with chronic illnesses erroneously believe that they do not have the same rights as others. There are protection and advocacy services in every state. Call them to find out what your rights are. Do your best to prevent advocacy stress. Any of you who have ever advocated for yourself will know what I mean. People with FMS may not handle confrontation well, and many of us have allowed others to abuse our boundaries in the past. It is difficult to advocate if you are stressed. If you are well prepared, you will lessen the advocacy stress.

Become familiar with your medical records. Know what people have said about you and your condition. You may pay dearly for your caregivers' lack of training in FMS and CMP. You never know when an "It's All In The Head" former diagnosis will jump up and bite you. Don't let the mistakes of others haunt you. You can have them changed, or at least be prepared with defenses should they be used against you.

Medical records do belong to the doctor or hospital where the records were taken. Many states give patients the right to get copies of their records, although you may have to pay a copying fee. In no state is a doctor allowed to refuse to *show* you those records. Laws in different countries vary. Never allow your medical records to be forwarded without knowing what is in them. Misdiagnosis, offhand remarks, misinterpretations, and prejudices of the past may be used to deny you care in the future. Insurance companies are always looking for ways to save money. They look for *cost* effectiveness, not *treatment* effectiveness.

In a worst-case situation, you may have to take your doctor to court to get a copy of your records, and you may not be able to understand them once you get them. Medical shorthand (abbreviations), medical terms, and poor handwriting can make your records search difficult. There are Web sites with medical abbreviations, but each abbreviation must be taken in context, because it may mean several things. In addition, many states allow doctors to destroy patient records after ten years, if you are not a current patient.

Decide What You Want and Need

Deciding what you want and need helps you set goals and be clear in your communications. For example, you may need

short-armed patients that they should use foam rubber pads or sponges to properly support their arms. Then, she had the dentist slump forward in his chair with his head tilted toward the ground, and she palpated the lateral border of the trapezius.

She found a TrP and induced a twitch that indented his back along the trapezius on both sides of the TrP. She sprayed the muscle, moving the stream of vapocoolant slowly and deliberately. After she palpated his trapezius, his skin was distinctly red. She said this was a histamine reaction. She scraped a fingernail over the skin of his back drawing a red "X," and said, "See, it stays there." And it did. She told him to take antihistamines for a couple of months and that should eliminate the problem.

Then she told him to stick out his tongue, and said it looked normal. She explained that the tongue and the mucosa of the mouth are pieces of the GI tract, and when there is a malabsorption syndrome (which can induce nutritional deficiencies and then myofascial syndromes), there is a film on the lining of the GI tract and on the tongue. She asked if he had had a blood vitamin test. He had. The only vitamin that was low was B12. She said that he need about 3 grams per day to correct a B12 deficiency. She asked him if he was anemic and he said no. She said he could still have a B12 deficiency. While it might not show up as anemia, as a folic acid deficiency would, it still might bring about sub-acute lateral sclerosis.

Someone in the audience asked, "When do you use injections?" She answered, "When the patient lacks motor coordination or for some other reason is unable to cooperate in properly stretching during the Spray and Stretch procedure."

Her demonstration was a practical as practical can be. Behaviorists have long taught that the best way to learn to do something well is to model someone who has mastered the skill. For relieving myofascial pain, there is no better model than Dr. Janet Travell, the master of myofascial therapy.

—Excerpted and adapted from: "The Master of Myofascial Therapy" by John C. Lowe, M.A., D.C., 1993. The *ACA Journal of Chiropractic* (November).

specific treatment. This is often the first place where you can gain experience in advocating. Perhaps you need a complete physical examination from your doctor. You may need to practice self-advocacy on your job for an appropriate accommodation in your work conditions. Perhaps a flare will cause you to demand the sick leave mandated by law but that your employer doesn't want to grant. Your advocacy may be to contact your state or federal legislators about health care programs that don't acknowledge FMS or CMP in terms of entitling those of us with those conditions to the same rights as those granted to people with other chronic conditions.

Get the Facts

To open doors, you must have your facts in order. There is a scene in the Tolkien saga, *The Lord of the Rings*, where everyone, even the wizard Gandalf, is baffled by a locked door. They know that a word or phrase will open the door, because on the door, written in runic letters, it says, "Speak, friend, and enter." They try every magical phrase they can think of, but nothing works. Then the light dawns. Gandalf says the word "friend" in several languages, and the right one works. To get doors to open in front of you, you need the right words behind you.

Your information must be accurate and up-to-date. Here are some ways you can do this:

1. Write down all important information. Everyone forgets things. Writing important information down and keeping it where you can find it helps.

2. Develop a personal medical file, and keep it updated and in good order. For instance, when advocating for appropriate physical therapy, go to your appointment prepared with references from this book, from *The Fibromyalgia Advocate*,[3] and from current informational newsletters with references from medical journals to show to your physician. If you are petitioning for sick leave when you are in flare, contact your state agency of protection and advocacy, or your attorney, to find out what your rights are. Make sure that your legal representative has read the section entitled "What Your Attorney Should Know" from the *Advocate*. Several attorneys have also made good use of my video to advocate for their clients.

3. Make phone calls. Many agencies have advocacy material. They are only a phone call, email, or letter away. Remember to note to whom you spoke, and the date and time. Keep a phone log of all important calls. The Internet is also a good resource. If you don't have a computer, you may be able to get access at your local library. Ask your librarian to help you research the information you need.

In addition to the references that appear in the Endnotes to the chapters in this edition, the following excerpts can help you and your legal representative find other medical references that may help you plead your case:

In the workplace, it is important to mix tasks for fibromyalgia patients. If one area is used excessively, that area will produce the most pain. Vary your tasks and the muscle groups used in your tasks. The more ways you can find to do a certain task, the less dangerous it will be for you to do that task repetitively.[4]

Musculoskeletal soft tissue injuries consume considerable resources in personal suffering, medical care, work absenteeism, and compensation benefits. The rate of return to work for workers who were provided with modified jobs was two times higher than for those with no such accommodation in employment. The employer's provision of a modified job is important in the prevention of continued disability.[5]

Myofascial pain was present in a hundred percent of work related musculoskeletal disorders.[6]

Insurance companies aren't yet aware that full-blown chronic myofascial pain and fibromyalgia are largely preventable. Their focus is not on prevention. We must change this. What is needed is physician training in the diagnosis and treatment of these conditions as early as possible. A great deal of pain could be prevented, as well as astronomical cost.

How to Do Research

Throughout this book, tiny numbers appear above some phrases and at the end of some sentences. These numbers mean that the quote or information preceding them came from a specific reference. Now you will learn how to use these references to provide formal documentation when you need it. If you want to find a specific reference, match the number after the sentence with the same number in the endnotes. Each chapter has its own set of endnotes. For example, consider the following quote:

Insurance companies haven't yet understood the economic importance of the lack of physician training in the diagnosis and treatment of myofascial TrPs. So many complaints could be treated rapidly and efficiently if the physicians understood what they were seeing. Patients with simple myofascial TrPs get well instantly when the TrPs are properly treated and the perpetuating factors

---

David Simons, M.D., Above and Beyond

David Simons, co-author of the definitive texts on myofascial medicine, was a pre-astronaut, the first man to see the curvature of the earth. He was suspended from a balloon in what amounted to a metal can, to find out what happens to someone at that altitude over a 24-hour period. On August 19, 1957, Dr. Simons viewed the earth from an altitude almost 20 miles above the surface of the earth, higher than any balloonist had ever been. He ran experiments and recorded biomedical, astronomical, meteorological, and electromagnetic observations. One problem after another plagued the flight, but still he chose to continue. He saw colors that had no name, and described them for the people waiting below.

"Where the atmosphere merged with the colorless blackness of space, the sky was so heavily saturated with this blue-purple color that it was inescapable, yet its intensity was so low that it was hard to comprehend, like a musical note which is beautifully vibrant but so high that it lies almost beyond the ear's ability to hear, leaving you certain of its brilliance but unsure whether you actually heard it or dreamed of its beauty," he said in the taped log of *Project Manhigh II.*

Craig Ryan, in *The Pre- Astronauts: Manned Ballooning on the Threshold of Space*, tells the story of Dr. Simons' flight and these quotes are from his book. "Simons would say later that the sunset from his vantage at the top of the stratosphere was the single most startling sight his eyes had ever seen."

"A curious reversal of night and day met my eyes,' he wrote. 'High in the atmosphere, where the sun still shot its rays, the ever-deepening blue sky was acquiring a greenish, sunset tinge. But below it, closer to the earth, was a giant demarcation line which looked like a faded rainbow arching from south to north across the eastern horizon. And beneath the line was the dark- ness of night covering the earth below. The daylit sky was above, the darkened sky below. And as the sunset progressed, the rainbow arch rose ever higher, drawing with it a curtain of blackness. Above the slowly changing colors was a layer of blue so clear that it was as if someone had lifted a veil from an ordinary blue sky to leave it polished and bright and clean with no scattered light to diffuse it.' Night fell, and he marveled, 'The stars glow like an animal's

are promptly dealt with. This would avoid the evolution into complex chronic pain states, saving a great deal of cost.[7]

If you look at the endnotes at the end of this chapter, number 7 reads: Pongratz, D. E., and M. Spath. 1998. [No title available]. *Fortschr Med* 116(27):24-29. [German] This article is unusual, because unlike most medical papers, it lacks a title. The first set of brackets indicates that the article is not English. The second set of brackets tells you the language in which the article is written. To see if an abstract, or summary, or the article itself is available, check on PubMed or one of the other free online services. PubMed is at http://www.ncbi.nlm.nih.gov/ entrez/query. You enter one or more terms to search the PubMed database. In this case, enter the authors' names "Pongratz D E, Spath M" on a search, you must omit the periods after the initials. Since there is more than one author, separate the names with a comma, and put them in quotes. When looking for other articles, you can use the title. To further refine your search, you can click the "limits" box and narrow it down as to the date or publisher. The publisher abbreviation in this instance is *"Fortschr Med,"* the volume number is 166, the issue is 27, and the page numbers are 24-29. If you read an abstract and think that it would be helpful to have the whole article, talk to your local reference librarian. You can often get these articles through an Interlibrary Loan.

If you don't have a computer, your local librarian can still help you, but in this case, unless you read German, you would want the abstract, and not the entire article. Your local library may give classes on the use of computers for searching libraries. There are many free medical data libraries. Besides PubMed, there is GratefulMed, and there are medical school libraries you can access by computer. There are also the computer databases of the National Institutes of Health National Network of Libraries of Medicine at the Web site http://www.nlm.nih.gov/

When you first glance through the references, you may think, who *is* this Dr. et al., and how does s/he know so much! "Et al." is not an amazingly prolific researcher. It's just shorthand for "and the rest of the folks on the research team." When you look up a subject, you need to know what kinds of key words to use. "Myofascial pain" may not yield the same results as "trigger point." Whenever you have more than one word, you need to put them in quotes. Most Internet library programs have a FAQ (frequently asked questions) sheet to help you learn how to access information. If you get a copy for a member of your medical team to read, don't forget to keep a copy for yourself.

Gather Your Support

It's much easier to advocate for yourself when you have the support of others. Nothing helps self-advocacy more than supportive friends. You can build your support by joining an FMS and CMP or chronic pain support group. If your FMS support group doesn't know about CMP, teach them. You may have the answer to many of their most distressing symptoms. Make sure that your support group is one that focuses on positive thinking, and is not a "grief group" that focuses on venting and complaining. The negativity generated by this type of group can drag you down fast. Find a group where you can share information and give and receive support.

Target Your Efforts

Who is the person, persons, or organization with whom you need to deal to get action on a particular matter? Speak directly to the person who can best assist you. It may take a few phone calls to discover which organization or specific person can help, or who is in charge, but it is worth the effort. Keep trying until you find the right person. Keep notes of your efforts to avoid duplications.

Express Yourself Clearly

Good communication skills are vital for effective self-advocacy. Learn effective communication skills so you can get your message across. It's not difficult. Just remember the following rules:

- Be brief. • Stick to the point. Deal with one issue at a time. • Don't allow yourself to be diverted, or to ramble on with unimportant details. • State your concern, what you want, or how you want things changed.
- Write down what you plan to say in advance, especially if you think that you won't remember what to say. • *Document everything*.

If you have a hard time communicating clearly or effectively, practice with a counselor or supporter. Read *The Tao of Conversation* (see Kahn on the Reading List) to hone your communication skills.

Assert Yourself Calmly

Stay cool. Don't lose your temper and lash out at the person with whom you are dealing, or at the character or organization for which that person works. This is often very hard for people with FMS. Your neurotransmitters and hormones may affect your mood, and your sensitivity may be enhanced. Everyone feels irritable when they hurt. Explain this briefly to the person with whom you are speaking, if you think it will help.

Speak out, and then listen. Respect the rights of others, but don't let them intimidate or abuse you. If you must go to an office, taking a supporter with you often helps. Be firm and

eyes.... I have a ringside view of the heavens—it is indescribable.'"

The book goes on to say, "He had prevailed over long odds, meager funds, a deadly storm, and near-toxic carbon dioxide levels. He was the first man to spend an entire night and day in the stratosphere, the first man ever to float down into a thunderstorm, the first man to ascend above 100,000 feet in a balloon. David Simons had just completed one of the greatest feats of endurance and perseverance in aviation history."

Of this material are heroes made. Dr. Simons later met Janet Travell, and he turned his descriptive talents to TrPs. Together they defined the field of myofascial medicine and gave us all a chance to rise above the world of chronic pain.

persistent. Keep after what you want. Always follow through on what you say. Dedicate yourself to getting whatever it is you need for yourself.

Face to Face

Speaking to someone in person is the most effective way to advocate for yourself. Here are some guidelines:

- Make an appointment—don't just show up.

- Bring a tape recorder and use it. Explain that you need it to help you remember. It is amazing how much more helpful people can be if they know they are being recorded.

- Plan what you are going to say and the points you need to make. Practice with the help of friends, tape recorders, or mirrors if you feel unsure of yourself.

- Dress neatly for the appointment, but don't wear yourself out. Do the best you can with the resources you've got.

- Be on time.

- State your message clearly and simply. How you say something often makes a greater impression than what you say. Tell the person exactly what it is that you want. Explain why you need it. Tell the person why it is in his or her best interest to respond to your request. Speak loudly enough to be heard without shouting.

- Expect a positive response.

- Listen to what the other person says. If you don't understand something, ask questions.

- If you feel you are not getting anywhere, tell the other person that you wish to pursue your issues further, and ask to speak to the person's supervisor.

- At the end of the meeting, restate any action that has been decided upon so you both understand each other clearly. For instance, you might say, "As a result of this meeting, you are going to order a glucose tolerance test for me." Or, "As a result of this meeting, I understand you are going to change my status to 'active.'" Thank the people you met with for their time and assistance.

- Send a follow-up note thanking them for meeting with you and summarizing any agreed-upon action. It's a nice gesture. It also acts as a reminder, and provides assurance that you both have the same understanding about the result of the meeting. It is also documentation.

Getting Action Through Letter Writing

Writing is a useful way to request information, present facts, express your opinion, or ask for what you need. Here are some suggestions:

- Make the letter short, simple, and clear. One page is best. Long letters may not be read and often don't stick to the point.

- It is acceptable to write the letter by hand if you don't have access to a typewriter or computer, but make sure it is understandable and legible. You may think it is clear and legible, but you are used to your own style of writing and already know what you are trying to say. You may have to print. Ask a supporter to read your letter and answer truthfully about whether it is clearly understandable and legible.

You may have a difficult time writing by hand because of TrPs. In that case, you may find it easier to write using a computer or word processor. Alternatively, perhaps a relative or friend could print a letter for you. If appropriate, send copies of your letter to others you want to inform, such as your legislator or advocacy agency. Put "cc" (which means copies circulated) at the bottom of the letter, with a list of the others to whom you are sending copies. Keep a copy of the letter in your file for future reference. It's a good idea to follow up a letter with a phone call. That way, you make sure the person got the letter, and you can discuss the situation further.

Advocating by Phone

You can initiate letters and visits with phone calls, if appropriate. The telephone is useful for gathering information, keeping track of what's going on, and letting people know what you want. Before you call, write down the essential points of what you want to say. Have extra paper and a pen handy, or your computer. Don't hold the phone to your ear with your shoulder. If you plan to write, use a speaker-phone, unless you want to be listening to your TrPs! Have any information you need (such as your doctor's name, address, and phone number) handy.

When calling, follow these guidelines:

- First identify yourself. Then, ask for the name and position of the person to whom you are speaking.

- Briefly describe your situation to the person who answers, and ask if he or she is the right person to deal with such a request. If this is not the right person, ask to be transferred to someone who is more appropriate. If that person is not available, ask that he or she return your call. If you have not had a response by the next day, call back. Don't be put off or give up because your call has not been returned. Keep calling until you reach the person you need.

- Once you have reached the appropriate person, make your request for action brief and clear.

- If the person cannot respond to your request immediately, ask when she or he will get back to you, or by what date you can expect action.

- Thank the person for being helpful, when that's the case.

- When a person has been particularly helpful, it is a good idea to send a thank-you card. This may help to open the door for further contact on related issues.

- Keep a written record of your calls in your file. Include the date of your call, whom you spoke to, issues addressed, and promised action.

- If you are not contacted when a return call is expected, if the promised action is not taken or the situation is not resolved, call the appropriate person or persons back. Persist until you reach the right person, the promised action is taken, or a satisfactory resolution is reached.

Computer Advocacy

There are pros and cons to computer advocacy. One of the pluses is that you can reach an agency at any time of the day or night and access information. You can often find exactly whom it is you need to contact, even if you can't contact them by email. You can also find out what services are available to you.

There are also minuses to computer access. Others may be able to keep track of which Web sites you visit. This may or may not be a problem for you. You need to be very sure of Web addresses, and type them carefully. There are a lot of very weird Web sites out there. For example, I was looking for a site on liturgical music. The site I wanted was run by a nun who calls herself "websister," but when I put that into a search engine, I received a list of sites I had absolutely no interest in visiting, none of which were run by musical nuns! A visit to the wrong site can result in embarrassing "spam" emails that you don't need and don't want. Keep deleting the spam, and don't try to reply. They never answer.

There is also a lot of misleading information out there on the Net, written by insurance company doctors and others who have their own financial interests at heart. Their articles are used as references by insurance company lawyers to try to deny you access to services you need and deserve. If you believe in yourself, believe in the rights you have, and learn to communicate what your needs are, you have the best chance of receiving the assistance for which you ask.

Nowadays, there is also a lot of information about FMS and CMP in the media. A lot of it is still incorrect or incomplete, but it is improving. Fibromyalgia has now been mispronounced by some of the top names in broadcasting. One by one, we are educating people about FMS and CMP. One by one, we are opening new doors. One by one, we are finding that the whole universe is spread out before us, and there is absolutely nothing that can hold us back. We are FMily.

In Conclusion

I feel very close to every one of you. I hope that you will find what you need in this edition of the *Survival Manual*, and that it will make your path easier. Although I can't be there to answer your questions individually, I can and do carry you all in my prayers and in my heart. God grant you love, healing, and peace.

May the Lord send Angels to watch over thee.
May their wings blow gentle breezes if you feel fevered.
May they wrap you in softness and warmth when you feel chill,
And may their halos light your path when all seems dark.
May they comfort you, cheer you,
And bless your days with joy and your nights with peaceful slumber,
And when comes the time for you to return
To the place prepared for you,
May they transport you with swift and gentle wings.

—Devin

Endnotes

1. Starlanyl, D. 1998. *The Fibromyalgia Advocate*: Oakland, CA: New Harbinger Publications.

2. McKay, M., and P. Fanning. 2000. *Self-Esteem*. Third edition. Oakland, CA: New Harbinger Publications.

3. Starlanyl. 1998. *Op. cit.*

4. Farrell, J., and G. O. Littlejohn. 1999. Pain, nature of task, and body part used in fibromyalgia syndrome. *J Musculoskel Pain* 7(1-2):279-284.

5. Crook, J., H. Moldofsky, and H. Shannon.1998. Determinants of disability after a work-related musculoskeletal injury. *J Rheumatol* 25(8):1570-1577.

6. Lin, T. Y., M. J. Teixeira, A. A. Fischer, F. G. Barboza, S. T. Immura, and R. Mattar, Jr.1997. Work-related musculoskeletal disorders. *Phys Med Rehab Clin N Am (Phila)*: 8(1):113-117.

7. Pongratz, D. E., and M. Spath. 1998. [No title available]. *Fortschr Med* 116(27):24-29. [German]

APPENDIX A

Resources

Agencies and Organizations

AARP 601 East Street, N.W., Washington, DC 20049. Web site: www.aarp.org. Pharmacy Service: Phone: 800-456-2277.

Academy for Myofascial Trigger Point Therapy is now the Pittsburgh School of Pain Management. Website: www.painschool.com

Acupressure Institute, 1533 Shattuck Ave., Berkeley, CA 94709. Phone: 510-845-1059. Web site: www.acupressure.com

American Academy of Environmental Medicine, 7701 E. Kellogg, Suite 625, Wichita, KS 67207. Phone: 316-684-5500. Web site: www.aaem.com

American Academy of Pain Medicine (AAPM), 4700 W. Lake Ave., Glenview, IL 60025. Phone: 847-375-4731. Fax: 847-375-4777. Email: aapm@amctec.com. Web site: www.aapm.com

American Academy of Sleep Medicine, 6301 Bandell Road., Suite 101, Rochester, MN 55901. Phone: 507-287-6006. Web site: www.aasmnet.org

American Association of Naturopathic Physicians, 8201 Greensboro Drive, Suite 300, McLean, VA 22102. Phone: 703-610-9037. Web site: www.naturopathic.org

American Association of People with Disabilites. 1819 H St., NW, Suite 330, Washington, DC 20006. 1-800-840-8844, 202-457-0046. Web site: www.aapd-dc.org. Information, prescription drug program, career center.

American Association of Professional Hypnotherapists, 2443 Ash Street, Suite D, Palo Alto, CA 94306. Phone 650-323-3224. Web site: www.aaph.org

American Center for the Alexander Technique, 39 W. 14th St., #507, New York, NY 10011. Phone: 212-633-2229. Email: acatusa@aol.com. Web site: www.acatny.org

American Chiropractic Association, 1701 Clarendon Blvd., Arlington, VA 22209. Phone: 703-276-8800. Web site: www.acatoday.com

American Chronic Pain Association, POB 850, Rocklin, CA 95677. Phone: 916-632-0922. Web site: www.theacpa.org

American Massage Therapy Association, 820 Davis St., Suite 100, Evanston, IL, 60201. Phone: 888-843-2682. Web site: www.amtamassage.org

American Music Therapy Association, Inc., 8455 Colesville Road, Suite 1000, Silver Spring, MD 20910. Phone: 301-589-3300. Fax: 301-589-5175. Email: info@musictherapy.org. Web site: www.musictherapy.org

American Occupational Therapy Association, 4720 Montgomery Lane, PO Box 31220, Bethesda, MD 20824-1220. Phone: 301-652-2682. Web site: www.aota.org

American Osteopathic Association, 142 E. Ontario Street, Chicago, IL 60611-2864. Phone: 312-380-5800. Web site: www.am-osteo-assn.org

American Pain Foundation, 111 South Calvert St., Suite 2700, Baltimore, MD 21202. Email: ampainfoun@aol.com. Web site: www.painfoundation.org: Patient information, education and advocacy organization.

American Physical Therapy Association, 1111 N. Fairfax St., Alexandria, VA 22314. Phone: 703-684-2782. Web site: www.apta.org

Arthritis Foundation, 1330 W. Peachtree St., Atlanta, GA 30309. Phone: 800-283-7800. Web site: www.arthritis.org

Biofeedback Certification Institute of America, 10200 W. 44th Ave., Suite 304, Wheat Ridge, CO 80033. Phone: 303-420-2902. Web site: www.bcia.org

Bonnie Prudden Pain Erasure, LLC, P. O. Box 65240, Tucson, AZ 85728-5240. Phone: 1-800-221-4634. Fax: 520-529-6679. Web site: www.bonnieprudden.com

Chronic Fatigue and Immune Dysfunction Syndrome of America, P. O. Box 220398, Charlotte, NC. 28222-0398. Phone: 800-442-3437. Email: info@cfids.org. Web site: www.cfids.org

DO-IT Program at the University of WA. Email: doit@u.washington.edu. Web site: www.washington.edu/doit. Resources, programs. (Disabilities, Opportunities, Internetworking, and Technology).

Dr. Vodder School—North America, P. O. Box 5701, Victoria, B.C. V8R 6S8. Canada email: drvodderna@vodderschool.com. Web site: www.vodderschool.com

Environmental Health Network, P. O. Box 1155, Larkspur, CA 94977. Phone: 415-541-5075. Multiple chemical Sensitivities; information, referrals, peer support, newsletter.

Environmental Illness (Gulf War Syndrome) Share, Care and Prayer, P. O. Box 2080, Frazier Park, CA 93225.

Federation of State Medical Boards, 400 Fuller Wiser Road., Suite 300, Euless, TX 76039. Phone: 817-868-4000. Web site: www.fsmb.org. Information on state laws governing prescribing of controlled substances for severe chronic pain.

Feldenkrais Guild, 3611 S.W. Hood Ave., Suite 100, Portland, OR 97201. Phone: 503-221-6612. Web site: www.feldenkrais.com

Focusing Institute, 34 East Lane, Spring Valley, NY 10977. Phone: 845-362-5222 or 800-799-7418. Email: info@focusing.org. Web site: www.focusing.org. Referrals, workshops, brochures, books, scientific journals.

Health Equations, Lynne August, M.D., P. O. Box 323, Newfane, VT 05345. Phone: 800-328-2818. Web site: www.healthequations.com

Herb Research Foundation. Phone: 800-748-2617. Nonprofit organization: information on herbs.

Hypoglycemia Association, Inc., P. O. Box 165, Ashton, MD 20861-0165. Phone: 202-544-4044.

International Association of Compounding Pharmacists, P.O. Box 1365, Sugar Land, TX, 77487. Phone: 800-927-4227. Fax: 281-495-0602. Web site: www.iacprx.org

International Association for the Study of Pain (IASP), 909 N.E. 43rd St., Suite 306, Seattle, WA 98105-6020. Nongovernmental affiliate of the World Health Organization (WHO). Phone: 206-547-6409. Fax: 206-547-1703. Email: IASP@locke.hs.washington.edu. Web site: www.halcyon.com/iasp

International MyoPain Society. Phone: 210-567-4661. Fax: 210-567-6669. Web site: www.myopain.org

Muscle Balance and Function (MBF), Eduardo Barrera, Gravity Werks, 3272 California Ave., Seattle, WA 98116; Dynamics of Physical Development Consultants, c/o Carolyn Brumfield, 1071 Bonita Drive, Encinitas, CA 92024. Phone: 760-634-3565. Web site: www.dpdc-mbf.co

Myofascial Release (John Barnes) Inner Awareness Audio Tapes, 222 West Lancaster Avenue, Paoli, PA 19301. 1-800-FASCIAL. Web site: www.myofascialrelease.com

National Association of Myofascial Trigger Point Therapists, 1541 Summit Hills Drive N.E., Albuquerque, NM 87112. Web site: www.myofascialtherapy.org

National Attention Deficit Disorder Association, 1788 Second Street, Suite 200, Highland Park, IL 60035. Phone: 847-432-ADDA. Fax: 847-432-5874. Email: mail@add.org. Web site: www.add.org

National Center for Homeopathy, 801 N. Fairfax St., Suite 306, Alexandria, VA 22314. Phone: 703-548-7790. Web site: www.homeopathic.org

National Center for Post-Traumatic Stress Disorder, V.A. Medical Center, 116D, White River Junction, VT 05001. Phone: 802-296-5132. Web site: www.ncptsd.org

National Family Caregivers Association, 10400 Connecticut Ave., Suite 500, Kensington, MD 20895. Phone: 301-942-6430. Web site: www.nfcacares.org

National Fibromyalgia Partnership. 140 Zinn Way, Linden, VA 22642-5609. Phone: 703-790-2324. Fax: 540-622-2998. (Flexyx tapes).

National Institute on Disability and Rehabilitation Research, U.S. Department of Education, ABLEDATA Database of Assistive Technology, 8630 Fenton Street, Suite 930, Silver Spring, MD 20910. Phone: 301-589-3563. Fax: 301-608-8958. Web site: www.abledata.com. Resource guide on ADA materials.

National Organization for Rare Disorders, P.O. Box 8923, New Fairfield, CT 06812-8923. Phone: 800-999-6673. Web site: www.rarediseases.org

National Self-Help Clearinghouse, 365 5th Ave., Suite 3300, New York, NY 10016. Web site: www.selfhelpweb.org

New England ADA Technical Assistance Center, 374 Congress St., Suite 301, Boston, MA 02210. Phone: 617-695-0085 or 800-949-4232. Web site: www.adaptenv.org. Information on the Americans with Disabilities Act.

North American Registry, Bowen Therapy Academy of Australia, P. O. Box 768, Lafayette, CO 80026. Phone: 303-665-2667. Fax: 303-665-2557. Email: usabowen@aol.com

Office of Equal Employment Opportunity. Phone: 800-669-3362. Free booklet on ADA.

Pharmaceutical Research and Manufacturers of America, 1100 15th St., N.W., Washington, D C 20005. Phone: 202-835-3400. Directory of Pharmaceutical Indigent Assistance. Web site: www.phrma.org

Reaching Across Countries: Young people with FMS or CFIDS, would you like a Pen Pal who understands? R.A.C. will find a correspondent somewhere in the world just for you. If you are under 25 years old and have one of these conditions, send your name, address and interests to R.A.C., P. O. Box 9204, Bardonia, NY, 10954, or write Lisa Cohen at brainfog@att.net

Social Security Administration. Phone: 800-772-1213. Web site: www.ssa.org

Social Security Claims Representatives. Phone: 800-431-2804. Web site: www.nosscr.org

United States Travel Service, United States Dept. of Commerce, Washington, DC 20230. Travel Tips for the Handicapped.

Well Spouse Foundation, 30 E. 40th Street PH, New York, NY 10016. Support groups, newsletter. Phone: 212-685-8815. Fax: 212-685-8676. Toll-free: 800-838-0879. Web site: www.wellspouse.org

Newsletters

AFSA Update: The American Fibromyalgia Syndrome Assoc., 6380 E. Tanque Verde Rd., Suite D, Tucson, AZ 85715-3822. Phone: 520-733-1570. Research.

Eagle Watch: Information on FMS and ME, Canadian perspective. RR1, Site 15, Box 10, Mindemoya, Ontario, P0P (P zero P), Canada.

Fibromyalgia Network Newsletter: Editor: Kristin Thorson. P. O. Box 31750, Tucson, AZ, 85751. Phone: 800-853-2929. Fax: 520-290-5550. Web site: www.fmnetnews.com: Information packets and other publications.

From Fatigued to Fantastic! A private health letter. c/o Jacob Teitelbaum, M.D., 466 Forelands Road, Annapolis, MD 21501. Phone: 800-333-5287.

Inland Northwest FM Association. Editor: Diana Langston. Inland Northwest FM Association, Wells Fargo Bank Bldg., 3021 S. Regal, #301, Spokane, WA 99223. Phone: 509-838-3001.

Journal of Musculoskeletal Pain. Publisher: Haworth Medical Press, 10 Alice Street, Binghamton, NY 13904. Phone: 800-342-9678.

National Fibromyalgia Partnership. Editor: Tamara Liller. 140 Zinn Way, Linden, VA 22642-5609. Phone: 703-790-2324. Fax: 540-622-2998. Email: mail@fmpartnership.org., Web site: www. fmpartnership.org

The CFIDS Chronicle. The CFIDS Assoc. of America, P. O. Box 220398, Charlotte, NC 28222-0398. Phone: 800-442-3437.

To Your Health and Healthpoints. Free resource catalogue and newspaper for FMS, CFIDS, arthritis, and chronic pain. To Your Health, 17007 East Colony Drive, Suite 105, Fountain Hills, AZ 85268. Phone: 800-801-1406.

Vulvar Pain Foundation Newsletter. The Vulvar Pain Foundation, 203½ North Main Street, Suite 203, Graham, NC 27253. Phone: 336-226-0704 (Tues. and Thurs.). Web site : www.vulvarpainfoundation.org

Products

Decent Exposures, 2202 115th N.E., Seattle, WA 98125. Phone: 800-524-4949 U.S. and Canada 9-9 PST. Pull-on/step-in sports style bras, with no hardware, in cotton, cotton-Lycra, and firm support cotton velour. They aren't cheap, but they custom-make large sizes.

Dome Company. Phone: 800-432-4352. Hand-eze support gloves. They must be sized to fit. Dome will supply a size chart to anyone who calls for it.

Gebauer Company, 9410 Catherine St., Cleveland, OH 44104. Phone: 800-321-9348 (216-271-5252 in Ohio). Ethyl-Chloride Vapocoolant Spray for Spray and Stretch. Fluori-Ethyl Vapocoolant Spray for Spray and Stretch (requires prescription).

The Grain and Salt Society, P. O. Box DD, Magalia, CA 95954. Phone: 916-872-5800. Celtic Salt, whole grains. Each bag of salt is labeled with the analysis by the Laboratory of Analytical and Hydrological Chemistry of Nantes France. (Celtic Salt is produced in Brittany, France.)

Hyrex Pharmaceuticals, 3494 Democrat Road, Memphis, TN 38118. Phone: 800-238-5282. Suppliers of over-the-counter guaifenesin. Email: hyrex@concentric.net

JC Penney, Special Needs Home Health Care and Easy Dressing Fashions, P. O. Box 2021, Milwaukee, WI 53201-2021. Catalog phone: 800-222-6161.

Keepers, Inc., P. O. Box 12648, Portland, OR 97212. Phone: 503-282-0436. Fax: 503-284-9883. Web site: www.gladrags.com. Glad Rags Cotton menstrual pads.

Liss Stimulator, MEDI Consultants, Inc., 265 Vreeland Ave., Patterson, NJ 07504. Phone: 973-278-0200.

Mother Wear. Comfortable clothing and products for nursing mothers. Phone: 800-950-2500. Web site: www.motherwear.com

Myofascial Pain Syndromes: The Travell Trigger Point Tapes. Williams and Wilkins, 800-527-5597. Daitz, Ben, M.D., with Janet Travell, M.D. No physical therapy department should be without this six-tape series.

Neuromuscular Electronic Stimulator (NMES unit called Focus). EMPI, 599 Cardigan Rd., St. Paul, MN 55126. Phone: 651-415-9000 or 1-888-FOR-EMPI. Web site: www.empi.com

OPTP (Orthopedic Physical Therapy Products). Physical therapy and rehabilitation products and resource books, including FMS resources and large balls. P. O. Box 47009, Minneapolis, MN 55447. Phone: 800-367-7393. Fax: 763-553-9355. Email: OPTP@worldnet.att.net. Web site: www.optp.com

Special Needs Project. Bookseller, offering book lists by topic. Phone: 800-333-6867. Web site: www.specialneeds.com

APPENDIX B

Reading List

Aron, Elaine N. 1997. *The Highly Sensitive Person.* New York: Broadway Books.

Barnes, John. 2000. *Healing Ancient Wounds: The Renegade's Wisdom.* Paoli, PA: Rehabilitation Services, Inc.

Carper, Jean. 1991. *The Food Pharmacy.* New York: Bantam Doubleday.

Cassileth, Barrie R. 1998. *The Alternative Medicine Handbook.* New York: W. W. Norton & Co.

Catalano, Ellen Mohr, and Kimeron N. Hardin. 1996. *The Chronic Pain Control Workbook.* Oakland, CA.: New Harbinger Publications.

Cohen, Don. 1995. *An Introduction to Craniosacral Therapy.* Berkeley, CA: North Atlantic Books.

Cohen, Kenneth S. 1997. *The Way of Qigong: The Art and Science of Chinese Energy Healing.* New York: Ballantine Books.

Copeland, Mary Ellen. 2000. *The Loneliness Workbook: A Guide to Developing and Maintaining Lasting Connections.* Oakland, CA: New Harbinger Publications.

———. 1999. *Winning Against Relapse: A Workbook of Action Plans for Recurring Health and Emotional Problems.* Oakland, CA: New Harbinger Publications.

———. 1998. *The Worry Control Book.* Oakland, CA: New Harbinger Publications.

———. 1994. *Living Without Depression and Manic Depression: A Workbook for Maintaining Mood Stability.* Oakland, CA: New Harbinger Publications.

Daoust, J., and G. Daoust. 1996. *Fat Burning Nutrition: The Dietary Hormonal Connection to Permanent Weight Loss and Better Health.* Del Mar, CA: Wharton Publishing.

DerMarderosian, Ara, ed. 1999. *A Guide to Popular Natural Products.* St. Louis, MO: Facts and Comparisons Publishing Group.

Dunnewold, A., and D. G. Sanford, PhD. 1994. *Postpartum Survival Guide.* Oakland, CA: New Harbinger Publications.

Egoscue, P., and R. Gittines. 1998. *Pain Free: A Revolutionary Method for Stopping Chronic Pain.* New York: Bantam Press.

Feinberg, R. A., and B. I. Feinberg. 1997. *Anatomy of an Injury.* Injury Specialists, 3565 Pennridge Dr., Bridgeton, MO 63044.

Flaws, Bob. 2000. *Curing Fibromyalgia Naturally with Chinese Medicine.* Boulder, CO: Blue Poppy Press.

Gallagher, Paul. *T'ai Chi Basic Conditioning and Internal Training Video.* P. O. Box 19835, Ashville, NC 28815: The Center for Personal Mastery.

Graham-Pole, John. 2000. *Illness and the Art of Creative Self-Expression.* Oakland, CA: New Harbinger Publications.

Hallowell, E. M., and J. J. Ratey. 1994. *Driven to Distraction* (ADD). New York: Simon and Schuster.

Headley, Barbara. 1997. *When Movement Hurts.* Boulder, CO: Innovative Systems for Rehabilitation (see Resources, distributor OPTP).

Hendler, S. S. 1991. *The Doctors' Vitamin and Mineral Encyclopedia.* New York: Simon and Schuster.

Huston, J. E., and D. Lanka, M.D. 1997. *Perimenopause: Changes in Women's Health after Thirty-Five*. Oakland, CA: New Harbinger Publications.

Kahn, Michael. 1995. *The Tao of Conversation*. Oakland, CA: New Harbinger Publications.

Kane, Jeff. 1991. *Be Sick Well: A Healthy Approach to Chronic Illness*. Oakland, CA: New Harbinger Publications.

Martinelli, Linda. 1996. *Poetry of Pain*. Lynnewood, WA: Simply Books.

McCaffery, M., and C. Paseo. 1999. *Pain: Clinical Manual* Second edition. St. Louis: Mosby.

McKay, Mattthew, Martha Davis, and Patrick Fanning. 2000. *Relaxation and Stress Reduction Workbook*. Oakland, CA: New Harbinger Publications.

McKay, Matthew, and Patrick Fanning. 2000. *Self-Esteem*. Oakland, CA: New Harbinger Publications.

Murray, Michael T. 1994. *Natural Alternatives to Over-the-Counter and Prescription Drugs*. New York: William Morrow and Company.

O'Hara, Valerie. 1995. *Wellness at Work: Preventative Health Practices for the Workplace*. Oakland, CA: New Harbinger Publications.

O'Neil, M. S., and C. E. Newbold. 1994. *Boundary Power*. Antioch, TN: Sonlight Publishing.

Osborn, Carol. 1997. *The Art of Resilience*. New York: Random House.

Pellegrino, Mark J. 1995. *The Fibromyalgia Survivor*. Columbus, OH: Anadem Publishing, Inc.

Piburn, Gregg. 1999. *Beyond Chaos: One Man's Journey Alongside His Chronically Ill Wife*. Atlanta, GA: The Arthritis Foundation.

Richardson, Cheryl. 1999. *Take Time for Your Life: A Personal Coach's 7-Step Program for Creating the Life You Want*. New York: Broadway Books.

Saunders, Cat. 2000. *Dr. Cat's Helping Handbook: A Compassionate Guide for Being Human*. Heartwings Foundation, P. O. Box 30712, Seattle, WA.

Sears, B. 1997. *Zone-Perfect Meals in Minutes*. New York: HarperCollins.

Shankland, Wesley E., II, with James Boyd and Devin Starlanyl. 2000. *Face the Pain: The Challenge of Facial Pain*. Columbus, OH: Aomega Publishing Co.

Shankland, Wesley E., II. 1996. *TMJ: Its Many Faces: Diagnosis of TMJ and Related Disorders* Second edition. Columbia, Ohio: Anadem Publishers.

Simmons, Gary. 1998. *Embrace Tiger, Return to Mountain: Spiritual Conflict Management*. 85 minute audio tape. Unity Village. ISBN 0871598272.

Skelly, M., and A. Helm. 1999. *Alternative Treatments for Fibromyalgia and Chronic Fatigue Syndrome*. Alameda, CA: Hunter House Publishing.

Spanos, Tasso. *Feeling Better Exercises*. Video tape. The Center for Pain Management, 1312 E. Carson Street, Pittsburgh, PA 15203. Phone: 412-431-9180.

St. Amand, R. Paul, and Claudia C. Marek. 1999. *What Your Doctor May Not Tell You About Fibromyalgia*. New York: Warner Books.

———. 2001. *What Your Doctor May Not Tell You About Pediatric Fibromyalgia*. Microsoft Reader. E-Book. Available at online bookstores.

Starlanyl, Devin J. 1999. *Worlds of Power, Lines of Light*, Devstar. P. O. Box 301, W. Chesterfield, NH 03466. $7.95.

———. 1998. *The Fibromyalgia Advocate: Getting the Support You Need to Cope with Fibromyalgia and Myofascial Pain Syndrome*. Oakland, CA: New Harbinger Publications.

———. 1997. *Chronic Myofascial Pain Syndrome: A Guide to the Trigger Points*. 2 hour video. Oakland: New Harbinger Publications.

Taylor, S., and R. Epstein. 1999. *Living Well with a Hidden Disability*. Oakland, CA: New Harbinger Publications.

Teitelbaum, Jacob. 1996. *From Fatigued to Fantastic*. Garden City Park, NY: Avery Publishing Group.

Uppgaard, Robert O. 1999. *Taking Control of TMJ: Your Total Wellness Program for Recovering from Temporomandibular Joint Pain, Whiplash, Fibromyalgia and Related Disorders*. Oakland, CA: New Harbinger Publications.

Vliet, E. L. 1995. *Screaming to Be Heard*. New York: M. Evans and Co.

Wright, J. V., and J. Morgenthaler. 1997. *Natural Hormone Replacement*. Petaluma, CA: Smart Publications.

APPENDIX C

Medical Care Providers' Reading List

August, L., M. D. *A Blood Test Evaluation of Physiology and Physiopathology: Physician Manual.* P.O. Box 323, Newfare, VT 05345: Health Equations.

Baldry, P. E. 1993. *Acupuncture, Trigger Points and Musculoskeletal Pain.* New York, NY: Churchill Livingston.

Cantu, R. I., and A. J. Grodin. 1992. *Myofascial Manipulation: Theory and Clinical Application.* Gaithersburg, MD: Aspen Publishers, Inc.

Finando, D., and S. Finando. 1999. *Informed Touch: A Clinician's Guide to the Evaluation and Treatment of Myofascial Disorders.* Rochester, VT: Healing Arts Press. (acupuncture)

Gershon, M. D. 1998. *The Second Brain.* New York, NY: HarperCollins. (the gastrointestinal system's own central nervous system and its role in disease and dysfunction)

Greenman, P. E. 1996. *Principles of Manual Medicine.* Second edition. Baltimore: Williams and Wilkins.

Hardie, D. G. 1991. *Biochemical Messengers: Hormones, Neurotransmitters and Growth Factors.* New York: Chapman and Hall.

Haworth Medical Press, 10 Alice Street, Binghamton, NY 13904. Phone: 800-342-9678.

International MyoPain Society: Phone: 210-567-4661. Fax: 210-567-6669. Web Site: www.myopain.org (membership includes *Journal of Musculoskeletal Pain*).

Jacobsen, S., and B. Danneskiold-Samsoe. 1993. *Musculoskeletal Pain, Myofascial Pain Syndrome, and the Fibromyalgia Syndrome.* Binghamton, PA: Haworth Press.

Lowe, J. C. 2000. *The Metabolic Treatment of Fibromyalgia.* Boulder, CO: McDowell Publishing Company.

Margoles, M. S., and R. Weiner. 1999. *Chronic Pain: Assessment, Diagnosis, and Management.* Boca Raton: CRC Press.

McCaffery, M., and C. Paseo. 1999. *Pain: Clinical Manual, 2nd edition.* St. Louis, MO: Mosby.

Mense, S., and D. G. Simons, with I. J. Russell. 2000. *Muscle Pain: Understanding Its Nature, Diagnosis and Treatment.* Baltimore: Lippincott Williams and Wilkins

Russell, I. J. 1996. *Clinical Overview and Pathogenesis of the Fibromyalgia Syndrome, Myofascial Pain Syndrome, and Other Pain Syndromes.* Binghamton, PA: Haworth Press.

Simons, D. G., J. G. Travell, and L. S. Simons. 1999. *Travell and Simons' Myofascial Pain and Dysfunction: The Trigger Point Manual, Vol. I: The Upper Body.* Baltimore: Williams and Wilkins.

Stimmel, B. 1997. *Pain and Its Relief Without Addiction: Clinical Issues in the Use of Opioids and Other Analgesics.* Binghamton, PA: Haworth Press.

Travell, J. G., and D. G. Simons. 1992. *Myofascial Pain and Dysfunction: The Trigger Point Manual, Vol. II: The Lower Body.* Baltimore: Williams and Wilkins.

Tapes

Myofascial Pain Syndrome: The Travell Trigger Point Tapes with Janet Travell, M.D. Set of six videotapes. Ben Daitz, M.D., ed. These tapes can be purchased from Lipppincott Williams and Wilkins, 351 West Camden Street, Baltimore, MD 21201-2436. Phone: 800-527-5597.

Myofascial Pain: An Integrated Approach to Diagnosis and Treatment, with Robert D. Gerwin, MD. Set of five videos (includes exam and injection technique). These tapes can also be purchased from Lipppincott Williams and Wilkins, 351 West Camden Street, Baltimore, MD 21201-2436. Phone: 800-527-5597.

For information on hands-on teaching in the diagnosis and treatment of myofascial pain, as well as seminars on musculoskeletal pain, contact: The Janet Travell Seminar Series, Pain and Rehabilitation Medicine, 7830 Old Georgetown Road, Suite C-15, Bethesda, MD 20814-2432. Phone: 301-656-0220. Web site: www.painpoints.com.

Starlanyl, Devin. 1997. *Chronic Myofascial Pain Syndrome: A Guide to the Trigger Points.* Oakland: New Harbinger Publications. Two-hour video.

Index

Waldie, Andrew, 238
walking casts, 55
walking exercise, 223
walking meditation, 245, 246-247
Walters, Barbara, 53
Wang, Kuan, 179
warm-up stretching exercises, 222
waste products, 20
water consumption, 224, 303-304
weight problems, 77, 298
weight training, 231-232
Wellbutrin, 269
Wellness Recovery Action Plan (WRAP), 156, 183-194; crisis plan, 191-192; daily maintenance list, 186-187; early warning signs plan, 189; effective use of, 192-193; functions of, 183; personal example of using, 193-194; supplies required for, 184; tools for developing, 184-186; triggers list, 188; worsening symptoms plan, 190-191. *See also* life management strategies
What Your Doctor May Not Tell You About Fibromyalgia (St. Amand & Marek), 145, 177
whiplash, 66, 206
Wiesel, S. W., 317
Winning Against Relapse (Copeland), 194
Wolfe, Frederick, 351
women: breast-related symptoms in, 131-132; fertility issues for, 127-128, 135; genital symptoms in, 132; hormone replacement therapy for, 133; lack of sexual desire in, 128-129; menopause and perimenopause, 138-139; pain during sexual intercourse, 97, 100, 130; pregnancy issues for, 135-138; premenstrual syndrome in, 132-133; responses to medications by, 127; vaginal dryness in, 131. *See also* gender issues
words: affirmative, 214-215; power of, 243
work: changing, 348-349; disability benefits and, 351-363; education and training for, 350-351; equal opportunity laws and, 348; inability to, 351; perpetuating factors related to, 54-55, 63; relationships at, 347, 348; risks in the workplace and, 343-347; shifting schedules of, 122; vocational rehabilitation and, 349-351
Worker's Compensation, 357
workplace issues, 343-348; aggravating activities, 343-344; computer use, 346-347; coworkers, 348; creating workplace changes, 344-345; employers, 347; environmental problems, 347; equal opportunity laws, 348; workstations, 345-347
World Health Organization, 9
worsening symptoms plan, 190-191
WRAP. *See* Wellness Recovery Action Plan
Wright, Mary, 164
writing: journal, 194, 195; letters of advocacy, 372-373

X

Xanax, 269

Y

Yaksh, Tony, 174
yeast problems: as coexisting condition, 48-49; die-off phenomenon, 155; fibrofog and, 205-206; flare and, 155
yo-yo effect, 59
Yu, Leepo, 179
Yue, Samuel, 39, 177-178

Z

Zanaflex, 269
Zilin, Rob, 287
Zofran, 269
Zoloft, 269
Zone diet, 125, 298-299

Some Other
New Harbinger Titles

Solid to the Core, Item 4305 $14.95

Staying Focused in the Age of Distraction, Item 433X $16.95

Living Beyond Your Pain, Item 4097 $19.95

Fibromyalgia & Chronic Fatigue Syndrome, Item 4593 $14.95

Your Miraculous Back, Item 4526 $18.95

TriEnergetics, Item 4453 $15.95

Emotional Fitness for Couples, Item 4399 $14.95

The MS Workbook, Item 3902 $19.95

Depression & Your Thyroid, Item 4062 $15.95

The Eating Wisely for Hormonal Balance Journal, Item 3945 $15.95

Healing Adult Acne, Item 4151 $15.95

The Memory Doctor, Item 3708 $11.95

The Emotional Wellness Way to Cardiac Health, Item 3740 $16.95

The Cyclothymia Workbook, Item 383X $18.95

The Matrix Repatterning Program for Pain Relief, Item 3910 $18.95

Transforming Stress, Item 397X $10.95

Eating Mindfully, Item 3503 $13.95

Living with RSDS, Item 3554 $16.95

The Ten Hidden Barriers to Weight Loss, Item 3244 $11.95

The Sjogren's Syndrome Survival Guide, Item 3562 $15.95

Stop Feeling Tired, Item 3139 $14.95

Responsible Drinking, Item 2949 $19.95

The Mitral Valve Prolapse/Dysautonomia Survival Guide, Item 3031 $14.95

The Vulvodynia Survival Guide, Item 2914 $16.95

The Multifidus Back Pain Solution, Item 2787 $12.95

Move Your Body, Tone Your Mood, Item 2752 $17.95

The Woman's Book of Sleep, Item 2493 $14.95

The Trigger Point Therapy Workbook, second edition, Item 3759 $19.95

Fibromyalgia and Chronic Myofascial Pain Syndrome, second edition, Item 2388 $19.95

Rosacea, Item 2248 $14.95

Call **toll free, 1-800-748-6273,** or log on to our online bookstore at **www.newharbinger.com** to order. Have your Visa or Mastercard number ready. Or send a check for the titles you want to New Harbinger Publications, Inc., 5674 Shattuck Ave., Oakland, CA 94609. Include $4.50 for the first book and 75¢ for each additional book, to cover shipping and handling. (California residents please include appropriate sales tax.) Allow two to five weeks for delivery.

Prices subject to change without notice.